Mental Health Social Work

D0076264

Mental health social work can be one of the most rewarding and one of the most frustrating areas of social work practice. Mental health is a key policy arena in which the involvement of service users has been particularly successful, and in which there are many new and controversial initiatives. Social workers must not only have a good knowledge of interventions and their evidence bases, from pharmacology to psychotherapy, but also be able to work sensitively and effectively with both clients and carers in a rapidly changing context.

In *Mental Health Social Work*, Colin Pritchard draws on his many years of experience in research, teaching and practice to explore key issues for social workers who want to work in the mental health field. Topics covered include:

- the multiple factors affecting mental health;
- the bio-psychosocial model of practice;
- key areas including depression, suicide, schizophrenia and personality disorder;
- the mental health–child protection interface;
- residential work;
- treatment modalities.

This important book presents essential information in a clear and accessible way and includes a series of case exercises to help the reader consolidate what has been learned. It will be invaluable reading for undergraduate social work students and for practising social workers.

Colin Pritchard is Professor Emeritus at the University of Southampton and Research Professor in Psychiatric Social Work at the Institute of Health and Community Studies, University of Bournemouth. He is an academic veteran of the social care field who has maintained a mental health practice while being an active and sometimes controversial interdisciplinary researcher.

Mental Health Social Work
Evidence-based practice

Colin Pritchard

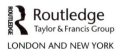

Routledge
Taylor & Francis Group

LONDON AND NEW YORK

First published 2006
by Routledge
2 Park Square, Milton Park, Abingdon, Oxon OX14 4RN

Simultaneously published in the USA and Canada
by Routledge
270 Madison Ave, New York, NY 10016
Routledge is an imprint of the Taylor & Francis Group

© 2006 Colin Pritchard

Typeset in Times New Roman by Prepress Projects Ltd, Perth
Printed and bound in Great Britain by TJ International, Padstow, Cornwall

British Library Cataloguing in Publication Data
A catalogue record for this book is available from the British Library

Library of Congress Cataloging in Publication Data
Pritchard, Colin, 1936–
      Mental health social work: evidence-based practice/Colin Pritchard.
      p. cm.
      Includes bibliographical references and index.
      ISBN 0-415-31902-1 (pbk.) – ISBN 0-415-31901-3 (hardback)
      1. Psychiatric social work. 2. Evidence-based psychiatry. I. Title.
      HV689.P65 2006
      362.2′0425–dc22
      2005025906

ISBN10: 0-415-31901-3 (hbk)
ISBN10: 0-415-31902-1 (pbk)

ISBN13: 9-78-0-415-31901-0 (hbk)
ISBN13: 9-78-0-415-31902-7 (pbk)

Contents

The emergency perspectives   147

10 Mental health social work with 'suicidal' people   149

11 Personality disorders and the psychiatric–child protection
     interface   182

12 Statutory mental health social work: care and control
     dilemmas and role of the Approved Social Worker   200

13 The accommodation dimension: housing and mental
     disorder   217
     REBECCA PRITCHARD

14 The vortex of mental disorder: the client speaks   241

     Bibliography   268
     Index   302

Figures

Tables

Preface

A personal journey – 'flying by the seat of your pants' to an evidence-based mental health social work

Social work's link with people described as mentally ill or mentally disordered goes back over a century, and it has always been a controversial association. This controversy initially stemmed from two disparate approaches to 'mental disorder'. On the one hand, medicine and psychiatry attempted to explain disturbed and disturbing behaviour by reference to discrete organic disorders. On the other hand, social work, with its roots in the social and behavioural sciences, appeared to offer an alternative explanation for this often stigmatised group of 'outsiders'. This book integrates the best of these two approaches and, from an evidence base, shows that people who experience what is considered a 'mental disorder' actually need input from both approaches to deal with phenomena that cross millennia, disciplines and cultures.

The mental health controversy reflects the redundant debate of 'nurture' versus 'nature'. For, according to a director of the Imperial Cancer Research Fund, even an 'organic disorder' such as cancer is a 'genetic predisposition awaiting an environmental trigger' (Bodmer and McKie 2000), as reflected, for example, in the changing morbidity and mortality statistics of cancer and neurological disease (Pritchard and Evans 1996, 1997; Pritchard et al. 2004a; Pritchard and Sunak 2005).

This illustrates the great Durkheimian insight that changing patterns of mortality reflect changes in society, while conversely, from physical conception, the social and emotional environment of the mother actually affects the baby's, infant's and child's physical development (McLloyd 1990; Aber et al. 1997; Hogan and Park 2000; Barker 2001; Barker et al. 2002; Rutter 2003). Thus, this book will offer a bio-psychosocial approach to understanding a core issue of humanity, the nature and development of the mind and human personality, and challenge a number of one-dimensional approaches. With our present knowledge, there is no one theory, school or technique that answers all questions about human behaviour, and this book is critical of both an overnarrow mechanistic medicine, as well as the over-simplistic global critique that can come from the social sciences.

Here is a confession. Initially, this book was planned as a textbook, one that could ask a question X and offer a straightforward answer Y, but this turned out to be impossible because practice experience and modern multidisciplinary research shattered any simplistic 'cookbook' framework, i.e. 'this is what to do in situation

X'. What this book does do is to share with you knowledge and techniques that may be appropriate to your client's or service user's needs. In the end, however, you will have to make your own decision about what is appropriate in the specific circumstances of working with a particular person at a particular time, because people are not like textbooks.

I learned this lesson in a seminal experience. After 15 years of working with vulnerable and troubled people, in 1970 I was close to burn-out and looked forward to an academic career, free of the pressures of practice. The late Professor Max Hamilton explained that, in medicine, 'if you teach a practice, you practice,' and this was invaluable advice. This meant that all the academics were also practitioners and, in a university department, all the practitioners were interested in user research relevant to the patient/client/service. After changing jobs, I had no client contact for over six months and, during a particularly successful seminar with post-graduate social work students, I suddenly realised that I was sounding like a textbook. To resolve this, I took up and continued with a small pro bono mental health practice, not only for the personal satisfaction that comes from service to others, but to remember just how hard, problematic, confusing, complex and sometimes downright scary mental health practice can be. Since then, I have been able to look students in the eye and genuinely commiserate with them when they share the problems they face daily in work with troubled and sometimes troublesome people.

This practice orientation has been reinforced in continued work with colleagues who share both academic and practice responsibilities and have been strongly influenced by modern medicine's efforts to develop a fully 'evidence-based practice' – an approach whereby a student or a trainee psychiatrist identifies a current practice problem and seeks to find a research paper that comes close to answering the patient's/client's problem. In about one-quarter of cases, there is no appropriate research paper, which means that we have to make judgements on limited information, not backed by research evidence. This should make us professionally humble, and reinforces the need to remember that we exist to serve our clients, which must entail that we include them in this service. Indeed, the first strength of the professional is to understand our professional limitations. On the other hand, the gaps in our practice knowledge can and do serve as a stimulus to research. For example, two initially disparate research topics, suicide and child protection, came from trying to answer questions to which no answers were available at the time (Pritchard 1999, 2004) and went on to create new practice knowledge that appears here for the first time.

We can never be satisfied with our knowledge for there is much we do not understand, especially in the field of mental health. However, one thing is known. Many, many people who seek our services have very often had a very bad deal in life, i.e. they often come from disadvantaged backgrounds, whether this be socioeconomic, social class, ethnic and/or intergenerational psychosocial poverty, not just economic, but also of mind and spirit. Therefore, in a continued pursuit of social justice, only the best is good enough for them, which means we must continue to seek to improve our service, asking the fundamental question: did it cure, improve or comfort the client/service user?

Social work, like medicine, seldom cures; like medicine, it often improves and, like medicine, it should always comfort. Sadly, medicine and social work sometimes fail this simple client-orientated test.

Another important aspect of work with people in the mental health field is the knowledge we need about ourselves, as much as about others. Nowhere is this insight better provided than through the great poets and playwrights as, generally, no matter how distinguished the research paper, if it is about people and cannot be found reflected in the great literature, then it is perhaps not all that important; hence, the sharing of these poetic insights throughout the book, for:

Canst thou not minister to a mind diseased. . .
Raze out the written troubles of the brain,
And. . .
Cleanse the stuffed bosom of that perilous stuff
Which weighs upon the heart?
(*Macbeth*, 5:3)

Shakespeare, about 400 years ago, showed that he understood something of the bio-psychosocial interactive nature of 'a mind diseased', yet 'Though this be madness, yet there is method in't' (*Hamlet*).

To reinforce further the authenticity of the practice text, case examples, all suitably anonymised, are offered to illustrate the complexities and intervention issues that emerge with the various types of mental disorder.

The book begins with our culture's evolving history of how we responded to mental disorder, and then considers philosophy – how we grapple with defining the mind and its ills. The concepts of mental disorder and the impact upon the sufferer and those around them are examined and the so-called 'minor mental disorders', which, at their worst, can be totally destructive of people's lives. As a balance to much medically orientated research, we take a critical look at modern clinical psychiatry and, in particular, the problem of its relationship with the pharmaceutical industry.

The book deals with the most 'familiar' of the mental health problems, mood disorders, as most people have experienced the ups and down, which at the extreme become dysfunctional and slip over into 'demoniac frenzy' and 'moping melancholy' (Milton). We explore in greater detail the syndrome known as schizophrenia and examine the very encouraging integrated bio-psychosocial treatment approaches.

A major chapter considers suicidal behaviour and crucially seeks to differentiate between suicide and so-called 'attempted suicide', now better described as 'deliberate self-harm', which is a reminder that the mentally disordered have shorter lives than the general population, as well as a high toll of suicide because of inadequately treated mental disorder (Harris and Barraclough 1998). The next theme is inevitably controversial because it explores that most unpopular concept, psychiatric 'personality disorder', which is admittedly defined in juxtaposition with 'social norms'. Here is brought together new research that highlights the psychiatric–child protection interface and the power of the media as the 'pendulum swings' between condemning feckless or overzealous practitioners.

Chapter 12 is written anonymously by a senior Approved Social Worker because, while maintaining a mental health practice for the last 30 years, I had no direct statutory responsibility under the Mental Health Act 1983, although occasionally dealing with 'psychiatric emergencies' on campus. To enhance further the practice authenticity of the text, we examine the often ignored issue of homelessness, written by a former Service Director for Centrepoint, Rebecca Pritchard, who is keen to highlight the mental health–homelessness interface.

The final chapter concerns examples of the psychosocial vortex that often surrounds mental disorder and, while maintaining anonymity, we hear the clients' voice on their experience, which better serves to aid our understanding and insight.

One overarching theme, which comes from the core values of social work, is the importance of the 'therapeutic relationship'. This is not just a pious statement as there is evidence that, irrespective of technique or approach, the ability to engage with the client, what some are calling the 'therapeutic alliance', is at the core of all effective interventions (Lazarus 1976; Pritchard *et al.* 1998; Pritchard and Williams 2001; Di Clemente *et al.* 2002).

The book draws upon classic and modern literature which provides special insights and shares many illuminating quotes. But, if the book had but two 'texts', the first would be about the need for up-to-date research in a field that is rapidly changing, hence Francis Bacon's comment, 'If a man will begin with certainties, he shall end in doubts; but if he will be content to begin with doubts, he shall end in certainties'. The second is a reminder that this is a text about practice, not groups or categories of people, but rather individuals and their families, and the great Quaker dictum of 'Seek ye the godhead in every person' (George Fox) is a reminder for all mental health practitioners that, at this moment in time, we are working with and for this person, in their situation, in their time.

I must acknowledge my indebtedness to numerous colleagues who, in different ways, have contributed to this book. I owe much to people who have allowed me the privilege of entering their lives, and who have so enhanced my life by teaching me something about human dignity and resilience, and to generations of students who have asked awkward questions at the Universities of Bath, Bournemouth, Bradford, Hong Kong, Leeds, Monash and Southampton. To social workers Alan Butler, University of Leeds, and Mike Kerfoot, University of Manchester, who have encouraged me to ask the biological questions to social scientists, and to psychiatrists David Baldwin, Christal Buis, Lars Hansen, David Kingdon, Robert Peveler and David Wallbridge, for encouraging me to continue to pose the awkward psychosocial questions in medicine.

There are some special acknowledgements, though my academic indebtedness is clear in the bibliography: Graham Reading, Senior Social Worker, helped me confront some of the realities of under-resourced services; Claire Pritchard,

Senior Social Worker with Children's Services Hammersmith and Fulham, gave advice on the psychiatric–child protection interface; and Rebecca Pritchard of Centrepoint taught me about the practice and organisational problems of the homeless–psychiatric interface.

I am very appreciative of colleagues in Routledge, Taylor & Francis, who have been so understanding and helpful in bringing this text to completion, especially Andrew R. Davidson of Prepress Projects for his patient forbearance.

Finally, and acknowledgements are often formulaic, but without the support, love, encouragement, humour and friendship of Beryl, my wife for more than 40 years, nothing worthwhile would ever have been accomplished, for her life-long professionalism was a steadfast example of what it means to be a caring professional.

Colin Pritchard

Part I
A psychiatric perspective

1 In the beginning

Cultural history and poetry of madness

> Babylon in all its despoliation is a sight not so awful as that of the human mind in ruins.
>
> (Scrope Davies 1783–1852, *Letters*)

In all cultures and in all times, the perception of madness, possession or mental disorder has created a conflict between fear and compassion (Porter 1993). Scrope Davies, viewing the ruins of a once proud empire, Babylon, reflected this ambivalence and the tragedy of the 'human mind in ruins'. This goes to the heart of the practice problem which, in a civilised society, should excite sympathy and a search for understanding. From the Old Testament, which feeds into the Christian, Islamic and Jewish faiths, we hear the psalmist hope that he will not be smitten by 'the moon at night' (Psalm 121). For to be 'moonstruck' was a description of madness that echoed well into the nineteenth century, seen in the word 'lunatic'. Hence, in 1820, the Lunatic Asylum Act sought to give refuge to the afflicted, not least in recognition that even the highest in the land, the late King George III, like King Lear, had admitted that 'I fear I am not in my perfect mind'. The term 'lunacy' was used as late as 1890 in the Lunacy Act, which was concerned with the compulsory admission of 'poor lunatics', and the term was not abandoned until the 1935 Mental Health Act.

The designation 'lunatic' reflected the assumption that the mad had been affected by malign lunar influences and, in this sense, was a diagnostic category. Another term which started as descriptive but became pejorative is 'asylum'. Originally meaning a place of 'refuge', a laudable concept for vulnerable people, the word and place rapidly became stigmatised.

Mental disorder remains one of the most stigmatised conditions throughout the world, even in modern Western societies (Shooter 2002). Our language and culture are still littered with earlier ideas that have become counterproductive, and the title of Kate Millett's book *The Looney Bin Trip*, describing the old 'asylums', was both a challenge and an evocation for sympathy, reminding us that:

> The old order changeth, yielding place to new; . . .
> Lest one good custom should corrupt the world.
>
> (Tennyson, *The Passing of Arthur*)

For example, another progressive piece of legislation was the 1913 Deficiency Act, which took the 'learning disabled' out of the old workhouses and gave them greater protection. Yet, no-one today would use the Act's language of 'moron, feeble minded or idiot' to describe another human as all civilised societies ascribe to one of the greatest monuments to human advancement, the United Nations Declaration of Human Rights 1948. True, the declaration's principles are often ignored, but it is a measure of how we should behave towards each other, when it asserts that all people are equal, irrespective of any 'category':

> Article 1: All human beings are born free and equal in dignity and rights. They are endowed with reason and conscience and should act towards one another in the spirit of brotherhood.

> Article 2: Everyone is entitled to all the rights and freedoms set forth in this Declaration, *without any distinction of any kind* such as race, colour, sex, language, religion, political or other opinion, national or social origins, property, birth or *other status* (my emphasis).

This book's search for an effective mental health practice is based upon this declaration. Since 1948, society has made great strides in recognising and renouncing discrimination against people of other ethnicities, religions, physical disability and differing sexual orientations, as well as beginning to recognise discrimination related to age, but there is a long way to go. In holding fast to our common humanity, the UN Declaration demands that we use the 'intellect and reason' with which we are endowed to respond to another's distress. This is heard in Robert Burton's (1577–1640) dramatic evocation of the wronged and manacled 'lunatic' in *Anatomy of Melancholy*:

> See the Madman rage downright
> With furious looks, a ghastly sight.
> Naked in chains bound doth he lie
> And roars amain, he knows not why!
> Observe him; for as in a glass
> Thine angry portraiture it was.
> His picture keep still in thy presence;
> 'Twixt him and thee there's no difference.

Although Robert Burton's great classic is limited by the confines of late Tudor and Jacobean science, his approach was essentially humane, and was coterminous with Shakespeare's great insight into the phenomena of the human mind, when he said:

> Though this be madness, yet there is method in't.
>   (*Hamlet*; commonly quoted as 'there is meaning in his madness')

Certainly, cultural factors have always fed a society's concept of madness or mental disorder (Pilgrim and Rogers 1998). This is seen in the example of 'delusions'. A popular cartoon image is of a deluded person believing they are Napoleon, yet I have never met such a person. But, among elderly patients, one could meet those who thought they were being persecuted by the Kaiser (Wilhelm II). Religious delusions are not uncommon, being taken over by God, the Virgin Mary or the Devil from those of a Christian culture; or the God Khali from those of a Hindu tradition; or Shaitan by Islamic people. Delusions reflect the contemporary culture, hence people express fear of 'extraterrestrial aliens', of being controlled by television or of persecution by spies reflected in the brilliant film starring Russell Crowe, *A Beautiful Mind*. This film was based upon the true story of a Nobel laureate, John Nash, who suffered from what we now designate schizophrenia. In the film, you initially enter John Nash's mind-set, so you believe, like him, that you are being kidnapped by the KGB, or was it the CIA?

It was Richard Titmuss who said, 'reality begins with history'. In order to understand why our culture reflects such dissonance, we need to be aware of the origins of ideas about madness and the often contradictory and conflicting themes that came from earlier religious and scientific thinking.

As early as the second century BC, we hear the 'pagan' Terence (195–159 BC) declaim that, 'Nothing in mankind is alien to me'. But the early Christian fathers found such acceptance of differences in others terrifying, as they feared that the mad were associated with witchcraft and demonic possession. Indeed, there was an association between possession and heresy in a society that increasingly demanded adherence to 'orthodoxy', a forerunner of modern totalitarian ideas. Saints Augustine and Jerome have much to answer for; and the arch-Protestant, Martin Luther, was quite convinced that his low moods came from the devil and is reputed to have thrown an inkpot at 'Old Nick'. These archaic attitudes litter Western culture and, weekly in the tabloids, there are examples of unwelcome or socially disapproved of behaviour being described as mad, psychopathic and/or coterminous with evil.

Even in the twenty-first century, when reason and science rule, the typical Hollywood film creates an immediate fearful rapport with its audience when, to a background of tremulous strings, amidst the Victorian gloom, we see a man with staring eyes, muttering meaningless expressions and rambling fears of persecution: 'They are here, don't let them get me.' Then, looking directly at the audience, he asks, 'Have you sent them?' And from his fear, we fear, as our subliminal cultural ambivalence about the mentally disordered is evoked.

We are still in the company of Euripides who said, 'Whom the Gods wish to destroy, they first make mad', echoing Davies' idea of the desolation and destruction that madness causes in humans. Yet, even in the Old Testament, not always associated with progressive ideas, we hear the call for a rational and knowledge-based approach in our dealings with each other, when Job declared:

Who is this that darkeneth counsel by words without knowledge?

(Job 38:2)

It is salutary to consider how relatively recent is our science that began to sever us from some of the old superstitions. For example, it was only in 1859 that Charles Darwin published his *Origin of Species* and, previously, the majority of humankind had few doubts that they were the centre of the universe. Yet, within a hundred years of Darwin, we have atomic power and rocket propulsion and recognise that our little planet orbits 'an unconsidered star at the edge of an unremarkable galaxy amongst billions of galaxies' (Greenpeace 1980). Indeed, we think nothing of recognising that some of these galaxies have distances across that we measure in thousands of light years (Bryson 2003), and even the late Pope, John Paul II, said that heaven and hell are not places but states of mind.

However, mental disorder has often been associated with apparent irrationality; hence, the contradictory issues of care and/or control have never been far below the surface. Furthermore, over the last 50 years, the pendulum has swung between 'certification', which proved a person was 'mad' and was not capable of reasoning and self-control under the 1890 Lunacy Act, to the major breakthrough of concepts about 'treatment', which was at the core of the 1959 Mental Health Act. This is still an important aspect of the present legislation, the 1983 Mental Health Act, although, unlike legislation concerning physical illness, 'mental disorder' still has elements of compulsion for a minority. The seminal breakthrough came in 1959, which was all about de-incarceration and treatment and the concept of 'care in the community'.

Younger colleagues who have never seen the horrors of the old mental hospitals, the old Bins, portrayed in Ken Loach's film *The Music Lovers*, can have little idea of what they became. By the mid-twentieth century, those well-intentioned places of refuge had become dreadful palaces of despair. It is hard to imagine the sum of human misery they accumulated. Under the 1890 Act, tens of thousands of people were de facto locked up for life because they had been 'certified' mad by a magistrate, not a physician, but no-one had considered how one 'proves' one's sanity or which, if any, people should be discharged. The main approach was for a patient to abscond and survive outside for seven days without committing a crime; this was then taken as evidence that the person was mentally competent and therefore 'sane'. The 'asylums' were simply overwhelmed by the numbers of people admitted. Without any provision for discharge, admission under certification had created a cul-de-sac. People understandably feared and resisted admission, and posed a threat to staff who were afraid they would abscond, so staff and patients were on 'different' sides, undermining any latent 'treatment' ideal. While numbers grew, resources shrank relatively. The overcrowding became so bad that many of the large county mental hospitals had their own TB hospital, as the incarceration took its toll in avoidable deaths (Jones 1959). In the old days, one would escort families to their dying relative in a psychiatric hospital's own TB hospital.

The idea of caring for people in the community was an incredible change. It was possible, in part, because of public confidence in the new psychotropic drugs. So that, within a little more than a decade, the number of people more or less permanently locked up in our mental hospitals was reduced from 220,000 to fewer than 70,000 in the 1990s, and now fewer than 30,000 (Department of Health 2002). It is a tribute to improved public perception, although it is still easy to evoke the old attitudes.

Both Mental Health Acts of 1959 and 1983 stressed 'care in the community', which closed the large institutions, creating 'psychiatric units' within the general hospital service. Although this was not perfect, it has gone a long way to reducing some of the stigma against the mentally ill, but there are still some areas that need improvement, not least adequate resources (Jones 1959; Pritchard *et al.* 1997a).

The 1960s and early 1970s were periods that coincided with challenges to established 'authority' and its nostrums and, specific to our interest, saw the burgeoning of anti-medicine and, in particular, an 'anti-psychiatry' movement (Szasz 1960; Laing and Esterton 1968; Illich 1971).

One such critic, Ivan Illich, had much to commend him, because he reminded medicine of the need to go back to its origins – that its art needs to be humane as well as science based – while the media-colourful Ronald D. Laing reminded us of Shakespeare's dictum that there is 'meaning in madness' and, therefore, we should consider the content of the person's apparent 'rambling' (Laing and Esterton 1968). However, Laing's work deteriorated into a diatribe of mystical metaphysics, although he was quite a good minor poet, but he left his science far behind. He later had to renounce his idea that psychosis, or the schizophrenias, was a form of clearer sanity, culturally and/or family induced (Sedgwick 1982). Sadly, some of his unsupported metaphysical theories were taken up by popular culture and can still be found in certain areas of psychobabble, where anecdote and conjecture get mixed up, ignoring the need for evidence-based practice (Skinner and Cleese 1994). One of many practice experiences that taught me to think a little clearer came from this period.

It concerned 'Alan', a nine-year-old diagnosed as autistic. He was 'typical' in that, while functioning at a severely learning-disabled level, he was a very handsome child, with none of the physical disabilities associated with the genetically linked learning disabilities, such as Down's syndrome. We were considering Alan for possible admission to an inpatient child psychiatric unit. His parents sat quietly and calmly with the consultant and me as Alan literally gyrated around the room in a startling exhibition of extreme autistic behaviour of a child who was obviously distressed at the strangeness of his surroundings.

The consultant and I, seeing the composure of the parents, were convinced that this was a classic example of 'refrigerator parents' outlined in the textbooks of the time. This was Leo Kanner's neo-Freudian theory that autism was essentially a lack of bonding between parent and child, mainly because the parent/s were cold and distanced 'refrigerator parents' – the dominant theory in the late 1960s and 1970s and still trotted out by some (Skinner and Cleese 1994).

At my subsequent home visit, I was surprised to find both parents being warmly playful with their younger child. Mrs 'Smith' saw my look and knowingly asked if I thought them 'refrigerator parents'. Now, frankly, nothing is more anxiety making for the professional than when one realises that the client knows as much or more than the therapist, and clearly the Smiths did. They explained that, from the much-wanted Alan's birth, it was Alan who did not react to them!

To all Mrs Smith's early expressions of concern to midwives, health visitors and the GP came the reassurance that all was well because Alan looked such a handsome baby and that she was being mildly overanxious, etc. The parents explained, 'Alan is ours and we love him. We've spent the last seven years trying to get help. But the only way for us to cope is to learn not to get upset at his behaviour. So we sit quietly whilst others panic and then they call us "refrigerator parents". How else could we manage him?'

As an aside, it is worth pointing out that this totally discredited idea continued to be disseminated by some quite eminent therapists long after it was discredited and disproved. For example, the late Robin Skinner, who had probably not conducted any serious research for years, in collaboration with the comedian John Cleese, perpetuated the idea in a book (Skinner and Cleese 1994) that continues to sell well on internet book sites. Since the 1980s, it has been known that the majority of those in the 'autistic' dimension are suffering from a neurological disability that impairs communication between the child and parent, not the other way around (Gilberg 1992; Rutter *et al.* 1994; Rutter 2000; Stoltenberg and Burmeister 2000; Cook 2001; Greenberg *et al.* 2001). The Smith parents, and many others like them, were right, not we 'experts'.

What we professionals, including Leo Kanner, a child psychiatrist of international repute, had *observed* was family and/or parents *reacting* to extreme, unfathomable behaviour of the autistic person, which no-one at the time could explain other than by theories that had no empirical confirmation. We experts were wrong. What they had seen was the *effect* of the condition on those around the child and put it down as a *cause*. It was a classic example of a false correlation. That assumes that, because A and B are present, one causes the other. I quickly appreciated that my then ego-dynamic theories were sadly limited, and that Laing's assertions that a person with a paranoid delusion was reflecting family strife was very attractive, but fundamentally flawed. The Laingians mixed up effect with cause, failing to differentiate between the 'form' of the syndrome and its 'content'.

The 'form' of the condition was those patterned 'signs and symptoms' of the condition, with its 'content' being totally culturally and person specific, as the person tries to make sense of the disruption in their thinking. Thus, the person first feels 'depressed' and then looks for reasons for this feeling from within their life situation. These ideas will be expanded upon later. But, to be fair, the 'anti-psychiatrists' were desperate to destigmatise mental disorder, but inadvertently switched the focus of 'blame' from the distressed person to their families. And Philip Larkin's 'They f*** you up, your mum and dad' is far too facile, appealing to old adolescent emotions in us, rather than looking hard at the *evidence*. That neglecting, rejecting, abusive parents do damage their children, with life-affecting psycho-socio-criminal consequences, is not in question (Pritchard 2004), but the majority of such people do not become psychotic (Pritchard and Butler 2000a). Moreover, careful reading of even the protagonists of 'child sex abuse causes schizophrenia' shows that it is a minority correlation, although it may explain the 'content' of some people's symptoms (Cheasty *et al.* 1998; Read and Argyle 1999; Hammersley *et al.* 2003; Spataro *et al.* 2005). Unhappy, miserable, disruptive lives, yes, as the cycle of deprivation, without adequate intervention, is given a further twist (Audit Commission 1996; Lyon *et al.* 1996), but these people do not necessarily develop one of the major mental disorders. Moreover, insightful novels such as *I Never Promised you a Rose Garden* mistook family conflict as causal, failing to appreciate that the majority of us who experienced an angry and turbulent adolescence nonetheless did not 'break down' into the structured syndromes that are the functional psychoses.

Practitioners will still find parents blaming themselves whereas, when you look into the family history, often the son or daughter experienced no particular family stress or scapegoating, and any family tensions emerged after the subtle and often catastrophic changes in the young person. However, as we will discuss later, there are often real 'trigger' stressors that can be linked to the first breakdown, because human behaviour is a mixture of *environmental events interacting with any genetic predisposition*. This is seen not only in the mental health field, but also in apparently more genetic-based conditions, such as cancers and neurological disease, as these physical conditions appear to require an 'environmental' trigger (Pritchard and Evans 1996, 2001; Bodmer and McKie 2000; Pritchard *et al.* 2004a; Pritchard and Sunak 2005). A key concept at the centre of our practice approach is the idea of the interactive influence of environment and biological endowment upon each other. The mistake is to assume the exclusivity of either. Time and again, it is the impact of the mental disorder that creates the family tension, not necessarily the other way around. Self-evidently, a negative psychosocial environment will predispose some to break down so, if there was previous family strife before the onset of the syndrome, then the advent of yet another stressor makes matters worse. One sees this reaction in families where an unexpected *physical* illness occurs. The majority of people go to great lengths to be understanding and supportive. However, for those undergoing marital disharmony, the impact of one of the partners having a serious illness can be the final straw, and they often blame the underlying tensions as the *cause* of the physical breakdown (Henwood 1998; Rowlands 1998; Pritchard *et al.* 2001, 2004b).

It is interesting to note that two major voluntary agencies concerned with mental health, Mind (the National Association of Mental Health) and the Schizophrenia Fellowship, initially reflected this divisive view of mental illness. Mind tended to blame either parents or the professions, whereas the Schizophrenia Fellowship had a sympathy for parents, who even today still carry the main burden of care and support for mentally disordered people (Leffley and Johnson 1990; Silveria and Ebrahim 1998; Pritchard 1999; Bustillo *et al.* 2001; Martens and Addington 2001). However, the impact of the anti-psychiatrists, who, in effect, ignored the inadequate underfunded mental health service, was to focus upon 'rights'. This led to the extant legislation, the 1983 Mental Health Act, which is very rights orientated, although currently under criticism (see Chapter 9) largely because the original critics forgot about the centrality of resources. Governments are happy to cede rights, as long as they can get away with minimal resources. Successive governmental apologists for underfunded public services trot out the mantra, 'you can't solve these problems by throwing money at them'. Indeed, who could not agree with Margaret Thatcher when she said, 'You can only have the services you can afford'. But, in terms of the proportion of its gross domestic product (GDP) expended on health, Britain does not afford as much as most of the Western world (US Bureau of Statistics 2004). It was shown as early as 1992 that, not only did the UK spend substantially less than the rest of the West, but matters were getting worse across health, education and social services in particular (Pritchard 1992c; Pritchard *et al.* 1997b; Evans and Pritchard 2000). When the last Conservative administration, while reaffirming its commitment to care in the community, gave a record £500 million to social services for their 'adult services', there were initial celebrations in the town halls. What most had failed to notice, however, was that in the early 1980s, 'mental health', because it deals with long-term problems, took 19 per cent of the NHS budget. Ten years later, mental health took only 11 per cent of the NHS budget. The difference between the two is not the half billion given to social services, but rather the three and a half billion that had cleverly been siphoned off (Pritchard *et al.* 1997b). Of course, it is right to expect 'savings' in the medium and long term for mental health services being community based, because this is a more humane and centrally efficient way of dealing with mental health problems. But these become ineffective if they are underfunded, so that front-line staff are often faced with an unfeasible task when there are insufficient resources to meet client needs.

The result of this is seen in recent evaluation of English local authorities' performance in the delivery of 'Social Care (C2) Adults'. Out of 154 local authorities, including the London boroughs, only four were graded 'good'. Forty-three local authorities were described as 'fair' whereas the rest were graded either weak or poor (Audit Commission 2004). Of course, politicians shuffle off any responsibility and blame the services, even though there is overwhelming evidence that, in terms of pound-for-pound expenditure, the British NHS is one of the most efficient in the world, in that it achieves far better clinical outcomes on a considerably lower financial input (Evans *et al.* 2001). In the mid-1990s, when the NHS was especially under-resourced, although cancer treatments had never been better, we had the lowest five-year cancer survival rates in the West (Evans and Pritchard 2000). But recent substantial funding for cancer services has meant that, in terms of the ultimate medical outcome measures, England and Wales has done better than the USA in reducing the death rate from cancers (Pritchard and Galvin 2006). However, this underfunding is not just a social service phenomenon, but occurs across the whole of the public sector. Hence, the current criticism of 'care in the community' and social services is targeting the wrong people – it is not the concept that is at fault, but rather inadequate funding and, it must be accepted, inadequate mental health training in social services, but this probably would not happen if managers did not have to cut corners. Yet, as the reduced cancer deaths have shown, improved resources do make a measurable difference (ibid.).

One longstanding problem that has bedevilled the mental health services has been the controversy centred on the concept of what do we mean by mental health or disorder, which is discussed in detail later. The initial difficulty was that our culture reflected the Cartesian separation of mind and body. This schematic dualism was initially very helpful in studying the human phenomena but, in sociological terms, it became reified, and what was essentially a metaphor became two seemingly concrete separate structures (Szasz 1960; Shilling 1996; Pilgrim and Rogers 1998).

Long after the Second World War, behavioural and mental disorder was seen as either 'organic', with a well-defined and demonstrated underlying physical problem, or 'mental', which simply meant, based upon the technology of the day, that there was no demonstrable physical lesion to account for the problematic and dysfunctional behaviour. This led to an artificial schematic approach of either 'organically orientated', where the patient was treated almost exclusively with pharmacological treatments, or 'psychological', particularly psychodynamic, where everything stemmed from the patient's past. At its worst, and it could be very bad, the 'organic' approach led to the chemical cosh to control behaviour and what my old professor, the late Max Hamilton, described as 'jug and bottle psychiatry'.

The paradox of the psychological approach was that families in desperate social need were offered a watered down psychoanalysis, 'and how do you feel about your mother?', whereas what they required was better education, housing and employment. Not surprisingly, when people's real needs were not addressed, they did not respond to either ineffective approach. Suffice to say, there has been an evolution in ideas about mental health, but one is tempted to assert that, amid all the explanatory research of human behaviour, if we cannot find it reflected in the great poets and playwrights, then it is probably not very important. For example, Shakespeare confronts the question of mind and body head on when he asks:

Canst thou not minister to a mind diseased
Pluck from the memory a rooted sorrow? [disease and stress interaction]

> Raze out the written troubles of the brain,
> And with some sweet oblivious antidote
> Cleanse the stuffed bosom of that perilous stuff
> Which weighs upon the heart? [behaviour patterns, symptom drug treatment
> and emotional reaction]

(Macbeth, 5:3)

The physician's answer is only that:

> Therein the patient
> Must minister to himself.

And, seeing the limits of the medicine of the day, the frantic husband, Macbeth, echoes many of today's patients and families when he says, 'Throw physic to the dogs, I'll none of it.' Yet, as we shall discover, the best evidence points to needing an integration of both approaches.

The classic mental disorders, described as 'functional psychoses' in many psychiatric textbooks, are recognised in every culture (Padmavathi *et al.* 1998; Banerjee *et al.* 2000; Patel 2000; Weisman *et al.* 2000; WHO 2000; Fabrega 2001). However, one of our problems is that, while some behaviour at the extreme is unequivocally 'pathological', for example when a loving mother drowns her child in order to 'save it' from the coming Armageddon (Stroud 2003), at another end of the continuum, a mother's anxiety leads her to behave in a way that most would see as overprotective. There is much in the argument that mental disorder is in part a continuum of emotions and behaviour (Bentall 1995, 2003). Nonetheless, the 'big three' mental disorders do exist, 'the schizophrenias', 'the depressions' and the 'manias', aptly described by Milton when he said:

> Demoniac frenzy [mania], moping melancholia [depression]
> And moonstruck madness [schizophrenia].

(Paradise Lost)

His great insight is marred by his acceptance of his time's assumption of cause, demonic possession, influence of the moon and disorder of the body's 'humours'. We should not, however, sneer at Milton's beliefs as, after all, we were wrong about the benefits of bleeding and the causes of autism, and the more we learn about the functional psychoses, the more we realise that they are far more complex that was first appreciated. What was wrong with Milton's attribution of madness was his limited science, for

> There are more things in heaven and earth, Horatio,
> Than are dreamt of in your philosophy [knowledge].

(Hamlet, 1:2)

Again, Shakespeare's insight tells us much when Hamlet's mother seeks to understand her son's apparently aberrant behaviour. Polonius answers:

> Since brevity is the soul of wit . . .
> I will be brief. Your noble son is mad.
> Mad call I it, for to define true madness,
> What is't but to be nothing else but mad?

Polonius then offers a rationale for Hamlet's behaviour, who

> Fell into a sadness, then into a fast
> Thence to a watch, thence into a weakness,
> Thence to a lightness and by this declension
> Into the madness wherein he now raves . . .
> (3:2)

Self-evidently, such a definition is culture bound but, as we shall see, it is a good description of the 'decline' into what we call schizophrenia as it describes the early confusion of the person, whose own reactive withdrawal and apparently disjointed thoughts, expressed in words, do not register as rational with the observers. Such a situation, then as now, can evoke a degree of apprehension and compassion at a 'mind in ruins'.

What our history, both social and scientific, should teach us is that we need to have an open mind for, as Bacon says:

> If a man will begin with certainties he shall end in doubts: but if he will be content to begin with doubts, he shall end in certainties.
> (*Advancement of Learning*)

My initial training was essentially 'organic psychiatry', which was very limited. Then followed a combination of psychoanalytic and sociological perspectives, which, while having some value, was also limited. On the one hand, the psychodynamic model was of little practical use to a range of clients, as the psychoanalytic theory suggested that it was the client who was 'resistant', not the limitations of the model or of an oppressive society. On the other hand, the sociological approach, while invaluable for the broader context, said little about the person with whom one was working. The development of a psychosocial behavioural approach, which combined some of the empirically established insights of the ego-dynamic (Pritchard and Ward 1974): the centrality of the importance of a client-specific rapport (relationship) as the vehicle for effective communication (Falloon 1993; Linehan 1993); culminating in the use of cognitive behavioural therapy (Kingdon and Turkington 2002), allied with appropriate psychotropic drugs (Baldwin and Birtwhistle 2002); leads to an integrated bio-psychosocial model of mental health social work. This offers the practitioner the widest effective approach to respond to specific client's needs and is empirically based research that is concerned with what works (Falloon 1993; Linehan 1993; Baldwin and Birtwhistle 2002; Warner 2000; Browne 2002; Hirschfeld *et al.* 2002; Kingdon and Turkington 2002).

How important is 'what works', that is, the issue of 'effective outcome'? Or is this but another passing fad?

It is admitted that measuring successful intervention, especially if one is concerned with prevention, can be difficult (Huxley *et al.* 1987; Pritchard 1999; Shepherd 2002). Yet it is central to practice for, if we get the mental health situation wrong, people die (Harris and Barraclough 1998; Pritchard 1996a, 2004; Pritchard and Bagley 2001), and this book pays particular attention to those life and death situations associated with mental disorder. These can end tragically, either when the person turns their distress and aggression against themselves, ending in suicide (Pritchard 1999), or in the often ignored child protection–psychiatric interface, which can end in the death of a child (Stroud 2003; Pritchard 2004). However, all these events are statistically rare, and even rarer is when a complete stranger dies, as in the case of Jonathan Zito's tragic death (Appleby *et al.* 1999; Shaw *et al.* 1999).

It should be stressed at the outset that the mentally disordered are far more at risk of harming themselves than of hurting others (Appleby 1997; Pritchard 1999; Appleby *et al.* 1999; Shaw *et al.* 1999). Nonetheless, we have to acknowledge the reality that family members and those who work with the mentally distressed, especially in the 'residential' situation, face a potential risk (Falkov 1996). Yet, with knowledge, understanding and reasonable care, although the risk exists, it is minimal. This is one reason why we stress the need for all practice to be evidence based.

This book will share with you a wide range of mainly recent or current practice-related research. Yet there is another particularly invaluable source of knowledge for the practitioner, the client. Because we are sometimes uncertain of what is going on, and mental health social work is difficult and demanding, we often fly by the seat of our pants and can always learn from our clients. We can continue to learn only if we keep an open mind, remembering that people are seldom like textbooks. Indeed, the good physician knows that, even when they get a classic case of a physical illness, they are seeing it demonstrated and mediated through the person's individual perspective and unique experience. Moreover, whatever intervention model the practitioner favours, it may not be appropriate with this particular person.

Perhaps the most important feature that we learn from those whom we would serve is the extent of human resilience, integrity, capacity and indomitable spirit in the face of often life-long disadvantage. One of the weaknesses of the 'medical model' is that it tends to focus upon signs and symptoms of 'problems' and weaknesses, often ignoring the strengths the person brings and the context in which they live.

We have already seen how the experts were wrong with regard to autism, because it was not just the individual experience of our 'Smith' family, but hundreds of families like them, who formed the Autistic Children's Society, which made the professionals re-evaluate their practice.

This was also seen in the case of 'Mr Barker', who 'wished to die' and who challenged my simplistic ideas about the rationality of suicide, which can be a major complication or concomitant of mental disorder.

'Mr Barker' was a successful businessman who faced the most horrendous situation and, apparently rationally and with careful preparation, attempted to kill himself, but was saved by a remarkable fluke. On recovering consciousness, he raged at the ward staff for their impertinence in intervening in his life. And after hearing his reasons for his suicidal behaviour, virtually everyone felt very sympathetic to him.

His son had just gone to prison after defrauding a 200-year-old family business; his daughter had been killed in a road accident three months previously; he was dying of terminal cancer with less than three months to live and his wife, who could not deal with the situation, had left him. Professor Max Hamilton, my old mentor, saw him and told him, 'in my book anyone attempting suicide is mentally ill'. Mr Barker's fury was set at nought when Max said 'under the law I can keep you here virtually as long as I like'. This high-handed approach had not ended. Max told Mr Barker that, if he agreed to take some antidepressants for six weeks, and see one of 'my nice young men' for two weeks, he would allow Mr Barker home. If not, not!

As one of the Professor's 'nice young men', I was furious and embarrassed, but agreed to take on Mr Barker, if only to free him from Max's less than gentle bedside manner. Some months later, Max showed me a letter 'which concerns you'. It came from Mr Barker and said 'Dear Professor Hamilton and Colin, thank you . . . the pain is just about manageable, they're saying perhaps I got another month . . . you were wise, life is precious, thank you again, I must have been mad . . .'.

Mr Barker taught me 'never despair' and be prepared to help someone to have another chance of life. On paper, Mr Barker appeared to have every reason to want to die in a controlled dignified way. Yet we had failed to appreciate what modern research shows, that people with physical disease can also have a treatable but accompanying psychiatric disorder (Mermelstein and Lesko 1992; Owen *et al.* 1994; Jones *et al.* 2002). Indeed, it is another case of mixing up effect with cause, for malignant disease actually makes people vulnerable to mental disorders that are found to be treatable (Duckworth and McBride 1996; Linden and Barnow 1997). Indeed, new work shows that fewer older people are dying from suicide than ever before, and that England and Wales in particular have had a big reduction in elderly suicides (Pritchard and Hansen 2005b). One possible explanation for this positive finding is that England and Wales have a specific psycho-geriatric service and, reflecting Durkheim, there is greater social cohesion for elderly people.

Every culture has descriptions of what is considered deviant, bizarre, unacceptable and sometimes dangerous behaviour. Whereas Hindu, Islamic and Western cultures have some attitudes and beliefs about 'madness' that are different, they share many common elements, in which there is a mixture of historical myth, religious ideas and science. This leads to a popular response, which oscillates between apprehension and compassion (Porter 1993). What is most impressive is not those minor cultural differences that are often overemphasised but, rather, the common elements. This was seen in an intriguing case study that led to a direct appeal to the president of a European state. Indeed, you might care to work out when and where the case took place.

The president, who was head of the Senate, was asked to determine the disposal of a senator who had murdered his mother. Asked what punishment the senator should receive, the president replied, 'If you have ascertained that Senator CC was so insane that he is permanently mad and thus incapable of reasoning when he killed his mother, and did not kill her with the pretence of being mad, you need not concern yourself with the question of how he should be punished, as *insanity is punishment enough* (my emphasis).

'At the same time, he should be kept in close custody. This need not be done by way of punishment, but as much for his own and his neighbours' safety. If, however, as often happens, he has intervals of sanity, you must investigate whether he committed his crime on one of these occasions and thus has no claims for mercy on the grounds of insanity.

'But, as we learn from you, his present treatment and care was in the hands of friends, confined to his own house. Your proper course is to examine those in charge of him at the time and determine how they were so remiss, to determine whether there was any excuse or negligence on their part.

'The object of the keepers of the insane is to stop them not merely harming themselves but from destroying others and, if this happens, there is a case for blame upon any who were so negligent.'

This real case study provides as good a rationale for a human rights approach to mental health and disorder as one could find. However, it raises the issues of the 'reality' of a psychiatric diagnosis, personal and professional responsibility, irrationality and any violence surrounding mental illness, and intervention, reflecting the constant tension between care and compassion and, at the extremes, necessary control. The president who wrote this perhaps showed greater than usual perspicacity for a politician as he mixed understanding, compassion and realism; after all, he did not want another tragedy, especially from such a high-profile figure. What would the press say if he or they got it wrong?

Have you worked out when and where the tragedy occurred?

There was no press when this was written, for the case occurred years before the British Lunacy Acts, even earlier than the eighteenth-century Age of Reason, even before the Tudors, with their burgeoning humanity. The president in question was the pre-Christian Emperor Marcus Aurelius (AD 121–180), perhaps appropriately known to history as the 'Philosopher Emperor', the subhero in the modern film *Gladiator*.

Marcus's letter reminds us that mental disorder is part of the human experience and has long posed difficult ethical and practical dilemmas. It will be argued that, holding fast to the human rights approach enshrined in the UN Declaration of Human Rights, allied to the best available practice-related research, we can offer a rational, compassionate and secure service to the person, their family and community. This will be shown in the following chapters, even though at times one feels to be 'flying by the seat of one's pants'.

2 What does mental health/ disorder mean?

Objectives: by the end of the chapter you should:

- understand the concepts of the mind and self;
- understand the cultural and historical roots of our attitudes to mental health and disorder;
- understand the problems surrounding defining mental disorders;
- understand the mood disorders from a psychiatric perspective;
- explore the schizophrenias from a psychiatric perspective;
- understand the strengths and weakness of the medical model.

For to define true madness,
What is't but to be nothing else but mad?
[Polonius in *Hamlet* 2:2 (Shakespeare, 1564–1616)]

This madness has come on us for our sins.
(Tennyson, 1809–1892, *The Holy Grail*)

Great wits are sure to madness near allied
And thin partitions do their bounds divide.
(Dryden, 1631–1700, *Absalom and Achitophel*)

Concepts of mind and self

Our title *Mental Health Social Work* carries an implicit positive message. The word 'health' implies a search for well-being that will enable a person to achieve their life goals. This reflects the great NHS Act of 1948, which rejected the 'sickness' model for its citizens because its founder, Nye Bevan, saw positive health, including social and psychological as well as physical health, as a social and a political goal (Foot 1978). Thus, social work and social care are part of that wider view of the 'healthy' state, which incorporates all aspects of the person and seeks to serve the citizen at every stage of their lives, rejecting any qualification based on gender, class, age or any 'other status' (UN 1948). No matter what may happen with the present structure of social services, there is the continuing recognition that the individual and their family may at different times require a 'personal social service' (Seebohm Report 1968). Indeed, it has been heard said that 'social work' as a term is so badly damaged by unfair media criticism that it needs 'rebranding', and why is the General Council of 'Social Care', not of 'Social Work'? Nonetheless, 'social work' is an integral part of modern British society and is implicitly part of an interdisciplinary approach to the citizen's general welfare, and is therefore multiagency. Fredrick Seebohm's great ideal for Britain was to provide a personal social service coterminous and complementary to the National Health Service. He aimed at a 'one-stop' agency for the family, rather than the multiplicity of agencies that previously existed. However, this 'generic' agency was mistakenly developed as a 'generic' social work service, whereas Seebohm always recognised the need for 'specialisation', in particular, for children, probation and mental health (ibid.). This is not the place to rehearse the policy developments of the past 30 years; suffice to say that the new General Social Care Council accepts the need for a comprehensive personal social service for individuals and their families, including mental health (Berry 2002). What do we mean by 'health'? The *Shorter Oxford Dictionary* (Clarendon Press 1987) defines it as:

1. Soundness of body: that condition in which its functions are duly discharged.
2. Hence: The general condition of the body, usually qualified as good, bad delicate, etc.
3. Healing, cure (1555).
4. Spiritual, moral or mental soundness; salvation.
5. Well being, safety, deliverance (1611).
6. A wish expressed for a person's welfare; a toast drunk in a person's honour (1596).

Thus, we see 'health' as a process, which has positive as well as negative aspects, such as good or bad health. Interestingly, the *Shorter Oxford Dictionary* includes the spiritual and moral along with the mental aspects of health, first noted in the seventeenth century (1611), whereas health activity, healing and cure were so defined almost a century earlier (1555), and a little later (1596) as making positive comment or regard, wishing a person 'good health'. Despite Descartes (1596–1650) separating out 'body' and 'mind', as he radically distinguished the mind as indubitable, 'I think therefore I am', and explained the body on the basis of mechanistic principles, nonetheless health was seen to have both corporal and mental aspects, as well as the 'spiritual'. This goes back to the Greeks, as they saw health as positive in both mind and body, and this integrative notion of health is a crucial basis for all mental health social work, as for general medicine.

With regard to the definition of 'mental', the *Shorter Oxford Dictionary* says:

1. Of pertaining to the mind.
2. Carried on or performed by the mind (1526).
3. Concerned with the phenomena of the mind (1820).

The *Shorter Oxford Dictionary* goes on specifically:

4. Pertaining to, or characterised by, a disordered mind; also
5. Arithmetic, the art of performing arithmetical operations within the mind . . .
6. Mental science (1860).

Here, we have another active or adjectival definition, as 'mental' is perceived and described as a process that is allied to notions of states of health and ideas of 'disorder'.

At the heart of the concept of 'mental health', therefore, is the dual process of mind and body. Within the norm of human experience, we all know how well or ill we feel, when either mind or body is transiently 'disordered' or underfunctioning, which is determined and experienced by the 'mind' – the sense of self.

Concepts of the 'mind', or *'nous'* in Greek, were also related to concepts of the 'soul', whereas 'self' is what the 'mind' recognises as its own. The origins and meaning of both 'mind' and 'self', which are at the core of ideas of normative health and the meaning of the human phenomena, have been at the centre of thousands of years of philosophical debate, which are essentially trying to understand what it is to be human. Hence, how we define mind, mental health and their 'disorder' will inevitably be controversial, because it gets close to central ideas about who we are, not only in relation to each other, but also the cosmos, with all those metaphysical and religious dilemmas and tensions.

Most of us struggle with philosophy but, before answering the question 'what does mental disorder mean?', we need to understand ideas of mental health that impact upon both 'mind' and 'self'. Hence, we consider the development of ideas about the nature of the self and mind, lest we fall into Polonius' circular trap of defining 'true madness' as 'but to be nothing else but mad'.

Humanity's search for meaning drew upon religion, philosophy and science, in that order, which were not initially seen in opposition. Humankind from earliest times recognised itself as part of the physical world, but claimed for itself an 'otherness', which seemed to separate and distinguish itself from other life forms. This philosophical search for truth quintessentially concerned the nature of human existence, so it is to be expected that differing perspectives will arouse passions of opposition for, even in science, 'heresy' is initially not tolerated, until the new heresy becomes the established doctrine. Bertrand Russell's *A History of Western Philosophy* (2000) is more than worth exploring if you wish to go further, and some of his insights are explored in the following pages.

One of the earliest Greek philosophers was Anaxagoras (500–432 BC), who saw mind as the centre and mover of all things. He anticipated Descartes in that he felt that the mind had no physicality.

Plato (428–347 BC) postulated that mind was the arbiter and judge of experience, both physical and non-physical. He stated that the mind contemplates and perceives life and the existence around it, of which itself is a part and apart and, without mind, we cannot understand existence or knowledge of existence.

Moreover, Plato saw knowledge as consisting of reflection, not impressions or merely incoming stimuli. This might be summarised in the dicta, 'Knowledge is perception' and 'Man is the measure of all things'.

Aristotle (384–322 BC), the first great empiricist, sought to differentiate body, soul and mind, the last being superior, essentially because it is the part of humanity that understands abstract ideas such as mathematics and philosophy. This was the epitome of what was best and morally highest in the human being and what distinguished us from all other living things. Moreover, it is human minds that produce social ethics for living, which to the Greek philosophers self-evidently meant the pursuit of the 'good life'. With a strong moral and ethical code for the times, and although such values were only attributable to the citizen, not foreigners, slaves, etc., it did place human thought and behaviour within a strong social context, with obligations to behave in a certain way.

Mind, or nous, for the Greeks was close to the modern concepts of the 'soul', but it was not until Spinoza, said by Russell to be the most 'loveable' of all the philosophers, because of his great ethical humanity, that 'mind' was placed at the centre, albeit with a religious connotation. Spinoza felt that the body belonged to the physical world, whereas the mind was an individualised fragment of 'God', reflecting the earlier Greeks, especially Zeno, who described 'God' as the 'fiery mind of the world'.

The eighteenth-century German philosopher, Immanuel Kant, whom many consider the greatest of the moderns, argued in his critique of knowledge that only mind exists in the absolute, whereas matter was palpably finite. In the twentieth century, the Frenchman Henri Bergson, with his very attractive concept of '*élan vital*' (vital spark), saw mind as memory, which gives shape to the individual, arguing that memory 'is just the intersection of mind and matter'. Russell, reviewing 2,000 years of the history of ideas, quietly and rightly jettisons the artificial division of mind and matter. Indeed, John Gribbon (2002) recently noted that 'whilst physics have been making matter less material' – just consider subatomic particles which show us that even the most dense material, diamonds, have more 'space' than matter – at the same time some branches of psychology 'have been making mind less mental' (Russell 2000). Moreover, as the distinction between mind and matter came into philosophy from religion, and for centuries before modern empirical science the distinction appeared to have validity, it still remains within the public consciousness as such, 'both mind and matter are merely convenient ways of grouping events . . . some belong only to the material groups, but others belong to both kind of groups and are therefore mental and material' (Russell 2000).

Yet, the 'common sense' view of mind, that it defines the self and the individual person, has its own complications. Ideas and emotions that we all have and feel are first and foremost attributed to our selves, but we 'know' they have a physical base in our bodies.

Hume wrestled with the idea of 'self' as an independent being. Being an empirical philosopher, he said 'when I enter most intimately into what I call myself, I always stumble on some particular perception . . . I never catch myself at any time without perception'. Therefore, Russell interprets Hume's ideas of the 'self' as a 'bundle of perceptions', which are concerned with knowledge and probability, of which one's self is a part, while Hegel explained this apparent denial of 'self' by stating that 'Reason is the conscious certainty of being all reality', thus the individual's mind perceives the world and others and has a consciousness of their own being and individuality. Hence, we are both 'object' and 'subject', the 'knower' as opposed to the 'known' according to Henry James. So to define madness is to assert something about the nature of humankind, of you and me, even if we accept in part that 'madness' is a degree, or a continuum, of an extreme state away from 'mental health', or 'normality', as defined by either ourselves or others.

As a practitioner, I am more comfortable with having firmer foundations, albeit not perfect, but a 'good enough' working model, until more or all is known. A seminal work came from the alliance of two unlikely collaborators, a 'Christian' neurophysiologist, Sir John Eccles, and the modern doyen of empirical philosophy, Sir Karl Popper. It was Popper who gave us the 'null hypothesis' idea that researchers should try to disprove their ideas, in an attempt to avoid bias, in the search for more objective truth. Their book *The Self and its Brain: An Argument for Interactionalism* (1984) seems to say it all. Based upon an in-depth study of a range of physiological and psychological experiments in both animal and human cohorts, we find sobering evidence that our genetic linkage to the 'animal' kingdom also has simple cognitive links. Using philosophical notions of mind, Popper and Eccles amply demonstrate the interaction between our sense of self and our neurophysiology in the activities of the brain. Their insights, moreover, came before the development of a range of neuroimaging techniques, such as CT (computerised tomography) and MRI (magnetic resonance imaging) scans, which show subtle structural changes associated with a range of neurological conditions that have psychological features as well as a core mental disorder, schizophrenia.

Other forms of scanning show physiological changes, that is how the structures and nerve cells are operating, and trace areas of neuroactivity associated with consciousness, emotions and perceptions. These are MRS (magnetic resonance spectroscopy), concerned with the concentration of metabolites and cell density, SPECT (single photon emission computerised tomography), PET (positron emission tomography) and FMR (functional magnetic resonance), which are similar and measure blood flow in the brain, indicating physiological activity, and can be associated with emotions. Truly, they are a set of technologies that leave one breathless (Dinan 1997; Malhi *et al.* 2000). Yet it should be emphasised again and again that the innate physiology and anatomical structures are themselves strongly influenced by environmental stimuli and go on being so (Bodmer and McKie 2000; Pritchard *et al.* 2001). Moreover, the classic interaction of pregnancy and social environment is increasingly demonstrated in research concerned with 'fetal origins of disease' (Barker *et al.* 2002), which also includes findings of adult mental disorders and initial low birthweight (Harrison *et al.* 2001; Thompson *et al.* 2001).

The marvel of the neurological is demonstrated in exploring current research in molecular biology, which is opening up to comprehension the way neurotransmitters operate at a subcell level. As you are reading this, there is incredible activity going on in the millions of neurones your brain contains, and as we try a little experiment together. Recall your first day at school – how long has that memory been there, how fast did it return, how detailed is your recall? As yet, no-one knows fully the answers to the questions we have just posed. Recently, in the foremost science journal *Nature*, a review of cutting-edge research on intra- and intercellular activity posed as many unanswered questions as it did explanations (Madden 2002; Kawahara *et al.* 2005; Swanson *et al.* 2005), and we have to resort to the 'poets' again and recall the children's writer Philip Pullman's description of us as beings for whom 'matter was made conscious'.

But to return to consideration of what is the mind. If the mind is the self, what does this do to the concept of our humanity or core ideas about ourselves when 'I fear I am not in my perfect mind'? Of all the anguish of despair in *King Lear*, nothing is more haunting than when he cries 'Let me not be mad, not mad, sweet heaven! Keep me in temper, I would not be mad.' The victim therefore reflects their cultural prejudice and fear, as madness appears to take away their humanity if they are no longer in control, for the UN declaration attributes us rights because we are 'endowed with reason and conscience'. If we have a disorder of the mind, does this not deny our humanity? It may popularly be thought so but, as will be argued, it is not the case at all. Nevertheless, there is good empirical evidence to support Lear's fear of madness as, almost paradoxically, victims of mental disorder take on the discrimination felt about the mad (Foucault 1965; Pilgrim and Rogers 1998), and a classic study of the impact of mental disorder upon women found that, of all the negatives associated with the experience, the initial referral to a psychiatrist was the most distressing, as it seemed to confirm in the mind of the client that they 'were mental' (Miles 1987).

This idea of a disordered sense of self was very much taken up by the anti-psychiatrists of the 1960s and 70s, as utilising the classic false correlation of two events assumed to be causal. This was the height of the 'Cold War madness', when thinking people took to the streets to protest that the irrational defence policy of nuclear weapons relied upon the mnemonic 'mutually assured destruction' (MAD). That is, Britain defended herself against nuclear attack by deterring the 'other side' from a pre-emptive strike. The extreme Conservative MP Enoch Powell pointed out that, because of the geographical size of Britain, three or four hydrogen bombs would have made most of Britain uninhabitable, not to menton causing millions of casualties; Powell described the position as suicide and therefore as a 'defence' totally illogical (Taylor and Pritchard 1982). In the 1960s, Laing (Laing and Esterton 1968) rhetorically asked who was 'maddest', 'Cold War' politicians or people who found the 'irrational' world so at odds with their 'real selves', their 'inner selves', that they withdrew from this 'mad' world?

It is this apparent 'irrationality', the loss of 'self-control' or control of the self, with its associated threat at the extreme of violence, which lies at the heart of individual and societal apprehension of mental disorder. It is not surprising that 'mad' and 'mental' are among the commonest insults in all our cultures, with our philosophical history of notions of the self and all sorts of archaic and superstitious ideas linked to religious beliefs about demonic possession and early rudimentary science.

But, as we shall see, the mind and therefore the self can lose its 'equilibrium' and can become disordered, but the origins are complex and essentially interactive. As the self and its brain becomes dysfunctional, the person and/or others feel that they can no longer meet their psychosocial responsibilities, and they are then defined as mentally ill/disordered or mad. Crucially, however, the experience and its meaning, be it apparently objective, as well as subjective, are profoundly influenced by the culture and psychosocial background of those involved.

Defining mental disorder

One 'cultural' problem is that knowledge and information are truly beginning to be globalised. For example, while what is recognised as disturbed and disturbing behaviour in countries such as India and China, apparently with very different cultural norms, physicians and psychiatrists from that culture, who have been trained in 'Western' medicine, utilise concepts of mental disorder (Lau 1989; Obafunwa and Busuttil 1994). The question then becomes: are they fitting round pegs into square holes, and can such concepts have cross-cultural validity? The answer is 'yes', there is a degree of cross-cultural validity, based upon one of the most prestigious and respected non-governmental organisations (NGO), the World Health Organization (WHO). From the 1960s to the late 1970s, the WHO was active in trying to bring together cross-national understanding of psychiatry in a search for research-based reliable classification of 'mental disorders', and they collaborated with an American NGO, Drug Abuse and Mental Health Administration, because of its considerable experience of working with multiethnic groups [cultural roots are still reflected in USA morbidity and mortality (Holinger 1987; Pritchard and Wallace 2006)]. The WHO successfully developed an invaluable clinical and research tool, the International Classification of Diseases (ICD) and, over the years, improved the system to have ninth and tenth editions based upon the work of physicians from all four continents. The value of an ICD was that there were standardised definitions related to specific diagnoses, which were based upon patients' symptoms and signs. It is readily acknowledged that there will be variations between individuals, and that the ICD classifications from the beginning were only considered as guidelines, but, and this is the crucial point, within each specific diagnostic category, there would be core elements that had to be present before the diagnosis could be made. The ICD-9 was still being used by the WHO up to 2001 (WHO 1979a), and it enables researchers to utilise standardised mortality data to compare a country's performance over time on a number of causes of death. Here is an immediate paradox, for in the apparent hard categorised world of medical diagnosis, there are implicit social factors, as all accept the Durkheimian idea that changing death patterns reflect social changes, be this in diet, clean water or improved services (Wilson 2002; Pritchard *et al.* 2004a; Pritchard and Sunak 2005). Thus, social scientists can use WHO data to highlight differences between the developed nations, for example to show conclusively that, despite marked improvements in the Indian subcontinent, baby and infant death rates are closer to Western pre-Second World War rates, reflecting the reality of economic factors upon health outcomes (WHO 2005).

The WHO, however, was not satisfied with the earlier ICD-9 in relation to 'mental health' and brought together scientists from a range of disciplines from a number of different psychiatric traditions and cultures to seek to improve the classification system. Based upon coterminous research, using a 'composite international diagnostic interview', which then went to field trials conducted in some 40 countries, with co-ordinating centres and directors in Brazil, China, Egypt, India and Russia as well as Western countries, it produced the tenth edition of the ICD. This means that a diagnosis in one country, using this system, is reasonably reliable across countries and across cultures. It is acknowledged that it is not perfect, and Bentall (2003) has major criticisms of the system, while we must never forget in the last analysis that every human being is different and unique as our DNA shows (Wilson 2002). Hence, even in the narrowest physical diagnosis, say of pneumonia or TB, there are psychosocial and cultural overtones, which are reflected in each individual's experience of their physical illness. Nonetheless, the system provides a framework, against which individual's patterns of behaviour can be assessed and hopefully understood. Nonetheless, the WHO acknowledged that 'there is no doubt that scientific progress and experience with the use of these guidelines will ultimately require their revision and updating' (WHO 2000).

Bentall, a very influential clinical psychologist, has major criticisms of these efforts to categorise people (Bentall 2003). Most thoughtful practitioners would agree with him that mental disorders/illnesses are along a continuum of 'normality' of psychological attributes or traits and that the individual moves along a functioning into a dysfunctional and often self-defeating state. Hence, we might all feel occasionally that things, events, people are 'against us' (paranoia) or that we feel down, miserable, low (depressed) or that we can feel particularly good with ourselves, pleased and energised (mania), attributes which at the extreme are recognised as 'madness', when the person appears locked into a persecutory state, or mute and depressed or explosively manic.

Nonetheless, bearing these qualifications in mind, there is some merit in exploring these mental disorders which have a relative global reliability and validity, although we shall return to Bentall's seminal work later.

The WHO use the term 'disorder' to imply 'the existence of a clinically recognisable set of symptoms or behaviour, associated in most cases with distress and interference with personal functions. *Social deviance or conflict alone, without personal dysfunction*, should not be included in mental disorder as defined here' (my emphasis). Interestingly, the WHO eschewed the term 'disease' or 'illness', thus avoiding any inference as to cause. Hence, even though they acknowledged that the term 'disorder' was not exact, it is preferable to the other two as it avoids inference as to cause, and is essentially therefore a descriptive term of patterns of human behaviour and experience that have been found in all cultures.

The traditional division between 'neurosis' and 'psychosis' has been maintained. The former concerns 'stress-related and somatic (body) disorders'. This is in contrast to 'psychosis', which mainly indicates the presence of hallucinations (disordered perception) and/or delusions (false beliefs), or gross excitement and overactivity or marked psychomotor retardation. The conditions associated with a known organic cause are grouped separately.

There are ten main categories of disorder listed, containing specific conditions that appear from research to be logically related to each other; these will be discussed separately as a baseline, not least to familiarise practitioners with 'psychiatric' concepts, and this paradigm is explored in the following chapters.

3 Defining mental disorder
A psychiatric framework

We start with the 'normal' concept of 'mood', that is a state of mind or feeling. The categories are listed and grouped as follows:

1 **Mood disorders** (F30–F39, ICD-10) which include:

    F30 Manic episode, extreme excitements.
    F31 Bipolar affective disorder – mania and depression.
    F32 Depressive episode – ranging from mild to severe.

2 **Schizophrenia, schizotypal and delusional disorder** (F20–F29)

    F20 Schizophrenia – the main group in which the person experiences hallucinations and delusions.
    F21 Schizotypal disorder – which include the mixed category of schizo-mood affective disorder.

3 **Organic mental disorders** (F00–F09)

    F00 Alzheimer's dementia.
    F02 Dementia in other diseases.
    F06,7 Dementia or personality disorder related to brain damage.

4 **Mental and behavioural disorders due to psychoactive substance use** (F10–F19)

    F10 Behaviour disorders related to alcohol (F11–F19), linked to various substances.

5 **Behavioural syndromes associated with physiological disturbances** (F50–F59)

    F50 Eating disorders.
    F52 Sexual dysfunction without underlying organic cause.

And, for us, still somewhat controversial, the 'personality disorders':

6 **Disorder of psychological development** (F80–F89)

    F80 Specific developmental disorders of speech and language.

F81   Specific developmental disorders of scholastic skills.

F84   Childhood autism.

7   Behavioural and emotional disorders with onset in childhood and adolescence (F90–F98)

F90   Hyperkinetic disorders.

F91   Conduct disorders.

F93   Emotional disorders with specific onset in childhood.

F95   Tic disorders (sudden jerky movement of face or limbs, apparently uncontrollable or impulsive).

8   Neurosis, stress-related and somatoform disorders (F40–F48)

F40   Phobic anxieties.

F42   Obsessive compulsive disorder.

F43   Reaction to severe stress – post-traumatic stress disorder.

F44   Dissociative (conversion) disorders.

F45   Somatoform.

9   Disorders of adult personality and behaviour (F60–F69)

F60   Specific personality disorders, including 'paranoid', 'dissocial', 'emotionally unstable', 'histrionic'.

F63   Habit and impulse disorders – pathological gambling, fire-setting, stealing.

F65   Disorders of sexual preference – not 'homosexuality', but fetishism, voyeurism, paedophilia, sado-masochism, etc. – all in today's 'cultural relativism' probably considered controversial.

The next categories might well be considered essentially related to impairment of neurological development.

Finally, a term which seems singularly old-fashioned, stigmatised and inaccurate, 'mental retardation', is still used rather than 'learning disability':

10   Mental retardation (F70–F79)
These are grouped from mild to profound.

The first seven broad categories might reasonably be seen to 'belong' to psychiatry and have links with medicine because, as will be shown, there is a range of evidence to show that these conditions have varying degrees of biological features, as well as psychosocial factors. The learning disability categories are now recognised to be reactive to underlying organic conditions. However, the more socially orientated description of 'learning disability' was found to be more useful in seeking to meet the needs of such people, rather than what became, irrespective of intent, the overly passive hospitalisation leading to inadvertent social exclusion.

The neuroses, while traditionally belonging to the psychiatric–psychological field, are a different category. They can be thought to be at the end of a continuum of human behaviour, spanning what might be assumed to be the 'normal', be it defined socially or as a statistical average or mode, to frank pathology of the psychosis.

The biggest problem, which requires further discussion, is that of the 'personality disorders', which is not to deny such characteristic adult patterns of behaviour exist, but raises the question of aetiology, namely are 'personality disorders' due to disadvantaged backgrounds, inadequate or abusive parenting, or were people born like that? This is a controversial issue as it reflects the reality of practice, and provides a range of professionals – psychiatrists, physicians, teachers, police and lawyers – with major dilemmas, which requires a chapter of its own.

Taking the ICD guidelines as a whole, there is value in considering the approach, providing throughout that we remember it was produced as a guideline for, without such a framework, we can become very confused and uncertain about what we are dealing with in the hurly-burly of daily practice.

So, building upon this framework, this chapters deals with the main functional psychoses and the 'signs and symptoms' of these mental disorders, and the following chapter with the more reactive neurotic conditions.

Mood (affective) disorders

The mood disorders reflect the first two of Milton's great triad of madness – moping melancholia and demonic frenzy – translated into depressive and manic disorders.

Depression

Most humans have relatively low moods occasionally, often for no apparent reason, and, on reflection, most of us appreciate that our mood fluctuates mildly during the day. Individuals are usually described as either 'morning' or 'evening' people, depending on the time of day when they have greatest energy. Yet, self-evidently, in certain circumstances, we will feel misery and depression, classically during a period of ill health or in response to a broken relationship or bereavement: a low mood, a sense of misery or a more prolonged feeling of depression is a natural reaction to misfortune and within the range of normal human experience.

Figure 3.1 best illustrates this continuum from 'normality' into the pathological and dysfunctional.

There are two forms of depression, still described in the textbooks. The so-called 'reactive depression' or 'mild depression', is in apparent response to external stressors, such as divorce, serious illness or bereavement. The second is 'endogenous depression', apparently arising from within but with no apparent appropriate 'cause'. However, one often finds that this form of depression is associated with a relatively mild trigger stress, but the person moves into a deep, pathological form of depression.

ManiaManiaManiaManiaManiaManiaManiaManiaManiaManiaManiaManiaManiaMania

HHHHHHHHHypommmmmmmmmmmmmmmmmHypommmmmmmmmmHypommmmMania

GGGGGGGoodGoodGoodGoodGoodGoodGoodGoodGoodGoodGoodGoodGoodGoodgggg

Midway – Equilibrium_____

LowIIIIIIIIIIIIIIIIIIIIIIIIIIIIIIIIIIIIIIIIIIIIIIIIIIIIIIIIIIIIIIIIIIIIIIIIIIIIIIIIIIIIIIIIIIIIIIIIIIIIIIIIIIIIIIIIIIIIIIIIIIIIIIIIIIIIIIIIILow

MMMiserablemmmmmmmmmmmmmmmmmmmmmmmmmmmmmmmmmmmmmmmmmmmmMiserable

DDDDDDDDDDDDDDDDepression Depression DepressionDDDDDDDDDDDDDDDDDDDD

Figure 3.1 The continuum from 'normality' into the pathological and dysfunctional.

While reactive and endogenous are useful broad categories, in practice someone with 'reactive' depression can sometimes appear as profoundly depressed as someone with 'endogenous' depression, and there is evidence that the so-called 'endogenous' depression is often 'triggered' by stressful events, but it appears to be the speed and profundity of the decline into depression that is different in quality from the reactive form.

What is useful, however, is that there appear to be clear patterns of depression which the ICD usefully outlines.

'Depressive episodes' are typical of all forms of depression but to varying degrees. The person suffers from a loss of energy, diminished activity and low mood, associated with some of the following symptoms. Four main areas of the person's life are affected – mood, cognition, physical symptoms and accumulative interaction – in descending order of misery.

A   Mood

    1   Low mood – a feeling of misery.

B   Cognition

    2   Reduced concentration and attention, both leading to feelings of slowing of thoughts: 'when I try to think, it's like thinking in treacle'.
    3   Reduced self-esteem and self-confidence.

C   Physical

    4   Subjects often complain of poor sleep – they may go to sleep but wake in the early morning and cogitate and worry.

5   Diurnal variation: subjects often feel worse in the mornings, and their misery may lighten later in the day.
6   Poor appetite, sometimes resulting in marked weight loss.

D   Accumulative interactive impact

7   Ideas of guilt and unworthiness – quick to self-blame.
8   Sense of helplessness and, along the depressive continuum, a sense of hopelessness.
9   No sense of a future, sense of futility and emptiness.
10 Ideas about death, thoughts of actual self-harm or suicide.

The key symptoms which should alert you to thinking about depression are a sense of misery, diurnal variation, poor appetite and lowered self-esteem. If these symptoms last for two weeks or more, then most psychiatrists would diagnose the person as suffering from 'depression'.

If one thinks of what the above symptoms must feel like to the person, it is not surprising, dependent upon the severity, that they show a range of psychosocial dysfunction. Such feelings will interfere with their sense of self, their interpersonal relationships and their social interactions and, if they are parents, may undermining their parenting skills. Crucially, dependent upon the severity, they cannot rouse themselves easily out of their all-pervading sense of misery. Moreover, it can be said that depression is 'contagious', as it inevitably involves and affects those people close to the sufferer. In practice, therefore, seeing a procession of depressed people can be very heavy on the worker, whereas for the partner or family member living with a depressed person, it can be even worse when, for a time, they are surrounded by the unrelieved gloom of the other person.

Depression is associated with 'deliberate-self-harm' (DSH), the term now used for 'attempted suicide'. However, DSH is the preferred term as it describes the behaviour, not the inferred intent or 'destination'. Depression is strongly associated with the finality of suicide and merits a chapter on its own.

Mild to moderate depression

This can affect the person in a milder version of the above, in that the earlier symptoms are present, and usually two or three are characteristically present.

In terms of onset, depression in all its form can occur at any phase of life, and it is now accepted that depression can affect children (Hill *et al.* 2004; Bellino *et al.* 2005; Hankin *et al.* 2005; Ladouceur *et al.* 2005). However, it tends to occur in the late teens, with peaks in the middle years (45+ years), hence sometimes described as 'involutionary' depression. Nonetheless, some people may not have a depressive episode until they are quite elderly, 70+ years.

Severe depression (without psychotic symptoms)

Usually the four key symptoms are present, plus three or four of the others. This leads to considerable distress for the person and those around them. Two opposite patterns can be recognised: either distress leads to agitation or, the reverse, energy levels deteriorate and cognition is markedly retarded, leading to slowness of thought, voice or reaction – the sufferer sitting painfully, overwhelmed in a sea of misery. A particular worry is a collapse of their self-esteem, associated with a lack of self-worth, hence 'I'm not worth it – don't bother about me – I'm not worth your time'. In a severe episode, suicidal ideas may be an issue.

Severe depression with psychotic symptoms

This is sometimes referred to as a 'psychotic depression'. Most of the ten symptoms are present and at their severest. The sense of guilt and unworthiness progresses into delusional or even hallucinatory states. The delusions may involve a sense of sin, responsibility for family, community or larger calamities: 'it was my fault X died – I caused his cancer'. Hallucinations involve the subject believing that they are dead, that they can smell their rotting bodies. At the extreme, sufferers can become mute and their whole being may be pervaded with an indescribable stuporised misery.

The psalmist puts it starkly:

> My God, my God, why hast thou forsaken me? . . . I cry in the daytime. . . and in the night season and am not silent. . . . I am a worm and no man, a reproach of men and despised of the people . . . I am poured out like water, and all my bones are out of joint: my heart is like wax. My strength is dried up . . . thou hast brought me into the dust of death.
>
> (Psalm 22)

Or, Milton again,

> Blackened midnight born hag.
> (*Paradise Lost*)

And to see a severely depressed person is to see someone 'wrecked amidst the ship-wreck of mine own self-esteem' (John Clare, *Ballad of Nottingham Asylum*). Hopefully, with modern treatment and the fact that people are more willing to seek help earlier than previously, you should never see the extremes of untreated severe psychotic depression.

Once experienced, it is hard ever to forget it, as it is a dimension of misery far beyond most of our imagining. We should always try to be aware of the emotional reality of the experience and show our recognition to the person. However, experienced practitioners know well that, even in the presence of the most severe depression, when the person seems totally 'out of it', later it becomes apparent that the mute and withdrawn person was sharply aware of what was happening around them: 'when you told me things would get better, I could not believe it then, but I remembered it later and was grateful.' Two brief diagnostic examples from practice follow.

'Mrs Dawson' was a 40-year-old upper-middle-class woman, with three children and a devoted and successful husband; she appeared to have no reason not to believe her life would continue in the very privileged way it had. Her first two pregnancies were not problematic but, following the birth of the third child two years ago, she experienced 'something of the baby blues'. This 'down period' lasted only a few weeks and all appeared to be well.

Mrs Dawson began to feel unwell but in a very unspecified way. She lacked energy, found her sleep was disrupted, found herself becoming easily irritated and agitated with everything around, including the children. Her 'help' suggested she see her doctor, but Mrs Dawson was angry and felt stigmatised. Nonetheless, she found herself tearful and felt 'floods of misery'. Her husband noticed her decline in libido, but she rebuffed any idea that there was anything wrong and insisted that she would 'pull myself together'. Over the next few weeks, Mrs Dawson's mood became more miserable, she lost appetite and weight, always felt tired and, while she could get off to sleep, found herself with early-morning wakening and unable to return to sleep, during which time she 'worried and fretted'. She looked grey, drawn and quite ill, and initially saw her GP for a 'check-up', fearing cancer. His enquiry whether there were any problems between her and her husband was fiercely denied and, as she 'didn't believe in psychiatry', she refused antidepressants. She rebuffed 'Mr Dawson's' solicitous concern because she felt ashamed. Mr Dawson was away on business for two weeks, during which time she became miserable, withdrawn, taciturn and depressed, and later admitted to serious thoughts of harming herself: 'I've failed "John", I'm not worthy of his love, he'd be better off with me out of the way.' On his return, Mr Dawson was alarmed at her deterioration as, especially in the mornings, she either sat motionless and inert or cried in an agitated way, distressed 'because I don't know why I feel like this'. Within a discernible period of six weeks, Mrs Dawson had collapsed from being a happy, competent, confident middle-class woman to being a 'washed-out drab'.

Mrs Dawson was a classic case of unipolar affective disorder when, apparently with little external trigger, she slid quite rapidly into a seriously depressed state. She was treated very successfully with antidepressants and made a good recovery. However, this case was also a good example of how depression in one person affects the other.

On meeting Mr Dawson, the social worker mentioned that it must have been a difficult time for him. This remark distressed him: 'you're the first person to ask about me. When my wife first became ill, I did not recognise what was happening and I thought my marriage was coming apart. It was the worst time of my life as I thought I'd failed her.' Mr Dawson's needs had been ignored, in part because he was a very competent person, but his experience reminds us that depression is 'contagious' and that it does not happen in an emotional vacuum and invariably affects those around the sufferer.

Mania

If depression is a collapse of the ego, mania is almost the exact opposite. Everything is elation, a sense of boundless energy, so sleep appears unnecessary, thoughts race, ideas tumble over one another, and the world and the individuals themselves are wonderful. There is an almost electrifying expansion of their self-esteem and an expansive egoism that even politicians seldom match.

1 Mood – positive and rising at the extremes to ecstatic.
2 Cognition – speeding of thoughts and speech, so that words and ideas come so quickly that the person is close to being unintelligible.
3 Physical symptoms – energetic, never seems to tire, rushing around and very agitated. Sleep – 'who needs it?'
4 Accumulative interactive impact of affect, with growing excitement, joy, elation, ecstatic expansion of sense of self; said a client: 'I was Father Xmas to the world and on a high and I knew the great secret.'

Considering what such a state must feel like hints at the problems surrounding the person. First, they tire and overwhelm those around them and, if their excitement grows, they can cause fear and anxiety in others, which may lead to inadvertent reactive violence, in part from our incomprehension of the person and the client's irritation that we do not share their joy and understanding.

They quickly become incapable of normal social functioning, not least because their attention span is all over the place. Everything seems to be a source of stimulus and, while easily excited, equally easily distracted and often worrying to others, become totally disinhibited.

There are three accepted patterns of 'manic-affective disorder'.

Hypomania

This is a mood disorder in which the phase of mania is a little less marked than a full-blown manic episode. It is similar in theme to mild or moderate depression, in that the manic episode is much milder. Indeed, a good example are those TV adverts with the salesperson talking twenty to the dozen, buoyantly good-humoured, exuding hail-fellow-well-met. Indeed, as we shall see, Jamison (1995) suggests that 'subclinical' hypomania can be a valuable attribute in many professions and is a good indicator of the notion of a continuum of mood. Indeed, some people, when faced with extra demands, can almost call upon their own 'manic phase' to give them extra energy.

Mania without psychotic symptoms

This is the manic phase described above, which usually has its first onset between the ages of 15 and 30. The collapse of social inhibitions, with grandiose behaviour, quickly leads to a breakdown in social functioning.

Mania with psychotic symptoms

An even more severe form of mania, which may include delusions of different identity, although whether the person thinks they are the monarch or whether they feel they are like the monarch is debatable. Some authorities suggest there may be auditory hallucinations, and sometimes it is difficult amidst the boundless excitement and energy to know, and it almost merges into schizophrenia (see below).

'Dr Evans', aged 60, had very severe mania, which, unusually, was very hard to control. Over the years, he had relapsed a number of times after stopping his medication, lithium, although sometimes he had gone more than a year without an attack. Because of his age, we were concerned about heart failure.

His home had changed within two days from being a comfortable middle-class dwelling to being a near wreck, as he had scribbled mathematical formulae over every conceivable surface. On seeing me, he offered me a thousand, million, million, million, million, million pounds. His humour was infectious and, while tiring, made one smile. Sometimes, he would make sexual references if females were about, which of course could easily be misunderstood if observers did not realise that he was in a manic phase.

His speed of thought was reflected in his rapid speech in which his words tumbled over themselves. Later, one began to realise that the mania was subsiding, as he almost wistfully repeated his largesse but 'you couldn't live long enough to spend it'.

Typically, however, Dr Evans suffered not just from mania but also from the reverse side of the mood disorder.

Again, the extremes of mania are rarely seen because of better and speedy treatment but, once experienced, never forgotten.

Mania, similar to depression, is infectious, especially with the person with hypomania as it is hard not to smile and share their good humour and good fortune.

However, untreated mania can lead to death, and I remember the sense of tragedy we all felt when a client with severe mania absconded and, two days later, was found dead in a ditch, having died essentially from exhaustion.

Bipolar affective disorder

Depression is sometimes described as 'unipolar affective disorder' as the disordered mood produces only the depressive syndrome. Some people suffer from a 'bipolar affective disorder', as did Dr Evans, which produces a period of depression, either preceded or followed by a period of mania: Milton's 'demoniac frenzy'; the raging madman of popular stereotype.

However, to see Dr Evans post-manic phase, almost a shadow of the being of two or three days previously, as he moved into the pain of the other end of the spectrum, was a graphic illustration of this cruel affective disorder, namely 'manic-depressive' or 'bipolar affective disorder'. The sufferer is torn between the two extremes of a disordered mood. In a week, such people can span the heights of ecstasy and the depths of hell as the hopelessness of depression tells them to 'abandon hope all ye who enter here' (Dante's *Inferno*); hence, depression might rightly be called psychic hell.

Manic depression

However, bipolar affective disorder is characterised by repeated phases as the person swings from a manic phase into a depressive one, at the extremes, at both ends of the continuum. However, recovery is usually complete between episodes, and there is a tendency for people with mania to have a corresponding depressive phase but perhaps not at the extreme of depression, in that manic episodes by themselves are relatively rare.

Kay Jamison, a Johns Hopkins University Professor of Psychiatry, has written a personal memoir of someone who suffers from a 'manic-depressive' disorder, which is deeply moving and graphic. Her personal story and 'text', *An Unquiet Mind* (1995), confronts the usual stigma surrounding mental disorder and provides a 'must-read' guide for all practitioners. Yet she asks herself the question, as her bipolar disorder is largely controllable, would she, given the choice, have preferred not to have had the disorder – she answers 'no' (p.12).

> Strangely . . . I would choose to have it. It's complicated. Depression is awful beyond words, or sounds or images; I would not go through an extended one again. It bleeds relationships through suspicion, lack of confidence and self-respect . . . the exhaustion, the night terrors, the day terrors.

Professor Jamison argues that non-sufferers cannot know what depression is like, even in part through having themselves experienced traumatic life events, e.g. divorce, bereavement. But these events, she says, are different because 'these experiences carry with them feelings. Depression instead, is flat, hollow and unendurable . . . People cannot abide being around you if you are depressed.'

She reminds us that de facto depression is 'catching, contagious, as if it affects and wears down everyone around the sufferer'. Yet, as our Dr Evans would say, 'the mania almost makes up for it, because then I live life differently'.

Jamison goes on to say that 'though the hypomanias and mania itself all have brought into my life a different level of sensing and feeling . . . finding new corners in my mind . . . incredible and beautiful . . . some grotesque and ugly and I never wanted to know they were there or to see them again'. Shades of Huxley's *Gates of Perception*, with its dangerous subliminal 'advertising' of psychedelic drugs, but she uses her personal experience to remind us how important it is never to lose sight of the humanity in the person, even within the worst disturbed and disturbing episode. Indeed, she took her personal insights and explored the minds of other possible manic-depressive suffers. She traces the lives of some great Western poets, Shakespeare, Byron, Kelly, Keats, etc., in her book *Touched with Fire* (1996), in which she demonstrates the likelihood that some were also manic-depressive sufferers, such as the irrepressible William Blake, who may well have shared Professor Jamison's experiences of near-psychotic hallucinatory and delusional ideas, which the evolutionary psychologists speculate 'contribute to the richness of human nature'. Yet, in a modern, structured world, this can be dysfunctional, as it can also be creative and assist human progress (David and Cutting 1994; Pinker 1998; Stevens and Price 2000). And the common view that 'madness is akin to genius' is echoed in Dryden 'Great wits are sure to madness near allied', which reflects both the evolutionary psychologist's view and that of Jamison that poets are 'touched by fire'. Indeed, the psalmist David might well also have known such joys and agony, for he exhibited the depths of depression and the ecstasy of oneness with the cosmos (Pritchard 2000).

The mood disorders highlight the modern notion of a normal continuum of personality traits, which at the extreme are experienced as dysfunctional and would appear to be pathological. While we will discuss ideas of 'causes' later, our approach, if not already obvious, has to be declared, namely human experience is multicomplex and influenced by the interaction of our physiology, psychosocial backgrounds and experience. So that, when the poet says, 'This madness has come on us for our sins', while we reject such a direct relationship, our practice experience has many examples of a person attributing their depression to the gap between how they would like to be and how they feel they are. The question is, does the genetic susceptibility we may carry make us more vulnerable to the 'slings and arrows of outrageous fortune'? It seems reasonable to accept that, as we 'inherit' the potential for depression from our family backgrounds and psychosocial circumstances, our physical attributes, genetically influenced, will either be an asset or a barrier to being able to respond to external stressors and enter into a degree of mood disorder, at the extreme a full clinical depression (Wildes *et al.* 2002; Coyne *et al.* 2004; Hill *et al.* 2004).

Yet 'moping melancholy' appears with or without apparent cause. Interestingly, the rapid growth of morphological (study of cells) and genetic research over the past 20 years suggests that there may be genetic components making people vulnerable to mood disorders (Souery *et al.* 2000; Massett *et al.* 2002; Klar 2002; Swanson *et al.* 2005). However, the morphological mechanism is still far from clear, and, in contrast to schizophrenia, there is not the firm evidence from twin studies for the case of depression (Cardno *et al.* 1999), while the old nature versus nurture argument is far too simple. Interestingly, it is the bipolar rather than unipolar disorder that appears to have the stronger genetic influence, although current research on affective disorders emphasises the environmental and genetic interaction (Johansson *et al.* 2001; Arias *et al.* 2002; Souery *et al.* 2000; Klar 2002). On reflection, this really is common sense, for we have all met children and young people who belonged to the most damaged and disruptive families, yet emerged relatively unscathed, while others, apparently in response to quite minor stress, succumb – what Rutter (1999) has described as 'inherited resilience'.

We turn now to perhaps the most controversial of the mental disorders, the disruption of the mind and its self, the schizophrenias.

4 Defining mental disorder

A framework for the schizophrenias

The schizophrenias (F20–F29)

This mental disorder is perhaps one of the most misunderstood in the arguments about cause and origins. Typical of the late nineteenth-century scientist categorising new phenomena, the term schizophrenia is derived from the ancient Greek: 'schizo' literally means split or fractured, and 'phrenia', pertaining to the mind. Sometimes, this has popularly been described as 'split personality', which the syndrome is not, and some mix it up with the so-called 'multiple personality', which probably does not exist without the external shaping of unconscious 'collusion' of the therapist, and the receipt of an attention-giving media (Stubner *et al.* 1998; Rieber 1999). The ICD describes schizophrenia as 'characteristic distortions of thinking and perception', and it is best considered as a disorder of thought patterns. While normal cognition is usually maintained, because of the accompanying hallucinations, which can affect any of the senses, and delusions that seem to 'explain' to the person what is happening to them, the person is invariably disturbed and disturbing. This reaction can itself create a response in those around the person, often adding to the interactive complexity and confusion.

The disorder impacts upon the sense of self as the person's core identity can be overwhelmed by the experience, and many of the secondary signs and symptoms stem logically from the core disorder of their thoughts.

There is often a process as the person moves or is drawn into this core psychotic disorder, which may last weeks or may occur suddenly within hours.

What have been described as the 'front-rank symptoms' of schizophrenia are a useful *schematic* way of exploring the phenomena.

Disordered thoughts

These may be slowed down or speeded up; thought 'blocking' occurs, i.e. when the person cannot think (although this is a common phenomena when one is asked a question and the 'mind goes blank'). Sometimes, the person can hear their own thoughts, or feels their thoughts are echoed in their head. They can feel that either the thoughts are intruded into them, i.e. do not belong to them, or their thoughts can be heard by others, sometimes described as 'broadcasting of thoughts'.

All or any of these features can be present. It can be argued that, with this primary thought disorder, the following four front-rank symptoms are a 'logical' reaction to the inner experience, as the person attempts to make sense of what is happening to them.

Disorder of perception and affect

This is often described as classic 'incongruity of mood' where the person might have an almost reversal of expected mood, laughs at something sad, expresses sadness at something amusing. There can be a more persistent incongruity of fatuous mirth at any comment made by another person. Sometimes, there can be a rapid switch of mood – labile is the term used – which may cause you to think of a bipolar disorder. However, by centring upon the thought disorder, it is easy to understand how easily both their perception of what is happening around them and their mood can be disturbed and, equally, how easily others misunderstand them.

Disorder of volition

Some textbooks use the concept of 'passivity feeling', where the person no longer feels fully in control of themselves, or feels that they are being controlled or, before this stage is reached, they feel a lack of purpose, inert and unable to deal with what is occurring around them. At the extreme, they can appear both emotionally and physically stuporised (in a stupor), which forms the basis of a so-called type of schizophrenia, catatonia (see below). For some authorities, to clinch the diagnosis either primary hallucination or delusion or both must be present.

Disorder of senses: hallucination

All five senses can be the site of a hallucination.

Auditory hallucinations are the most frequent. The sufferer actually hears voices. Sometimes they start 'at the back of your mind like someone whispering, then you can tell the words, "you're a bastard, bastard". The voice is in your head, you can't get away from it and it terrifies you, oh no, not again, not again' was the description given by 34-year-old 'John', who had had two previous episodes of schizophrenia. Just imagine if this was you, as an idea, a thought, a voice expressing the most intimate hostility was happening to you; not surprisingly, such an experience is very disturbing.

Visual hallucinations, contrary to popular belief, are relatively unusual. When they do occur, it seems like a disturbance of vision as objects or people's faces are surrounded by a 'van Gogh'-like penumbra. For some, this can be visionary-like and may be associated with visionary-like delusions (see below). However, 'seeing things' such as snakes or fearsome animals is more likely to be associated with the extremes of chronic alcoholism, such as Korsakov's syndrome, or may be the result of mind-changing drugs such as LSD (Duwe and Turetsky 2002).

While Aldous Huxley in his *Gates of Perception* wrote somewhat blithely about the experience, in our own caseload we have known two deaths from 'bad trips' literally years after the last known intake of LSD. Recently, modern brain imaging techniques have highlighted visual hallucinations associated with certain forms of dementia and neurological disease, which raises fascinating questions about the bio-psychosocial interaction of visual hallucinations and the underlying anatomy and physiology (Hermanowicz 2002; Silberstein *et al.* 2002; Walker and Stevens 2002).

Taste and smell can also be the sites of hallucination, which can easily become the source of the idea of being poisoned. However, as with visual hallucinations, these hallucinations may well have an underlying organic base, such as epilepsy, and a physician should always rule out such a differential diagnosis.

Sensation, that is touch, can also be involved in a hallucination. This often runs with the idea or delusion of being infested with some crawling horror, or impenetrable itch. In the few cases I have known, hallucinations involving touch seemed to involve another person, if they had a close partner. All involved the person having ideas of alien infestation, a delusion which was then shared by their partners. When this occurs, there appears to be a shared psychotic state, described in the textbooks as *folie à deux*, madness of two, usually in the presence of a dominant person and a vulnerable one, such as a young adult and a parent, or a symbiotic relationship of a dominant man over a compliant woman (Cypriano *et al.* 2000; Raulin *et al.* 2001; Seiger *et al.* 2001). This is a rare situation, but can be very fraught, as suicide of one or both the sufferers is a real possibility.

Primary delusion

Delusions are defined as a false belief, but we must always give due acknowledgement to the emotional reality of the patient's experience. Moreover, delusions are always time and culturally influenced, and some believe that they are a form of logical explanation and attribution by the sufferer of what they are experiencing. Therefore, an 'intrusion of thoughts' might well easily lead to the idea of external malign or even alien forces. Moreover, we should remember Polonius' view 'Though this be madness, yet there is method in't'; indeed, one of the useful aspects of the anti-psychiatrists (Laing 1960; Laing and Esterton 1968; Sedgwick 1982) was to remind us that the thought-disordered person was attempting to communicate with us. It was as if one side of the two-way radio was faulty and the person with schizophrenia made utterances that were not so much nonsense but rather a 'word salad' of unintelligible jumbled-up words. If one knew the person or, as one should always do, listened carefully, we could often understand the person and certainly the emotions being expressed.

I was called to the university's children's nursery as a man had entered and was distressing mothers and children. On arriving, it was obvious that he was operating under some delusional ideas, although he was expressing real concern for the children and 'wanted to help – to protect them and keep them from harm'. I engaged him, giving overt recognition to his concern but was able to show that (a) the children were safe with staff and some of the mothers and (b) inadvertently he was causing alarm. While this confused him, he was willing to leave the building, which he had initially refused to do, which had caused the original alarm. When we got outside, he was confused and sat on the wall and said 'I am here for the children but you have hurt me . . . I can not be blamed for the evil that is around them . . . why don't you persecute them not me who wants to help'. I realised that he had felt wronged by my intervention, only in his thought-disordered confusion, he could not express this other than by showing his hurt feelings.

There are four common broad types of delusion. Classically, those surrounding religion, across the cultures, are evident as the person expresses beliefs that their God or some divine personage speaks to them, or has a special purpose for them (Lau 1989; Goold 1991).

Possibly associated with passivity thinking are those persecutory delusions, 'it, something, they' are against the sufferer. For example, this may be the Devil if a Christian, Shaitan if Muslim, or the God Khali if from a Hindu background. What is common across all three cultures is a supernatural personage persecuting them.

What might be described as 'science fiction' delusions, which overlap with persecutory delusions, occur when the sufferer is being spoken about on the TV or radio, is in contact with extraterrestrial beings, or their thoughts are being broadcast on microwaves and the like.

Finally, in what might be described as depersonalised delusions, the sufferer believes that he or she contains or has been taken over by another person, a notion that has elements of the persecutory and science fiction. Indeed, sometimes these delusions are quite patterned and systematic and form the plot for modern novels and plays, centring on misidentification. The sufferer is convinced that there is a personal double of a significant person close to them, or that another person has been taken over by impostors, robots or aliens (Ellis and Lewis 2001). This subset of schizophrenia is called the 'Capgras syndrome' and, although not common, is, once seen, never forgotten. Although 60 per cent of cases described are associated with schizophrenia, another intriguing dimension of this whole field is that the remaining 40 per cent can be associated with a range of organic disorders or brain trauma (Edelstyn and Oybode 1999; Breen *et al.* 2000; Marantz and Verghese 2002; Rentrop *et al.* 2002). Yet even here there are cultural influences; for example Capgras syndrome occurs more often in Maori people than in Caucasian New Zealanders, but we do not know why (MacKirdy and Shepherd 2000).

Positive and negative types

Modern textbooks are increasingly ignoring the classical types of schizophrenia and describing it in two broad types, which schematically fall into schizophrenia with 'positive' and/or 'negative' symptoms. The positive type occurs with florid symptoms, with marked sudden onset, clear indications of delusions and hallucinations but with shorter episodes and more often a good recovery.

Negative-type outcomes produce more passive symptoms, dulled affect and withdrawn, odd mannerisms, and social impoverishment as if the person had not developed a sufficiently robust independent personality before the ravages of the condition wore them down. Negative symptoms can often be secondary to late-onset schizophrenia, especially if they have had more than three or four schizophrenic episodes.

Classical types of schizophrenia

Simple

Onset usually occurs before the age of 20 and is characteristically insidious. Commonly, the family retrospectively describe deterioration in the young person's behaviour over the previous 6 or 12 months, e.g. staying in bed, inability to meet minor social demands, progressive oddities of behaviour, truculence, withdrawal, etc. Often, this is initially put down to 'typical' adolescent' behaviour. It is essential to appreciate that this is more than a transitory mood and that, in terms of maturity, the person has gone backwards as his or her personal performance declines. There can be an early slide into negative symptoms of blunting of affect and loss of volition, although clear-cut delusions and hallucinations are less frequent.

'Frankie' was nearly 18 when first seen by the consultant psychiatrist. Until she was 14 years old, she had been a bright, intelligent, albeit quiet teenager who enjoyed most things appropriate to her age. Frankie began to be 'a little difficult – obstructive' said her mother. 'I thought it was the teens sheens, until we realised that she'd gone backward in everything. Her work, her dress, and she used to be very keen on fashion, and got silly and babyish.' Over the past six months, 'Frankie' became withdrawn, occasionally fatuous to other people and, in an odd way, grandiose. She refused to get up in the mornings, began to neglect herself. Typically, her parents assumed she was being a difficult teenager, and the parents were very alarmed at the social worker's suggestion that she might need psychiatric help and, initially, they withdrew their request for service. Within two months, however, the parents realised that there had been further deterioration and that she was 'very unconnected'.

Frankie's illness was typical of early-onset simple schizophrenia, with the key signs that there appeared to be a break in her personality development. Later, there were signs that she had some thought disorder, with thought blocking and odd interpretation of what was said to her.

The parents were very self-critical: 'I blame myself, I should have realised that something was wrong.' The parents sought to attribute a cause or trigger for Frankie's condition but, until her simple schizophrenia emerged, there were only the usual minor family tensions of boundary setting and clash of generation boundary disputes. Later, it transpired that there was a maternal great-aunt who had probably had a schizophrenic-type illness some years before and Frankie's reactions were disproportional to any distress from peer pressures.

Hebephrenic

Hebe was the Greek goddess of youth, and thus the diagnosis of hebephrenic schizophrenia reflects both the time of onset and the frequent apparent prankiness and manneristic behaviour. It usually affects people in late youth, often with very florid symptoms: very thought-disordered, rambling speech, with inappropriate and unpredictable behaviour. The earlier the onset, the less good the outcome, as earlier 'negative' symptoms are a corollary of impaired personality development.

'Graham' was 22 years old; his first schizophrenic episode followed a minor employment crisis, when he changed from being a 'very average lad' into a very disturbed young man. He expressed bizarre and uncoordinated ideas, laughing fatuously and sometimes threateningly in a half-joke physical challenge, which, if misunderstood, could have led to reactionary violence from others. He had 'ideas of reference', he related everything on TV to himself, claiming that David B and Mrs B were in love with him, that he had 'the secret of life which will make England win the World Cup', and then his speech and ideas would wander off in unintelligible way, which made it very difficult to pick up his emotional state.

Paranoid

This is said to be the most common form of the schizophrenias, and is characterised by delusions of persecution which are often accompanied by 'command' hallucinations, in which the person is told and directed as to what to do. These can be especially distressing and frightening as sufferers often hear a voice commanding them to do certain things, not infrequently to kill themselves. Equally alarming can be command delusions to hurt someone else in order to protect themselves. Some textbooks suggest that this paranoid type has a later onset but, as the condition is quite systematic and stable, it may be that the ideas come from events in the person's life (Read and Argyle 1999). Conversely, the later the condition affects the individual, the less damage is done to the developing personality, and sufferers establish a more mature personality, enabling them to deal with the problem better, which is the converse of the 'simple' type.

'Mr Harris' was a 45-year-old successful businessman and a pillar of the local community. Some six months previously, his usual impeccable politeness and attention to detail deserted him, and there were a number of unexpected minor quarrels with a range of people. It was noticed that he would retire into his office even earlier than his usual early start and appeared to be reluctant to see anyone, even though he appeared to be managing his work. Later, it was recalled that, up to a week before the 'incident', he appeared preoccupied, and a number of observers thought that they had heard him muttering to himself. Mr Harris's description of what occurred is illuminating. For some weeks, he had felt very uneasy for no particular reason; he was quite sure that his staff had turned against him and were making unfounded complaints to Head Office. He recalls being disturbed by hissing sounds, which threatened to 'overwhelm my thoughts'. He knew there was something wrong but 'couldn't put my finger on it'. He was called to a meeting at Head Office and was driving himself, when he noticed a car trailing him. 'Suddenly I knew. It all became clear. It was the IRA trying to kill me.'

Mr Harris then drove his car into the frontage of a branch of his bank to 'escape his killers'. Fortunately, no-one was seriously hurt, but he exemplifies the late onset of paranoid schizophrenia and the relatively sound personality, which enables the late-onset person to cope with these abnormal experiences. He later produced a whole series of reasons why the IRA should want to injure him, in a very complex set of delusions, including the Royal Family, MI5 and MI6 and 'the Russians in cahoots with Colonel Gaddafi', which is typical of the systematised deluded ideas, probably a rationalisation of the psychotic experience, but all very current and culture specific. In that sense, therefore, there may well be 'method in his madness'.

While it must be stressed that mentally disordered indivduals are a much greater risk to themselves than to others (Pritchard 1999), the presence of patterned paranoid delusions in particular can be associated with the potential for violence (Monahan *et al.* 2005) and, while the strongest positive correlation for current violence is a history of previous violence (Hartl *et al.* 2005), it is in those interactive situations where the presence of a mental disorder is not understood and the person misinterprets others as being a risk to themself that violence can occur (McNeil and Binder 2005). Consequently, where paranoid ideas exist, special care has to be taken, and serious consideration has to be given before the therapist is alone with the person, unless there are security measures in the room. It is rare, but it happens, especially in the 'homelessness' situation (ibid.) and, if the worker is anxious about the situation, they should terminate the contact as gently as possible and gain some external advice. A recent actuarial model that predicts violence is valuable, but it must be remembered that, like all predictive instruments, it is only a guideline, albeit one of the best, and that none can ever be 100 per cent foolproof (Monahan *et al.* 2005).

Catatonic

Catationic schizophrenia is characterised by marked motor changes, mainly of stupor and inertia, with automatic obedience, but at the extremes can also include hyperactivity. Ideally, one might go through a career and never see this, as it is thought to be associated at the extreme of passivity feelings of untreated schizophrenia. Also, such catatonic states were seen in the worst examples of severe institutionalisation in the previous large mental institutions (Goffman 1961). The erosion of the 'big bins' of the inter- and immediate post-war years was such that there were incredibly overcrowded wards, with virtually no staff–patient interaction. I saw the effects of a famous project to reactivate 'mute schizophrenics', such were the numbers in the 1950s and 1960s. Hall and Baker (1971) introduced a behavioural token economy unit on a large back ward with men who not been known to speak for an average of 25 years. In retrospect, it was appreciated that the 'active ingredient' that reintroduced speech with the patients was that staff were tangentially given incentives to engage with their patients, in effect for the first time in many years. I had known the ward more than 15 years previously and visited to see the transformation. It was an impressive example of (a) the accumulative impact of warehousing mentally disordered people and (b) the power of active interactive personal relationships.

I was approached by 'Ivor', a man in his late 50s who had been in hospital more than 30 years. Ivor was the ward 'kicking post' as, following a fracas between patients, the loser would go and kick Ivor. Everyone bullied Ivor and, worse, we students were shown 'classic catatonia' as he was put through his paces of total passivity as his limbs were placed in statuesque postures. This was contrasted with another long-term inmate, 'Freddie', whose echolalia was demonstrated. That is, we would say something and Freddie would repeat it , such as 'am daft Freddie'. Even the most insensitive student recognised that this was a hideous form of Pavlovian conditioning – such were the back wards of the 1960s. On my return to the ward, at first I did not recognise Ivor, who spoke to me as he remembered that I had spoken to him and given him things in the past: 'You were an attendant here, you used to give me chocolate, how are you now?'

This was deeply moving because here was a man who had shown no emotional response whatsoever, yet could recall simple human contact years before, reminding us that the person always remains, even within the most severely psychotic state, whether or not it is biologically or environmentally induced.

When visiting long-term psychiatric hospitals in Romania just after the fall of the Ceauşescu regime, I again saw examples of institutionally created catatonic states, the accumulative impact of neglect and the simple warehousing of mentally disordered people, devoid of human stimulus (Pritchard 1991). However, recently I saw a 'natural' catatonia in a 45-year-old man, whose mother was desperate to keep him out of hospital by avoiding seeking help when 'Michael' refused his medication. He entered a psychotic state lasting for more than 12 months. His mother contacted us only when he finally refused to eat as she was alarmed at his physical deterioration. Such situations are very rare and, hopefully, today few front-line workers should expect to come across a person in a catatonic state.

Schizoaffective disorders

It had been thought that the schizophrenias and the affective disorders were completely separate conditions and that possible manic attacks or depressive symptoms within a schizophrenic state were reactive to the particular situation. Within this syndrome, either element of the affective disorder can predominate, depression or mania, which makes treatment and intervention more difficult, not least as the individual seems to slip across and between these categories. What is certain is that it causes distress to all around them.

Modern brain imaging and rapid advances in the last decade in genetic and neurocognitive research demonstrate that life is far more complex than simple diagnostic categories or unidimensional environment or genetic factors (Green 1998; Cardno *et al.* 1999; Cannon *et al.* 2000, Ebstein *et al.* 2000; Nolan *et al.* 2000; Freedman *et al.* 2001; Noyes 2001; Swanson *et al.* 2005).

It is now established that the schizoaffective syndrome really does exist in a patterned way, probably reflecting the polymorphic nature of the genetic component in the schizophrenias. But, even from the physiological field, critics warn of oversimplification and overemphasis on genetics. Twin studies have been invaluable in demonstrating that there is often a genetic 'predisposition', but the psychosocial features of being a twin, and the subtlety of genetic components in relation to personality traits, rather than gross conditions of such large categories as schizophrenia, make it difficult to differentiate the familial and environmental factors. That is, other than to state the obvious, that both interact and make a contribution to the schizophrenic state (Delisi *et al.* 2000; Torgersen 2000). Indeed, one of the most important British twin studies into the link between genetics and mental disorders reminds us that, while the schizophrenic type of disorders have quite strong heritability, apart from the bipolar affective disorders, there is as much environmental influence as genetic in the remainder of the affective disorders (Cardno *et al.* 1999). Indeed, in a number of neurological diseases, which have much tighter signs and symptoms, it is clear that even in studies of monozygotic (identical) twins, environment as well as genetic susceptibility contributes to the development of such diseases as Parkinson's and motor neurone disease, as well as psychotic states (Vieregge *et al.* 1992; Graham *et al.* 1997; Greenberg *et al.* 2001; Hay *et al.* 2001; Wirdefeldt *et al.* 2004).

Medical mode

In many sociological texts, the term 'medical model' is almost a pejorative term and purports to be a paradigm used by most physicians, which sees humans as essentially physiologically determined. 'Behaviour' is 'medicalised' with the implicit assumption that there are underlying physical problems causing the problematic behaviour or functioning when, in all probability, there are equally psychosocial aetiological factors (Szasz 1960; Goffman 1961; Illich 1971; Pilgrim and Rogers 1998). To be fair, this is a parody of a parody. As early as 1977, Anthony Clare, an eminent psychiatrist of the day, was busily pointing out that 'modern psychiatry' included and recognised the importance of the psychosocial and, in effect, suggested that a unidimensional physician or psychiatrist was an example of poor medical practice. A brief look at the curriculum of the Royal Colleges of General Practice and Psychiatry shows a very heavy loading of the applied psychosocial sciences (Royal College of Psychiatry 2005). The trouble is that this simplified idea of the 'medical model', and its undoubted limitations, persist in the minds of non-practising sociologists, although of course all professions, medicine and social work, can have their arrogant and self-opinionated practitioners. Some sociologists with 'practical' experience of ill health, both physical and mental, are especially scathing in their criticisms of an oversimplified social origin model of ill health (Sedgwick 1982; Shilling 1996), but they are often in the minority.

Irrespective of the weaknesses, one redeeming feature of medicine, which I wish our discipline would adopt, is that their art is science based, continued in the search for an evidence-based practice. This is exemplified when under- and post-graduate medical students identify a clinical problem and then look for the best research evidence to treat the person. Not infrequently, we find there is no firm evidence. It is equally important to know that the best information available does not fit the particular patient. Then, as with all professions, judgements have to be made on limited information as to the best course of action. This applies to social work when we seek to know how any evidence applies to the specific case of those complex mental health and child protection situations. The evidence-based practice approach teaches that we can usually improve on current best practice, which also reminds us of the limits of our knowledge and the need for further research. This latter point cannot be emphasised enough. For example, without firm empirical evidence, we would still persist in the centuries-old practice of 'bleeding', because false correlations convinced the practitioners of the day that it was efficacious. That is, a person would be ill, but not terminally; they would be bled and, if they were fit enough to recover from both infection and the bleeding, the physicians of the day claimed success, loudly applauded by an ignorant but grateful clientele. Indeed, to modern readers, Queen Victoria's father, the Duke of Kent, died because he was killed by his overzealous fee-receiving doctors, who kept bleeding him after every slight improvement in his fever. They virtually bled the poor man to death (St Aubyn 1991).

So what is the 'medical model' at its best?

Medicine is a multiscientific-based art, which seeks an individually focused response to a person's distress. It draws upon the physical and biological sciences for the 'form' of the condition, and the 'content' draws upon the psychosocial and behavioural sciences for possible aetiology of the condition.

The 'form' element is mainly based upon five inter-related physical factors: human anatomy (the body's structure); physiology (how the body works); pathology (the nature of change in the body or the impact of the injury on the body); process (how these pathological changes develop without intervention); and the diagnosis (the known category that accounts for all the previous evidence).

The physician listens to the person's description of their problem, the symptoms, and observes and 'tests' for any external 'signs'. The physician then tries to relate what the patient is saying to what they have observed, including physical tests ranging from simple pulse, temperature and blood pressure to blood pictures and a range of scanning.

The task then is one of scientific deduction of setting the information against what is known generally about the possibly relevant anatomy and physiology. Then, what is known about the pathology, i.e. the damage to either structure or functioning, be it trauma, infection, viral or bacterial, or toxaemias, poisons, too much alcohol or smoking. The last, incidentally, relates to having one's own personal environmental pollution factory, and the addiction that is tobacco smoking is doubly tragic when you visit an oncology clinic and find one in seven patients aged under 35, all of whom never thought that it 'could happen to them' (Pritchard and Evans 2001).

The process is what is known about the uninterrupted impact of the pathology upon the person and becomes the 'prognosis', namely what happens if there is or is not an intervention or treatment. Of course, not all illnesses kill, few do, but cumulatively various body systems can be negatively affected, which is why smoking emerges as a contributory factor in virtually all the body's systems.

Finally, the information is collated and a 'diagnosis' is made, which should ideally account for both symptoms and signs, and an indication of whether the person requires treatment.

The over-riding 'contextual' theme for medical practice is, of course, public health, classically seen in the massive reduction in infective diseases, as food, water supply and sewage disposal raised the standards of hygiene. So that measurement of death rates reflects the classic sociological insight of Emile Durkheim (1868) that, when there are changes in patterns of mortality, these will be reflected in changes in society (Pritchard and Evans 1996, 1997; Pritchard and Baldwin 2002), be it improvements in public sanitation or a worsening of the employment situation, pressures on the 'new man' (Platt 1984; Pritchard 1992b–e, 1996a–c; Pritchard and Evans 1997; Pritchard and Hansen 2005a,b), or the accumulative impact of multienvironmental pollution (Pritchard *et al.* 2004a; Pritchard and Sunak 2005). Indeed, it is fair to say that more progress has been made in the reduction of disease by public health preventative programmes than by any treatments, perhaps antibiotics apart.

It is an extremely successful model for dealing with many human conditions, and few of us would want anything different if we had, for example, pneumonia, meningitis, appendicitis, subarachnoid haemorrhage or the cancers, the death rates for all of which have fallen directly related to medical intervention.

However, if you or your client is feeling miserable, overexcited, hearing strange voices or having 'odd ideas', then the model appears to have some limits, yet it can be still relevant.

The problems start, as we observed earlier with Descartes, with an artificial division of mind and body, which was as much about not having the technical tools to measure the physical associations with mental and cognitive states. This has now improved and, not surprisingly, we find there is an interaction between disturbed mental states and observable physical changes in the brain (Green 1998). However, such interactions might as well be triggered by external stimulus, for example we know that children brought up in emotionally abusing homes, with high levels of anxiety, have actual subtle brain changes (Hogan and Park 2000; Kendler *et al.* 2000; Kallen 2001; Moss *et al.* 2001; Thompson *et al.* 2001; Grgik 2002).

So it is not a question of whether it is 'nature', the physiological, versus 'nurture', child rearing, nor the genetic endowment versus the psycho-socioeconomic environment, but rather a combination of all these factors interacting with each other.

Bentall (2003) is rightly concerned with issues of diagnosis and determining what, if any, are the 'boundaries' between madness and sanity, mental disorder and normality.

He overfocuses upon the historical issue of how fixed are these boundaries and the mistaken use of psychiatric diagnoses as being water-tight categories. But he makes the mistake of wanting such firm categories, when he knows they do not exist, criticising modern psychiatry for its imperfect past and forgetting that, in one sense, all disease is along a continuum of health to ill health to death. This is true for infections, as the body initially fights off an infection with a greater or lesser degree of success. The person becomes ill at a point of discomfort or dysfunction; so too with the mentally disordered person.

I am very sympathetic to Richard Bentall's position, not least for his seminal work on people with schizophrenia (see Chapter 9). The danger is in creating 'straw men', i.e. distinctive extreme positions, for while the jug and bottle psychiatrist does exist, they are increasingly rare, as he knows full well, when he calls upon the work of integrationalists such as Claridge *et al.* (1996), Jamison (1995) and Kingdon and Turkington (2002), etc. Bentall makes great play with Robert Burton's great sixteenth-century insight that ' 'Twixt him and theè there's no difference' and the classic narrow line between 'insanity and genius'. Indeed, Professor Kay Jamison, a Harvard psychiatrist who herself experienced a serious bipolar affective disorder, highlighted that some of the great poets were also bipolar, while as Ludwig (1994) pointed out in his review, many creative people have had quite serious and long-standing periods of severe psychological/mental disorder. The life of John Nash, the mathematician and Nobel laureate, was portrayed in a very successful film, *A Beautiful Mind*, in which the audience was taken into the mind-set of the person and they believed that he was being manipulated by unscrupulous criminals, yet he was, in fact, mentally ill. His wife described their turbulent times together when asked how could he believe in such preposterous ideas. Nash summed it perfectly, 'because the ideas about the supernatural beings came to me in the same way that my mathematical ideas did'.

All diagnoses are guidelines of patterns of experiences, signs and symptoms. The value of a diagnosis is that it is often linked with a pattern of process and prognosis, but always individually shaped within that person's bio-psychosocial situation. This in turn is linked to what is the best treatment, ideally research based, to deal with the signs and symptoms the person is experiencing. The model does not always fit the person, for we are seldom like the textbooks, but their guidance is the best we have. Of course, if we are in the hands of arrogant professionals, who are afraid to demonstrate the highest form of professional integrity, i.e. acknowledging the limits of their knowledge and expertise, indeed being willing to say, 'I do not know', then we are all in trouble. The paradox is, of course, that we the patient feel very uneasy when, at a time of need, 'the expert' disclaims any expertise or certainty about our condition. Medical doctors often have great difficulty in getting patients to listen to their professional limitations; often the patient would rather not know. My wife, after more than 30 years in neurosurgery, will tell of case after case where she wanted to explain the details and difficulties, but the patient and/or their relatives would say de facto, no thanks, we prefer to rely upon you; in effect, they did not want to know. Indeed, in three consecutive cohorts of neurosurgical patients, it was demonstrated that literally two-thirds of patients and their carers preferred to 'rely upon the doctors and nurses'. Interestingly, the third who had a better psychosocial outcome were those designated 'the dependent' group (Pritchard *et al.* 2001, 2004b,c).

Dare one say it, as students, we prefer to have a clear-cut answer but, in the world of practice reality, all, beginner and experienced therapist alike, often fly by the seat of our pants. The danger would be if we always did this and ignored the evidence that has come through over the past decade or two of what works.

The best practical way forward in this bog of confusion, theory and counter-theory is to consider that we are essentially dealing with the content and form of a person's life.

The 'content' consists mainly of that individual's psychosocial factors within the context of their culture, influenced by and reacting upon the 'form', which is the biological and physical endowment and attributes of the person.

The 'content' is easy to grasp: it is those features in an individual's life that they identify as their memories, life experiences and to which they attribute their lives and identity. Hence, no matter how classic the form of a disease or condition, it will always be a unique experience, as it is mediated through an individual's life experiences and understanding.

The key practice conflict occurs when a less aware psychiatrist focuses only upon the 'form' of the syndrome, and the social worker or psychologist only values the 'content' of the syndrome, which is the specific life situation of the person involved. In the field of mental health, 'form' and 'content' are essentially complementary, but often appear as opposites. Pharmacological treatments are helpful in dealing with some of the changed neurotransmitters, the form of the syndrome, whereas we need a psychosocial approach to deal with the 'content' of the syndrome, the personal experiences, the changed nature of interpersonal relationships, the social ramifications of the impact and meaning of their mental disorder.

What is well established is that the 'content' of the person's mental disorder reflects the intimacy and uniqueness of their lives, whereas the 'form' and pattern of the disorder reflect the pattern that is common throughout the world. In modern mental health social work, nursing, medicine and psychiatry, to be effective, we need to address both.

This is linked to issues about 'causes' and treatment outcomes, which will be discussed at greater length but, sufficient to say here is that, if a person suffering from one of the major mental disorders is not receiving help for both form and content aspects, then they are receiving a less than optimal service. As we shall see, there is considerable evidence supporting the benefits of an integrated approach to most of the different types of mental disorders (Granholm *et al.* 2003; Hopper and Barrow 2003; Lenroot *et al.* 2003; Malm *et al.* 2003; Miklowitz *et al.* 2003a,b; Wagner *et al.* 2004; Biondi and Picardi 2005; Bragin *et al.* 2005), and failure to provide both is a dereliction of our duty to the mentally disordered.

Arguments about resources are another matter. The seldom noticed problem with evidence-based practice is that there is evidence that sometimes the information is unwelcome to a government department that is more concerned with keeping costs down than with meeting the citizen's rights under the UN Declaration of Human Rights (Pritchard 2001, 2004). Hence, at the centre of any practice must be the appropriate use of a 'model', be it medical or psychosocial, to ensure that we bear in mind James Baldwin's dictum, 'are you part of the solution or part of the problem?'

An important contextual theme, however, is that of culture, and it must be remembered that the bulk of research is still Western orientated.

Cultural factors

The part cultural factors play in how a society attributes or 'defines' mental disorders is important. As we saw, the seventeenth-century Milton's view of 'Moonstruck madness' was a description of the schizophrenias, but these conditions, unlike the mood disorders, are generally outside the normative experience of most people. Indeed, when a person who has experienced a schizophrenic episode seeks to describe it to others, they invariably resort to metaphor, 'the nearest I can get to it is to say it's like a living dream, only you don't know what is real, until you're convinced it is, and then you're half aware that you're in a different world to other people, but it's them that don't understand' said one client sufferer – shades of John Nash and *A Beautiful Mind*.

Yet, despite the evidence that there is a degree of inherited predisposition with the mental disorders, they are expressed, experienced and perceived in the individual's culture.

Two PhD colleagues of mine approached cultural factors in mental disorder from entirely different perspectives, one a priest and hospital chaplain, the other a psychiatric consultant in Hong Kong, yet both ended by finding similar features (Goold 1991; Lau 1996). Goold explored religious ideas in three groups, acute admission to (a) a psychiatric ward, (b) a surgical ward and (c) a non-patient general control group. The control group did not report much concern with religious ideas, whereas the two patient groups did, as both reverted back to cultural stereotypes and sought comfort and reassurance in traditional religious ideas. Indeed, the only difference between the acute psychiatric and surgical patients was, if they had negative thoughts about themselves, be it depression or paranoid ideas, this was reflected in their ideas about religion; thus, they interpreted their newly aroused religious ideas with thoughts of guilt and sin. Lau had similar groups of patients and controls in Hong Kong Chinese and examined, by age and education, people's attribution of the causes of mental illness. Both psychiatric and surgical patients tended to revert to traditional ideas of cause, even the younger patients had incorporated traditional ideas, alongside their Western-educated views of mental disorder, demonstrating the all-pervading nature of cultural ideas.

The most dramatic example of how deep-seated are cultural influences upon mental disorder came from two unexpected sources. It was found that Westernised Asian countries such as Hong Kong, Japan, Singapore and South Korea had gender and age patterns of suicide more like mainland China than the Western nations (Pritchard 1996a; Lau and Pritchard 2001; Pritchard and Baldwin 2002), and Russian attitudes to suicide still reflect traditional Russian Orthodox theology, rather than Marxist–Leninist views, after more than 70 years of being a secular, anti-religious state (Wasserman *et al.* 1994; Tilson 1998).

As mentioned earlier, in multicultural Britain, delusional ideas and the experience of hallucinations reflect the person's social and ethnic background. The psychotic episodes experienced by a young person reflect the prevailing times and culture. Frankie and Graham mentioned David Beckham and Posh Spice, but it would be highly unlikely for them to mention either Napoleon or Josephine – indeed, if they did, in all probability, they would be faking. Similarly Mr Harris interpreted his psychosis as being due to the IRA.

These cultural features are very important, and in the 1970s well into the 1990s, these led to poor psychiatric practice and an inadvertent racism (Fernando 1988; Thomas *et al.* 1996; Harrison *et al.* 1999, 2001; Fernando *et al.* 2000), as different kind of behaviours were misinterpreted. On the other hand, we can be overly 'ethnic' focused and miss the key patterns of a mental disorder in our efforts to be inclusive.

'Mr Kemmal', 49 years old, was a very successful businessman and a pillar of the local Race Relations Board. He began to express some odd ideas to family, friends and some Caucasian colleagues. Unfortunately, their response confirmed for him that they were against him because of his success and religion. His work and his relationships with those around him deteriorated quickly over the next two months, but no-one dared to suggest he should seek help because it would be so badly received by Mr Kemmal and his family. In the last month of his life, he was expressing overt delusions and suicidal ideas, which of course were virtually anathema to his religion, as suicide is expressly condemned in the Koran. Mr Kemmal felt tortured by the fear of what was to come and, to protect his family, he killed them all, including himself.

This was a tragic case of busy pressurised professionals not having an open mind. In effect, recognising what they were seeing, but missing Mr Kemmal's patterned response, they simplistically assumed that racial harassment was the dominant reality. This is always difficult for, despite real progress in Britain over the past 20 years, prejudice and expressions of prejudice still come from a minority of the indigenous population (Thompson and Pritchard 1987), and are an all too frequent experience for those who come into contact with readers of certain tabloids.

'Lal' was a 30-year-old unemployed Asian bank clerk assigned to the caseload of a student who sought to assist with employment and tackle any racial harassment. Lal's family had been driven from Uganda in Idi Amin's ethnic cleansing in the 1970s. While Lal was still a schoolboy, he experienced the distress of his parents, especially his mother's depression, and they were all shocked by Lal's older brother's suicide within a year of coming to the UK.

Initially, Lal made a very good adjustment, quickly speaking with the local accent. He proved to be a popular and successful cricketing student and gained good 'A' levels. It was his decision not to go on to university, in part because his father had died, and he felt unable to leave his mother, who had spells of intermittent depression, with severe withdrawal. He obtained a job in a bank and was highly thought of, gaining promotion, but he left to join a friend in an independent business venture. Everything went wrong and Lal lost his investment and, after a number of temporary dead-end jobs, he had not worked for three years. His morale was rock bottom, which the student felt was perfectly understandable, and the expressions of 'I wish I was dead – I wish I'd never been born' were construed as metaphor. The student was challenged to think of an alternative explanation for both Lal's feelings and behaviour, other than him being a victim of discrimination. When the student began to think in terms of racial harassment, she discovered that 'Lal' was contemptuous of this idea, showing prejudice as he recognised that they were 'thickos, stupid inadequate people, not worth troubling your head about' and he always gave them a wide berth to avoid 'any aggro'. She began to listen to what Lal was truly complaining about, that he was depressed, ashamed, guilty and was so relieved that the student was not shocked at his serious suicidal ruminations.

This was very nearly a disastrous case, because the student was observing the 'form' of what might be there but had got taken up with the 'content' and, moreover, had imposed her own preconceptions, seeing Lal's behaviour as a reaction to racial prejudice, whereas he was suffering from a psychotic depression. This is a common fault that we are all inclined to, no matter how experienced or inexperienced, but we need to be aware of it, otherwise we try to fit our client into our theoretical model, rather than be open-minded and see what there is to be seen in a client-specific way.

The above case experience is ten years old, but new research highlights how the stigma surrounding suicide can create a 'collusion' between the Islamic client, their family and Western professionals, as they deny any suicidal ideas because it is culturally unacceptable, because suicide is condemned in the Koran (Surah 4:29). Yet new WHO data (2005) from former Soviet Islamic countries are showing that, of nine Islamic countries that reported suicide deaths, Kazakhstan, Kyrgyzstan and Turkmenistan had higher suicide rates than in England and Wales (1998–2000) and Uzbekistan was close to the Anglo-Welsh levels, strongly suggesting that suicide, at least in these Islamic countries, is a reality, which is being denied (Pritchard and Amunullah 2006).

Prejudice and discrimination sadly exist in all cultures, so that, even in 'age-revering' China, we find passive discrimination in terms of a disproportionately high elderly suicide rate and a de facto sexism that makes Britain look perfect (Lau and Pritchard 2001; Pritchard and Baldwin 2002). While institutional racism has now been recognised and outlawed by the findings of the Macpherson Report following the tragedy of the murder of Stephen Lawrence, institutional ageism is only just being acknowledged as equally demeaning and undermining a person's human rights and dignity. The more recent racial killing of Anthony Walker in Liverpool shows that such bigots still exist in our society.

Another cultural influence upon mental health is seldom spoken about, but it could be argued that it is even more pervasive than issues of ethnicity, namely, social class (Browne 1987; Browne *et al.* 1990; Pritchard and Clooney 1994; Kmietowicz 2003; Brugha *et al.* 2004). Sadly, this is an almost unpopular and old-fashioned issue, yet recent research confirms the long-known social class treatment bias against non-middle-class people with mental disorders (Howard *et al.* 2004; Kahn *et al.* 2005); indeed, it could be argued that the same 'middle-class' cultural misunderstandings about people from ethnic minorities, especially African-Caribbean, are very similar to the misunderstandings and miscommunications that occur between professionals and non-middle-class people (Bhui *et al.* 2005). However, while there are clear physical health disparities between the social classes (Taylor *et al.* 2003; Singh *et al.* 2004; Kahn *et al.* 2005), in terms of frequency of mental disorder, against expectations, there are no social class differences: as many people in 'upper' socioeconomic groups have psychiatric problems as in 'lower' socioeconomic groups (Breslau *et al.* 2005; Thoits 2005).

Of course, these social class biases occur from the onset of the citizens' lives. Poverty is as much inherited as is wealth but has very little to do with genetic endowment, seen in the cycle of poor pre- and antenatal care, nursery, primary, secondary and tertiary education; not being able to break out of the socioeconomic group. Working-class people have poorer opportunities to improve their situation and are often alienated by the education system, which in turn undermines their talents and skills in the marketplace and so the cycle of disadvantage rolls on (Farrington 1995; Audit Commission 1996, 1998; Pritchard 2001) and, at the extreme, can kill (Judge and Benzeval 1993; Kmietowicz 2003; Taylor *et al.* 2003; Singh *et al.* 2004).

The final cultural factor is that of gender. That women through the centuries and even today have been discriminated against is not in doubt (see for example St Paul's comments about women in the epistles), but here is another paradox. In the field of mental health, it is men who are a victim of sexism, for men suffer from machismo! For example, men are culturally more reluctant to seek help for personal and physical problems; men are likely to be victims of violence from other men; men are less likely to be offered talking treatments unless they are educated and, because of our indoctrinated macho attitudes and our hormones, in the crisis of mental disorder, we are far more likely to die from suicide, as the mentally disordered male is more likely than a woman to use a more lethal method of self-harm (Pritchard 1999; McHolm *et al.* 2003). Indeed this 'crisis of machoism' has affected all the major Western countries as youth and young

Table 4.1 Suicide rates in the UK 2002 by gender and age (per million)

| | *Age (years)* | | | | | | | |
	15–24	*25–34*	*35–44*	*45–54*	*55–64*	*65–74*	*75+*	*All ages*
Male	82	173	179	148	115	87	104	108
Female	24	40	41	45	40	34	37	31
Ratio	1:3.4	1:4.3	1:4.4	1:3.3	1:2.9	1:2.6	1:2.8	1:3.5

adult suicides have never been higher (Gunnel *et al.* 2003; Pritchard and Hansen 2005a). This is seen in simple statistics of the latest suicide figures for the UK up to 2002 (WHO 2005). There were 3,124 male and 942 female suicides in the year, a ratio of one female to 3.3 males. Table 4.1 shows rates per million by gender and age.

Male suicide can be seen to exceed female in each of the age bands. Moreover, as suicide continues to be strongly associated with mental disorder (Harris and Barraclough 1997; King *et al.* 2001), it is an important indicator of the seriousness of inadequately treated and supported mental disorder. In addition, the total of 4,066 suicides not only exceed the tragic death toll of 11 September 2001, but is 40 times the rate of the extreme consequence of child abuse, a child dying violently (Pritchard and Butler 2003; Pritchard and Lewis 2006). Despite this, suicide seldom attracts the same media attention. However, as will be seen in Chapter 7 on suicide, the current pattern of suicide is very different from that of 20 or 30 years ago.

With regard to the mental disorder, however, factors such as gender, age, ethnicity and social class mean that mental disorders can never be seen in a unidimensional framework. There are always cultural overlays upon even the most clear-cut physical as well as mental disorders, as well as complex bio-sociopsychological interactive factors. Bearing these features in mind, we turn to the less clear-cut mental disorders, but no less important, the 'minor mental disorders' and explore the extent of both the 'serious' and the 'minor' mental disorders.

5 The 'minor' mental disorders

Extent of mental disorder?

Before exploring the 'minor mental disorders', it would be helpful to take a final contextual view of just how big a problem the mental disorders are in the general population. Fortunately, we have some very sound estimates, which provide a clear indication of how extensive they are. This can be shown by exploring some brief patient statistics on England and Wales shown in Table 5.1. This was based upon a 10 per cent household census survey and reflects the respondents' 'experience' of mental disorders (Jenkins *et al.* 1998), as people responded to the symptoms listed in the survey. This is especially useful because, as it was anonymous, people, especially men, avoided the stigma of having to admit to these experiences.

The figures are quite startling as more than 2.7 million people said they had experienced above 'normal' anxiety and depression in the past year, and more than 5.9 million people described a range of 'other neurotic disorders'. However, it must be stressed that many people described more than one set of symptoms. Thus, approximately 150,000 people described having functional psychosis, and as many as 450,000 as having some form of obsessional neurosis; the really big

Table 5.1 Household survey (Jenkins *et al.* 1998): 12-month prevalence of adult mental disorders (16–64 years); rates per 1,000 translated into number of people (UK population aged 16–64)

	Males		Females	
Problem	Rate	Number	Rate	Number
Mixed anxiety and depression	54	1,020,060	94	1,745,956
Depressive episode	17	321,130	25	464,350
Generalised anxiety	28	528,920	34	631,516
Phobias	7	132,230	14	260,036
Panic disorders	8	151,120	9	167,166
Other neurotic disorder	123	2,323,470	195	3,621,930
Obsessive–compulsive disorder	9	170,010	15	278,610
Alcohol dependence	75	1,416,750	21	390,054
Drug dependence	29	547,810	14	260,036
Functional psychosis	4	75,560	4	74,296

numbers involved states such as 'generalised anxiety'. It should also be stressed that this did not mean that these people always felt like this, but had experienced such distress during the year.

The later analysis, which shows the numbers of people actively seeking help from the psychiatric services, is given in Table 5.2. These are the actual numbers of people consulting an adult psychiatrist, which is a practical 'definition' of serious mental disorder in that the person required treatment and care beyond the dominant 'mode' of treatment, i.e. from the general practitioner (GP) in the community (Department of Health 2002).

Table 5.2 shows how, between 1992 and 2000, first attendances rose from 245,000 to 282,000 people, a rise of 15 per cent, representing 0.7 per cent of the Anglo-Welsh general population as new severely mentally disordered people. By definition, if they are referred to a consultant psychiatrist, they are considered to be beyond the capacity of the GP. Moreover, the caseloads of the community psychiatric nurse (CPN) rose from 475,000 to 586,000 people by 2000. This represents 1.4 per cent of the general population, who probably experienced a 'severe' mental disorder. Add to this number 2.3 million men and 3.6 million women who in the national household survey (Jenkins *et al.* 1998) reported 'neurotic' symptoms, the so-called 'minor mental disorders', representing 14 per cent of people in the general population. Thus, it would be fair to say that, despite the limits of

Table 5.2 NHS and personal social services statistics on mental health, 1993–2000 (Department of Health 2002)

Resource	1992/3	2000	Difference (%)
No. of first outpatient consultant appointments	245,000	282,000	15
No. of people with learning disability	5,000	7,000	40
No. of people receiving community psychiatric nursing	475,000	586,000	24
No. of people receiving community learning disability nursing	44,000	57,000	30
Hospital bed-days (millions)	14.0	11.2	−20
Community bed-days (millions)	2.4	4.4	83
Average daily available NHS beds	12,800	9,640	−25
People in staffed residential homes	36,290	43,660	20
People in voluntary residential homes	13,940	18,180	30
People in private residential homes	12,680	18,850	49
NHS beds for patients with mental health and learning disability	41,300	34,900	−15
Private elderly patients	19,330	21,490	11
Private non-elderly patients	4,860	7,280	50
First attendance, day care, mental illness	66,000	55,000	−17
First attendance, NHS day care, old age psychiatry	35,000	33,000	−6

defining 'mental disorder', such a proportion of people in the general population shows that mental disorder is part of our culture, albeit an unwanted one, and in this sense is not alien from most people's wider experience.

However, the often derided policy of 'care in the community', which sought to reduce the incarceration of more than 250,000 people in our old mental hospitals, now sees an average annual population of only 39,600 inpatients in the psychiatric units of our general hospitals (ONS 2005), barely 15 per cent of the previous 1960s concentration. Ignoring the substantial 'savings' on reduced numbers in hospital, the benefit to people of avoiding the stigma and trauma of admission is almost incalculable. Overall, this must be seen as a very positive outcome, reflecting well on all aspects of the mental health services.

If we took all the neurotic group, this would represent nearly 12 per cent of all men and 19 per cent of all women in the general population, in addition to the 75,580 men and 74,296 women who, over the past 12 months, reported symptoms of the functional psychoses. The Jenkins team explored the social factors statistically significantly more often associated with reported mental disorder and found that among unemployed people the rate was more than double (2.26), among the 'economically inactive' it was 71 per cent higher, among lone parents it was 56 per cent greater, among people living alone 48 per cent more and among people in rented accommodation it was 33 per cent higher (Jenkins *et al.* 1998). Indeed, even among young people less than 26 years old, more than 13 per cent had a 'non-clinical' depression, particularly among the unemployed and non-partnered (Bynner *et al.* 2002). Bearing in mind that clients of Probation and Social Service had an estimated 25 per cent and 40 per cent of mental disorder, respectively, puts this into perspective (Pritchard and Cox 1990; Ford *et al.* 1997; Pritchard *et al.* 1997b). Nonetheless, there is a considerable degree of mental suffering in the general population, not just in those who formally seek help from the mental health services (Jenkins *et al.* 1998; Bynner *et al.* 2002).

The neuroses

As we saw, it is the 'minor' mental disorders that make the greatest demand across the services. In terms of frequency, they far outweigh the major psychoses, representing a considerable range of psychic distress in the general population. Consequently, there is a danger in using the term 'minor neuroses' as if they are unimportant to the people involved

With regard to the 'neuroses', in an effort to formulate these problems, it is noteworthy that they take up more ICD pages than the major psychoses. However, while single focused 'pure' neurotic states exist, we will explore the more common ones, which often overlap.

Anxiety states

The essential feature is anxiety, which can be as wearing for the family of the sufferer as for the sufferer themselves. This is not to belittle the person, but the anxiety gets diffused and has a tendency to interact and trigger other social and psychological situations. It usually accompanies, to a greater or lesser degree, other neurotic states, and is often linked with mild depression, to the extent that there is a subcategory in the ICD of 'mixed anxiety and depressive disorder'.

Of course, all human beings get anxious – those who do not have another kind of mental disorder – but it is a question of extent. It is best seen as a 'continuum' disorder, and when the anxiety becomes dysfunctional will depend on the individual and those around them.

Phobic disorders

These can centre upon a particular area. Fear of spaces is one of the best known, i.e. 'agoraphobia', which can range in its severity; at the extreme, the suffer is virtually housebound. Three elements are present: a degree of autonomic (physical) symptoms, such as palpitations, sweating and/or tremors; anxiety related to crowds, open spaces or travelling; and the person's reactive response, i.e. avoidance mechanisms, which is often a predominant feature – hence the person becomes housebound.

Sometimes, the 'trigger' for the phobia is quite specific, for example spiders, snakes, dentists, injections; indeed, virtually anything can become the subject of a phobia. The trigger is usually learned in early childhood or following a crisis and is reinforced by the person's environment. Anxiety and the autonomic symptoms invariably follow the presence or the threat of the noxious idea.

Social phobia

Social phobia partly overlaps with 'agoraphobia', and there is increasing evidence to show that it is more pervasive than first thought, and might be a better designation of more disparate phobic problems. Social phobia affects between 7 and 12 per cent of adults in their lifetime (den Boer and Slaap 1998; Baldwin 2000). Again, the three key elements are present.

Panic attacks

These can either occur alone or follow an extreme anxiety or phobic situation. They can be alarming as, if they are prolonged, they invariably involve serious palpitations, leading to chest pains and a choking feeling; not infrequently, they lead to a call for an ambulance, as the panic spreads to those who witness the attack. It is, of course, a situation in which one feels helpless, fearing that the person is having a heart attack. However, calming down the situation is always a good course of action, and separating the person from others who might maintain or raise the tension is usually another good move, and helps the assessment/diagnosis as the person begins to breathe easier.

'Michael' was 42 years old, with longstanding neurotic difficulties. He was a 'life-long loner', shy, diffident and had to hide his intellectual prowess from his working-class peers. He was gay and had great difficulty in coming to terms with his sexual orientation, not least because he shared a cultural homophobia. His interest centred upon 15- to 17-year-old boys, and the illegality of his sexual targets added to his all-pervading anxiety, even though he decided to become celibate. He actively avoided all new 'social' situations if he could. He had 'learned to cope by drink and drugs – cannabis actually', mainly alone, but this took its toll, so that he could only relate to others when heavily in drink, which he used to 'buy' company, and he virtually lost a small fortune this way.

He became periodically depressed, but this improved when he became a mature university student. Unfortunately, his drinking became 'dependent' and incapacitated him from work, which had been as a solitary security guard: 'it suited me I didn't have to meet people'.

The memorable feature about Michael was the sudden and devastating impact of an anxiety attack when he virtually went into shock – pallor, near collapse, thready pulse, palpitations, cold sweats, and this in response to my rather clumsy questioning in an interview.

The other feature Michael reflected is increased use by psychiatrists of the concept 'dual diagnosis'. This invariably concerns substance abuse and either a depressive or a severe neurotic syndrome. The concept has been found to be useful because, by treating the associated or possibly underlying psychic distress, the substance misuse often becomes more manageable (Baldwin 2000), not least because, in one sense, the substance misuse is a form of self-medication or a counterproductive way of coping. This probably accounts for a considerable degree of comorbidity of all the mental disorders and substance misuse, including of course alcohol (Ball *et al.* 2000; Noyes 2001; Agosti *et al.* 2002; Enoch and Goldman 2002).

Substance abuse

This is another area of controversy in that, for some, it might be described as an alternative lifestyle, even though the use of some substances, cannabis, heroin, crack cocaine, etc., is illegal. While it is accepted that tobacco, another addictive substance, kills far more people than any illegal use of drugs, there can be serious consequences from the misuse of any drug, even cannabis. This latter drug was found to be associated with schizophrenic syndromes in former Swedish national servicemen. This was based upon a series of studies among those who had used the drug frequently and regularly over a number of years, even though they had no first- or second-degree relatives who had had schizophrenia (Zammit *et al.* 2002). This is not the place to rehearse the arguments for or against decriminalisation, although we cannot resist highlighting the massive change in the prevalence of the cancers over the past 20 years, especially among young women whose lifestyle has changed markedly in comparison with their mothers and, indeed, relative to their male peers, in which increased use of the addictive tobacco has made a major contribution (Pritchard and Evans 1996). While the impact upon the child of the substance-using pregnant mother is complex to determine, it is nevertheless strongly associated with a whole range of psychosocial, neurological and behavioural problems (Verdoux 2002). The presence of either heavy alcohol use or illegal drugs invariably makes a difficult situation worse (Agosti *et al.* 2002).

The ICD describes nine 'discrete' combinations of mental disorder with various substances, alcohol, opioids, cocaine, etc. It is clear that there are certain patterns with some of the more addictive drugs associated with hallucinations. However, the useful part is in the description of acute and chronic intoxication, the dependence state and the withdrawal state.

With respect to dependency, it revolves around a cluster of physiological, behavioural and cognitive phenomena, in which the outcome is desire or indeed an overwhelming need to take the psychoactive drug, including alcohol. People respond in a highly idiosyncratic way to even the simplest form of pharmacy, for example aspirin, a truly excellent drug, which to aspirin-allergic people is literally poison. Hence, a substance-dependent person's reactions are likely to be very individualistic, and this makes it problematic for the therapist, as there is often a degree of marked instability and unpredictability, even in clients one assumed one knew well. The desire for the substance becomes virtually compulsive, with all the disturbed cognition, which the user may well genuinely regret within hours of extreme behaviour, including violence. That is until the next time the cravings become overwhelming.

The 'alcoholic' syndrome, with reccurring dependency, leads in the later stages to pathological physical changes: as the person's tolerance rises, they need greater and greater quantities of alcohol to gain their buzz. It is sad to behold and, with changes in lifestyle, we are now seeing relatively young people with marked physical symptoms, including increased levels of fatal cirrhosis of the liver (Rossol 2001; WHO 2001–5). However, over the past ten years or so, there has been an increasing crossover between alcohol and substance abuse, the so-called 'polysubstance abuse', which is associated with rises in hepatitis C and links to sexually transmitted diseases and HIV infections, which reflect not so much dual diagnosis but a considerable degree of comorbidity (Norstrom and Skog 2001; Noyes 2001; Rossol 2001; Agosti *et al.* 2002; Kim *et al.* 2003). Indeed, as there has been a convergence of behaviour between men and women, we now see larger proportions of women with polysubstance abuse and its complications than ever before (Greenfield 2002; Kim *et al.* 2003). With regard to both major and minor mental disorders, very often a degree of alcoholism and substance misuse goes hand in hand with the primary mental health problem, apparently as a form of self-medication, as occurred with 'Michael' to help him deal with his panic attacks and anxiety states. Indeed, some critics of the drug industry might well point to the addictions that have evolved from the use of prescribed drugs.

The 'withdrawal state', the so-called 'cold turkey', is almost as distressing for observers as for those who are experiencing it. At the extremes, it can end in convulsions, but the positive aspect is that it is time limited, being dependent upon the amount of the drug in the person's system. Indeed, as we shall see later, substance misuse and the rest are associated with suicidal behaviour, which can end fatally.

Of all the problems most frequently associated with substance misuse, perhaps the commonest are those defined as 'personality disorders'. Under the ICD rubric, they are classified as 'Disorders of adult personality and behaviour', and this is perhaps one of the most controversial areas of misunderstanding between social work and psychiatry. Before trying to resolve these issues, let us first sketch out what the international field of mental health (WHO 1979b) means by personality disorder.

Disorders of adult personality and behaviour

Personality disorders

The ICD attempts to define people whose persistent patterns of behaviour and characteristic lifestyles impact adversely upon others and their own lives. Some of these patterns occur very early in the development of the child, discernible in childhood in fact, and appear to be 'a result of both constitutional factors and social experiences, while others are acquired later in life' (ibid.). They are essentially defined by behaviour and the person's response to other people. This infers a set of social values against which the person's behaviour is being assessed, which has been acknowledged by psychiatrists since the 1970s and the ICD itself (Clare 1977; WHO 1979b). Indeed, it is this social dimension that makes the concept of personality disorder so very different from the major mental disorders; although they might be seen as an extreme variation of psychic experience, the functional psychoses clearly result in behaviour that is internationally recognised as abnormal.

A key factor in understanding 'personality disorders' is that, by the ICD definition, in effect, there are two broad categories, first those who were assessed as problematic from childhood, inferring a constitutional and social interaction, and the second group who develop the problematic behaviour as teenagers or young adults. In effect, this suggests that some personality-disordered people were born with such a susceptibility, which was reinforced by their life experience, and the others, who developed the patterned behaviour, were more influenced by environment than any predisposing endowment.

There is evidence for the continuation of problematic behaviour in childhood, especially disorders of conduct, running on into later adolescence and young adulthood (Rutter *et al.* 1999; Messerschmitt 2002). While such behaviour is problematic for those around them, there is evidence that, apart from the exceptional extreme, many described as personality-disordered experience a range of subjective distress as well as problems in personal and social relationships.

The key elements appear to be marked dysharmonious attitudes and behaviour, which is patterned and long standing (sometimes described as 'they don't learn from their mistakes'); the behaviour is often maladaptive and pervasive in a range of personal and social circumstances, and often associated with significant occupational problems. Such people have been described as 'psychopaths', inferring 'mental derangement' (WHO 2000), whereas in the USA, the term 'sociopath' has been coined, placing the focus on the person's behaviour towards society, rather than inferring a psychological problem.

Perhaps the most useful way to look at personality disorders, or psychopaths, is to consider the condition as the end of a continuum so, while we can all feel selfish or behave so, we do not cross a boundary where our behaviour would be totally self-centred, with a callous disregard for others.

Dissocial personality disorder

This is the 'typical' psychopath or sociopath, characterised by a total indifference to the feelings of others, totally self-centred, almost appearing to be unaware that others might object to their often overt verbal and physical aggression. Often there is gross and persistent irresponsibility, with a total disregard for social norms and, especially important, an inability to sustain enduring personal relationships. They have great difficulty in tolerating even the mildest frustration with an associated very low threshold for the expression of aggression, which often ends in violence. Not only do they appear to be incapable of any remorse or feelings of guilt, or profit from previous experience, but they are extremely hard to work with as they invariably blame others, with, for example, egocentric rationalisations of why a man struck his female partner: 'she knows I've a temper, I'm a proper man, you can't mess with me, she was winding me up, I warned her, it was her own fault and if she hadn't have gone on, the kid wouldn't have got hurt'. This 'explanation' came from 23-year-old 'Neil' on being questioned by police and social services following his brutal attack on his female partner of six months, in which he kicked and fractured the ribs of his partner's three-year-old child. Both his victims required hospitalisation. This was typical of him as he had a string of violent convictions from a very early age, as well as a multiplicity of other crimes, including sexual assault, and his three spells in prison did little to improve his post-discharge behaviour. We will return to the cases of 'Neil' and others like him when we explore the child protection–mental health interface. Sufficient to say, the 'dissocial personality disorder' is found far more often among men, although not exclusively so. Irrespective of 'cause', experienced practitioners will recognise such patterns of behaviour in clients of most of the community agencies, especially the police, probation and child protection.

Paranoid personality disorder

As would be expected, this person is characterised by an excessive sensitivity to being 'got at', and is suspicious, overly so, often without any reasonable justification. This can lead him or her into combative situations, with a tendency to bear grudges and be preoccupied with their status and concerns over 'conspiratorial' activities and their 'rights' but less concerned about others. Self-evidently, there appears to be a link or overlap with paranoid schizophrenia; indeed, some suggest that this pattern of personality is along the continuum through an unfulfilled paranoid schizophrenia to a final breakdown (Bentall 1995, 2003).

Schizoid personality disorder

Along the continuum, this might appear to be a person with passive symptoms of schizophrenia. They appear cold, detached, with flattened affect and poor libido, solitary, having few relationships, preoccupied, introspective and withdrawn.

This should not be mistaken for the more specific Asperger's syndrome; they may appear somewhat autistic, but not with the clumsiness and marked features of Asperger's.

Histrionic personality disorder

This is characterised by high drama and self-dramatisation, a very suggestible personality, shallow and labile affect, and rapid swings of feeling from love to hate for the same person within minutes. The unwary practitioner can easily be drawn in and flattered by such an individual's apparent rapid response, but my heart sinks when new clients tell me within minutes how wonderfully understanding I am and that they have been waiting for such a therapist all their lives. This is sometimes reflected in their relations with other people who have tried to help them. At each positive response, the patient raises the stakes until, exhausted, the other person fails to meet the increased emotional demands, at which point the patient moves on, complaining of being misunderstood and rejected.

Patients with histrionic personality disorder can be attention seeking and may be quite coquettish, irrespective of the gender or sexual orientation of the recipient. Such individuals are often crudely described as 'drama queens'; both men and women may be affected, but there is a preponderance among women.

Histrionic personality disorder can be associated with 'dissociative disorders' with somatoform (physical) symptoms, classically the 'hysterical' conversion disorders. This leads to the manifestation of invalid physical symptoms, often of paralysis, e.g. 'glove and stocking' paralysis. However, although the subjects do not appear to feel pain, the numbed/paralysed area does not fit the known distribution of normal neurology. Histrionic personality disorder is more often found among people from simpler and less educated cultures, again classically with 'hysterical blindness'. These clients, at the first meeting, are likely to tell you that you are the therapist for whom they have been waiting, that at last someone understands them. They are appealingly 'childish' and unaware you might be mildly flattered by their obvious regard and hint of seductiveness. Before you know where you are, they will insist that you have promised them the earth, and how could you be so callous as to deny them what they need. If this sounds 'unprofessionally' harsh, it is not meant to be, but these people can be very manipulative, a word that most professionals seek to avoid, lest they appear to be making moral judgements. They can be helped, providing you are not overwhelmed by their practised art of building you up, only to reject you because you have failed to live up to their fantasy.

In these days of litigation, the worker needs to be extremely careful and self-aware so that they are not drawn into the client's manipulative fantasy, which might well lead to an allegation of sexual impropriety.

'Olive', 38 years, was referred to the child guidance clinic because of the alleged bizarre sexual behaviour of her six-year-old daughter. I was young and inexperienced and followed Olive's story, which became more and more extreme, and the initial interview with Olive's husband did not reassure, for his rejection of her allegations was initially thought to be hiding possible sexual abuse. 'I'll tell you now, its a load of xxxx bull, she's making it up, its one of her stories, she'll have you running around till you don't know whether you're coming or going. I've seen it before, you don't know' was the husband's dismissive response. A belated liaison with Olive's GP confirmed her history of changed GP, house moves, list of bizarre complaints about schools, all of which proved to be unfounded, but characterised by Olive's almost ecstatic excitement at being the centre of attention. A multidisciplinary case conference helped to clinch the 'assessment/diagnosis', as more experienced colleagues reassured me that they too had learned and suffered at the hands of Olive. The tragedy for Olive and her daughter was that the mother's behaviour over time, and Olive's distress, led to short but acute periods of rapid-onset misery, and made them ostracised by neighbours, family and the services.

Other forms of personality disorders are defined by the main characteristics. 'Anankastic' indicates the precise, cautious, perfectionist, rigid, pedantic conscientiousness person, sometimes described as the classic Freudian 'anal personality', a phrase whose utility lies only in its well-known parameters, rather than any adherence to Freudian theories about personality development. In effect, there is little evidence to support such theories (Kleine 1978); invariably, there are better alternative explanations than a personality fixated at less than 12 months old.

Other types are 'anxious personality disorder' and 'dependent personality disorder', each characterised by either anxiety or overdependency.

One category of particular use is that of 'borderline personality', where several of the problems of emotional instability are present in a patterned way, which often leads to intense but short-lived unstable relationships, characterised by the dominant theme of the overarching personality disorder, be it dissocial, paranoid, schizoid or histrionic.

It is this imprecision which leads to criticism of the concept, and not just from those of a social science orientation (Lewis 1955; Clare 1977; Barker *et al.* 1998; Szasz 2002), not least because the 'disorder' seems to be at one extreme of a continuum of ordinary personality traits and lacks the value of a traditional medical diagnosis, which excludes other conditions. Hence, a pain in the chest will be due to heart or lung pathology, with associated consequences which may be obscure but the diagnosis with other symptoms of secondary affected organs can always be traced back to the underlying pathology. Whereas personality disorders are, if anything, overinclusive.

Yet, despite the weaknesses inherent in genetic studies related to personality, i.e. the degree to which the environment influences any genetic predisposition (Torgersen 2000), there is considerable evidence to show that personality traits and whole patterns of personality both exist and have some genetic loading in most countries in the developed world (Ebstein *et al.* 2000; Nishiguchi *et al.* 2001; Bahlmann *et al.* 2002; Fu *et al.* 2002; Siever *et al.* 2002). Moreover, many of these patterns of behaviour appear to have their origin in childhood, not just as reactive, but again with genetic weighting (Rutter *et al.* 1999; Messerschmitt 2002).

Nonetheless, most of us from the social and behavioural sciences feel a little uncomfortable with the idea of a fixed personality disorder, in part because it suggests an intractability, and judgements are made on how 'different' the person is from a stereotyped idealised social norm. This can be seen in a startling historical comparison. In 1924, Winston Churchill fought a by-election in Dundee and was severely harassed by large crowds of disgruntled working-class voters, who had returned him as a Liberal before the First World War. He and Mrs Churchill felt very hurt and misunderstood and could not understand the ordinary Dundee women's anger and heckling of Mrs C, who had attended the political rallies, wearing strings of pearls – all real of course – nor why the voters were unsympathetic to Churchill, who had made special efforts to get to Dundee, despite having just risen from his sick bed. He published 'proof' of this in the local papers, certified by his three physicians, Lord Dawson, Sir Crispin England and a Dr Hartigan. This was, of course, the norm for the Churchills (Jenkins 2001); in contrast, most of Churchill's constituents were lucky to have one doctor, let alone three. Such is the weakness of tacitly assuming 'social norms'. Hence, to describe behaviour as a 'disorder' that is along a continuum is criticised as a 'medicalisation' by psychiatry of a spectrum of social behaviour (Pilgrim and Rogers 1998; Szasz 2002).

In part, this is because we think of much unwelcome behaviour, such as theft and vandalism, as reactive to adverse circumstance. Indeed, there is little doubt that the cycle of psycho-socioeconomic disadvantage is associated with a whole raft of antisocial behaviour (Audit Commission 1998), in which 'crime' might well be seen to be a 'rational alternative market response' to their disadvantage (Pritchard and Cox 1990; Pritchard 1991, 2001; Pritchard and Clooney 1994; Pritchard and Williams 2001). However, such a 'social reactive' position does not explain why the vast majority of 'poor' people do not continue in a life of crime, are not persistent thieves or vandals, are not wife-beaters and perpetrators of domestic violence and do not neglect and abuse their children.

The value of the concept of personality disorder lies in the recognition that there are characteristic longstanding patterns of behaviour that are found in certain individuals whose lives and the lives of those around them are disturbed, with differing degrees of distress. The 'personality disorders' are not like the functional psychoses, with strong biochemical markers (Ingraham and Kety 2000; Freedman *et al.* 2001), which differ from non-disordered people, but nonetheless the patterns and form are identifiable. The degree to which the person and others around them are damaged seems to be associated with age as, for example, the violent offender is less violent the older he gets. It appears that the dissocial personality-disordered person mellows relatively over time, or they 'grow out of it' as they exhibit a degree of maturity (Home Office 1994; Ebstein *et al.* 2000). What sticks hard with social workers, however, is that, under the Mental Health Act 1983, the concept of personality disorder is defined as either 'treatable' or 'untreatable'. The idea of 'rejecting' a person, giving up on them, strikes hard at the social work ethic of valuing all, rejecting none and purposeful acceptance of the individual (Plant 1968; Pritchard and Taylor 1978; Davies 1995). Yet from the field of mental health, Linehan (1993) has developed a very promising line of intervention, 'cognitive dialectic behaviour therapy', which is part of the growing 'school' of 'cognitive behavioural therapy' (Kingdon and Turkington 2002), more of which later. Social workers would find this a very compatible approach, especially as the 'dialectic' in the modality really refers to establishing a relationship with people who have little experience of positive regard or self-esteem-boosting relationships.

The concept of personality disorder can be useful when jettisoning the idea that it is an 'illness', rather than a disorder, which infers nothing about aetiology. Moreover, a simple analysis of long-term cases of any of the major social work agencies reveals people whose pattern of behaviour has got them into trouble since childhood (Pritchard 1992c; Farrington 1995; Ford *et al.* 1997; Pritchard and Butler 2000a,b; Ebstein *et al.* 2000). Yet social work has never tried to categorise behaviour with which most practitioners are familiar. It is as if we are afraid to quantify qualities of personality and behaviour, lest we appear to be judgemental. The danger here is that we are less able or willing to determine risk of violence, be it to another adult or against a child. Of course, our clients, service users, have never fitted the textbooks exactly, but that should not make us blind to the discernible patterns that are present. For example, the first 'extreme' dissocial 'psychopath' I worked with was typical in every way of the ICD description except that he was 'socialised' to his group.

'Peter' was a charming 45-year-old industrialist, who had been sent to prep and public school from the age of six, then away to university and the army; he ran his family business, and his family, with 'military discipline'. His son had been admitted to the regional adolescent unit and, on my first home visit, he 'gave the servants the afternoon off'. He expressed delight in meeting a 'chap', an ex-serviceman to boot, and his offer to talk cricket and arrange a ticket to the local football team was almost irresistible. 'Trouble is my boy can't decline his Latin verbs, damned nuisance because he's our only fella (in a family with four girls) and he's got to be able carry corn, what?' His wife who was present hardly said a word, nor did he expect her to, but one trusted one's intuition, a very dangerous thing to do and, on my next home visit, I arrived early in order to interview 'Mrs Peter' alone. It transpired that 'Peter' would drag the naked 11-year-old son from one bathroom to another, with a loofah stuffed in his mouth 'to stifle the screams', sobbed 'Mrs Peter', as his father cursed him 'you will learn your Latin verbs you little bastard xxxx' and plunged him into first a cold and then a hot bath.

I was very frightened on Peter's return, as it was with great difficulty he restrained himself from assaulting me. Nonetheless, we were able to negotiate a new situation for the son, but any suggestion of involving the police for the assaultative abuse was recognised to be counterproductive.

Peter was that rarity, but one does meet them, a person with a 'socialised' personality disorder, who is quite callous about other people's feelings, whose only mediation is their social persona. Later, we had some sessions with 'Peter' for his transient depression, but he rejected any further offer of help as 'it might be useful for the puerile and weak', but not for this sad man.

One could almost pity a man who de facto had been rejected at six, bullied and abused by a school residential system that Utting (1997) recognised can be so damaging. Change Peter's background for a prison rather than boarding schools, and he would be likely to have been a familiar case in many statutory agency caseloads.

If social work applied some simple research methodologies to that practice knowledge which surrounds us all, we too might find benefit in recognising patterns of behaviour, which require a very special response, particularly in the child protection–mental health interface.

Part II
Bio-psychosocial perspective

6 Critique of unidimensional medicalisation of mental disorder

So far, we have tried to provide a framework to understa[...] omenon of 'madness' that has drawn heavily upon the evidence-[...] modern medicine, concerned quintessentially with the humani[...]s. This is essentially an integrative bio-psychosocial approac[...] fore of practice, relevant to any of the fields of 'human care'. [...] ploring the psychosocial aspects of mental disorder, we need t[...] serious look at the criticisms of the bio-pharmacological asp[...] c care, especially by those who offer a mainly unidimensiona[...] care of mentally disordered people.

After years in the mental health field, I am more than aware of the inconsistencies, sloppy thinking and sometimes downright poor practice that passes as 'mental health' for people, who both historically and currently, are actively stigmatised and discriminated against (Burton 1590; Phillips *et al.* 2002; Schulze and Angermeyer 2002; McSween 2002; Marwaha and Livingston 2002; Luchins 2004; Kahng and Mowbray 2005; Thoits 2005). Sadly, irresponsible media reporting still perpetuates these hangovers of medieval thinking even today (Corrigan *et al.* 2005). Such prejudices cross international boundaries and ethnic groups, and also include a range of health care professionals, with unfortunate, albeit inadvertent, effects upon the person and their family (Katschnig 2002; Llerena *et al.* 2002; Schulze and Angermeyer 2002; Wancata 2002; Thoits 2005).

General psychiatry, when not practised well, faces a number of problems. These are:

1 the rigidity of its categories and overemphasis upon form rather than content, or indeed virtually ignoring individual content;
2 the issue of ethnicity and a tendency for a social class-biased unidimensional treatment approach;
3 problems of 'control' and compulsion;
4 the dilemma of the influence of the pharmaceutical industry upon treatment and, crucially, medical research.

Yet it can be argued that modern, integrated psychosocial psychiatry is one of the most exciting parts of medicine. Psychiatry, like mental health social work, is concerned with the core issues of the human phenomena, as mental disorder is the 'meeting place' of all the medical sciences, biochemistry, neurosciences, genetics, as well as the social and behavioural sciences, demonstrated in the curriculum of the Royal College of Psychiatrists. Other relevant areas of study are the history of humankind and its cultures, hence the intellectual as well as the practice excitement – the whole of humanity is our field of study and practice, hence we can call upon Shakespeare, the Bible, the Koran, the Lord Krishna, Omar Khayyám, as well as the psychosocial, biological and neurosciences.

Diagnostic rigidity

Perhaps the prevailing, albeit underlying, problem in psychiatry emerges in part because psychiatrists want to be identified with 'medicine' per se. The 'high-tech' glamour of cutting edge medicine, of neurosurgery and cardiac surgery, appeals, whereas traditionally there has been a degree of 'stigma' because psychiatrists are associated with a stigmatised 'out' group, the mentally disordered. Indeed, little more than 100 years ago, psychiatrists were known as the 'mad doctors'. The more up-to-date and well-integrated psychiatrists can smile at this because they know that even cutting edge medical research, as reflected in recent *Nature* reviews, almost poses as many questions as it answers (Madden 2002; Swanson *et al.* 2005), and they appreciate the essential psychosocial component in people's lives, which is part of their treatment approach (e.g. Kingdon and Turkington 2002). But there can be a tendency to be rigid about the concept of 'diagnosis'. Any open-minded practitioner knows, whether they are in general medicine, surgery or psychiatry, that the 'classic' signs and symptoms of a disease always vary to a degree between patients and, in fact, human beings are not mechanistic, although some medical textbooks make us seem as if we are. Therefore, when it comes to conditions, syndromes, disease or disorders that are manifested in people's emotions, perceptions and behaviour, the variations, relative to clearly physical disorders, can be quite marked. The problem arises when some psychiatrists see the disease model in a rigid way and assume that a pattern of emotions, perceptions and behaviour can be viewed as a rigid diagnostic category, and they assume that treatment x (usually a psychotropic or mood-stabilising drug) is the answer. Then, if they ignore either the precipitant or stressors surrounding the period of disorder, they wonder why their patients do not respond as well as the 'textbooks' imply, and they either increase the dosage or add another drug in the worst kind of 'jug and bottle' psychiatry.

The importance of predisposing as well as precipitant stressors in mental disorder cannot be overstated, although these are both bio-physical (genetic predisposition) as well as psychosocial. Here, we fly the flag for an integrative bio-psychosocial view of human development, behaviour and pathology, which means that all aspects are components in mental disorders, which span a continuum from 'normal' behaviour to extreme dysfunctional behaviour. Where the diagnostic paradigm is helpful is in understanding the person in their situation. On the one hand, this does not ignore those biochemical research findings associated with the schizophrenias or the mood disorders, nor does it under- or overplay the psychosocial antecedent or reactive behavioural outcomes.

A brilliant critical review of psychiatry came from everyone's favourite clinical psychologist, Professor Richard Bentall (2003). Professor Bentall's great contribution to mental health was to highlight how, when mental disorders emerge, they are related to people's personality and backgrounds. Thus, a person who was somewhat introspective, self-doubting and with low self-esteem met a concoction of problems, then blamed themself and presented as 'depressed', whereas another personality type blamed other people, then presented as paranoid (Bentall 1990, 2003; Bentall *et al.* 1989, 1991; Kerr 2003; Lee *et al.* 2004; Rankin *et al.* 2005).

Bentall is particularly severe on the so-called 'father' of scientific psychiatry, Emil Kraepeline, who sought to categorise mental disorders along lines similar to neurology and coined the term 'dementia praecox', which Manfred Bleuer later developed into the phrase 'schizophrenia' fractured persona. Bentall was a little unfair, not least because he takes Kraepeline out of his historical times of nineteenth-century German science, but Bentall was quite right when he saw that Kraepeline's approach, putting psychiatry at the heart of 'physical' rather than 'psychosocial' medicine, would be popular with a branch of medicine a little uncertain of its status. Bentall's fundamental belief is that:

> We should abandon psychiatric diagnosis altogether and instead try to explain and understand the actual experiences and behaviour of psychotic people. By such experiences and behaviour many of the kind of things psychiatrists describe as 'Symptoms', but which might better be labelled 'Complaints', such as hallucinations, delusions and disordered speech . . . once these complaints have been explained, there are no ghostly diseases remaining that also require explanation. 'Complaints' are all this is.
>
> (Bentall 2003: 141)

Thus, in essence, he does not deny the dysfunction or distress they cause, but Bentall sees mental disorders as an extreme 'normative' reaction to a particular set of circumstances and stressors. I think he goes too far along the psychosocial route, but is an invaluable counterweight to the overly organically orientated psychiatrist, not least because he is often cleverer than they and he offends the medical hauteur, *amour propre*, that is prized by many modern psychiatrists, especially from the cognitive behavioural therapy (CBT) field, to which he has made an important contribution (Craig *et al.* 2004; Tarrier *et al.* 2004; Brown *et al.* 2005).

Integrated conclusions

Despite the controversy surrounding the origins and development of mental disorders, there are some general evidenced-based conclusions that can be made about their nature, which integrates the disparate research strands across the biogenetic, psychosocial and cultural.

An emerging new school of psychology, the 'evolutionary psychologists', draws upon a range of interdisciplinary research that takes cognisance of new research and techniques in brain imaging and molecular biology and greater understanding of neurotransmitters, cognitive and psychosocial studies, and places the person within their culture and times (Wilson EO 1975, 1998, 2002; Wilson G 1998; Buss 2003). At the core of the 'evolutionary psychology' perspective is the realisation that humankind, in evolutionary terms, has not changed for thousands of years, and the ancient Sumerians, Egyptians, indeed, Cro-Magnon man and the cave painters at Lascaux of 15,000 years ago are biologically the same as humans today.

Therefore, a range of psycho-socio-physiological mechanisms is inherent in our psyche and behaviour, with certain evolutionary advantages, the only 'trouble' being that relatively modern humankind has only been significantly urban dwelling for a little more than 300 years. The theory is that, when these mechanisms become out of tilt or balance, then the person has problems. Thus, flight or fight mechanisms would be essential to the survival of the person but, in our modern world, such a mechanism is less vital, and indeed in many modern social situations, inappropriate.

Within primitive groups, including village living, of 500 years ago, 1,000, 2,000, 3,000 years ago, social arrangements would evolve hierarchically, and therefore require a degree of 'submission' to avoid conflict in a world where, if aggression was manifested, it could often end fatally. Therefore, an ability to be 'submissive' in certain situations had evolutionary advantages, although again in some modern situations would be inappropriate.

Equally, high activity and aggression would have advantages and interact with various social arrangements, would demand adjustment and an eventual equilibrium for social living to continue successfully, whereas although drive is still required today, overt aggression is, apart from a 'war' situation, social anathema.

These social factors are especially vital to humans and primates, and carry enormous evolutionary advantages, which eventually evolved into specialist roles for men and women and differential economic activities (Wilson G 1998). Indeed, it might be said that a human person cannot really function effectively outside the 'group' and that, like primates and a number of other mammals, human beings are essentially social beings, as well as biological (Wilson 1975, 1998). Such a position therefore demands an understanding of the inevitable interactive influences of genetic predisposition and the physical results, i.e. someone born a male has different hormones, inclining to x type of psychosocial behaviour, modified by individual bio-psychosocial circumstances and cultural norms. This is dramatically seen on recalling your own pre-puberty feelings and behaviour, when suddenly another person was 'sexualised' for you, which came essentially from your hormones but was dependent upon your circumstances, and changed your bio-psychosocial life for ever.

Brune (2002) argues that evolutionary psychology and evolutionary psychiatry are a metatheory that integrates all aspects of human mammalian behaviour. However, the relatively recent modern *Homo sapiens* have inherited and have to cope with a series of almost 'hair-trigger' mechanisms, which, in our urban, intensively populated world, means that most of the time we have to leave these responses behind or, more importantly, modify them. In evolutionary psychiatry, it is postulated that, for either genetic or particular psychosocial circumstances, these mechanisms become rigid and counterproductive, which would even fit R.D. Laing's (1960) 'psychedelic' ideas. Thus, the flight and fight mechanism might well underpin a 'post-traumatic stress disorder' (Silove 1998) or a panic reaction (Battaglia and Ogliari 2005), whereas the 'submission' response becomes locked into a depression (Pilmann 2001). The influential Professor G.W. Browne links this to his seminal work on social class and depression (Browne 2002). The high activity and/or aggression has been linked to attention deficit hyperactivity disorder (ADHD) and mania (Brody 2001), although of course the former may well be 'environmentally chemically' linked (Pritchard and Sunak 2005) but, if the individual cannot control either, they become very rapidly socially isolated and/or excluded.

Polimeni and Reiss (2003) make a strong case for schizophrenia 'evolving' out of communication confusion, related to the perhaps only truly unique aspect of human beings, namely our predisposition and power of speech. Here, the 'psychology' and 'psychiatry' aspects of the evolutionary model cross over into the biogenetic and the anatomical structures in the brain related to speech. Some theorists have suggested that the genetic mutation that led to humans developing speech, which gave us enormous evolutionary advantages, came at a cost of some genetic predisposition to 'speech/thought' disorder, in other words schizophrenia (Pinker 1998; Warner 2000; Buss 2003).

A neurological structural theory of schizophrenia is associated with Professor Crow (1997) from the Maudsley, and there is some fascinating empirical imaging evidence to support this (Narr *et al.* 2001; Barrick *et al.* 2005; Chance *et al.* 2005) based upon either case–control research or post-mortem studies. In brief, it has been found that there is an asymmetry of the brain around the area concerned with speech, with some brain volume loss, which worsens as the condition progresses (Ho *et al.* 2003). The Maudsley Family Study, which looked at this, found strong indicators of a genetic link in a study of patients, their first-degree relatives and a control group (Sharma 2001). However, while the patient and relatives might have shared similar asymmetry, most relatives were free from schizophrenia, indicating the need for a trigger or stressors, which completes the loop: genetic predisposition, bio-psychosocial circumstance and a triggering stress factor/s to develop the syndrome. The strength of the imaging technology means that, instead of examining only post-mortem brains, we can now investigate structure, volume and blood flow in living people. However, while there is theoretically no reason why the anti-psychotic drugs might influence brain volume, it remains an unknown, whereas it is conceivable that stressors may, over time, create a physiological feedback that may impact upon brain volume. We just do not know but here is evidence of the bio-psychosocial interaction but, as usual, new information raises further interesting questions.

Consequently, in view of the fact that the mood disorders have only a slight genetic weighting, but it is considerably stronger with schizophrenia, it can be said that, while anyone in certain 'depressing', repetitive, 'submissive', demoralising situations could become 'depressed', there would be a need to have a genetic weighting before one developed schizophrenia.

The logic would be the greater the genetic weighting, the less severe the psychosocial stress required, or vice versa. The schizo-affective disorders would sit somewhere between this, whereas the minor mental disorders are, in 'evolutionary psychiatric' terms, the result of faulty mechanisms, meeting predisposing psychosocial circumstances. The personality disorders are probably again a combination of endowment and family attachment problems, possibly even some neurological developmental delay, with subsequent inability to respond appropriately.

Some 'organic' orientated psychiatrists might feel that the structural neurology and genetic importance is being underplayed. Yet, all one has to do is to look at twin studies on a range of well defined physical conditions to find that even with monozygotic (identical) twins, concordance rates seldom exceed 60–70 per cent and are often even lower (Vieregge *et al.* 1992; Graham *et al.* 1997; Wirdefeldt *et al.* 2004). With regard to the 'psychiatric' disorders, while a genetic element is demonstrated, many concordance rates are lower than 50 per cent (Cardno *et al.* 1999; Kendler *et al.* 2000; Greenberg *et al.* 2001; Hay *et al.* 2001; Holmes *et al.* 2002).

This integrative model seems to be able to incorporate all the main research fields and give a reasonable account of the general development of the mental disorders, and an explanation for the unique and highly individualistic response and experience of sufferers.

There are, however, other problems in psychiatry which require understanding, and these are explored, with the aim of showing that, although psychiatry has its weaknesses, it also has much to offer people experiencing mental disorders.

7 Other problems of psychiatry

The person, whether designated client, patient or service user, is the sum of all these approaches. For the 'proper study of mankind is man', and psychiatry and mental health social work are at the frontiers of new knowledge, understanding and techniques to reach our troubled and sometimes troublesome fellow citizen, as well as the development of self-understanding.

It must be admitted that the busy psychiatrist sometimes fails to respond to the specific individuality of the client, focusing only upon the 'form' of the condition for 'diagnostic' purposes; yet failure to consider the person's 'content' can actually be damaging. For example, failure on the part of the physician to ask about the accommodation of a person with schizophrenia may well end up with them being homeless (Scott 1993). Failure to consider the impact of the mental disorder upon the person's family negates any effective treatment, because the psychiatrist may undermine the most important psychosocial support the person has, namely their family, and such insensitivity may contribute to relapse and the need for readmission (Kingdon and Turkington 2002). But this is bad psychiatry, and we should not dismiss the whole of psychiatry because of poor practice. As with the media stereotype, we should not be dismissive of British social work, e.g. the Victoria Climbié inquiry, which was 'bad social work' allied with poor professional supervision and management. This is not typical of the majority of child protection, as the evidence points to the British child protection system being one of the most effective in the world; fewer children die from violence in Britain now than since records began – so much for media perception (Pritchard 1996c, 2002; UNICEF 1999; Pritchard and Butler 2003; Pritchard and Lewis 2006). So too with psychiatry, and some critics really do create 'straw men' in their polemics against psychiatry, e.g. equating Nazi Germany's treatment of mentally ill people (Myer 1988) with modern British psychiatry, or quoting physicians from the 1851 slave states of pre-Civil War USA as typical of prevailing attitudes (Pilgrim and Rogers 1998). This is being less than balanced. Indeed, it is as accurate a description of modern psychiatry as the accusation that social workers are 'child slavers', a complaint heard levelled at British child protection officers from people from traditional societies, who cannot understand when we 'take children away', especially when it is a male child!

Notwithstanding, in the 1970s, the anti-psychiatry movement fiercely and, to some extent, justifiably criticised psychiatry for 'colour blindness'. Psychiatrists failed to account for the person's different culture and lifestyle, resulting in disproportionate numbers of compulsory hospital admissions of people from ethnic minorities, especially people from an African-Caribbean background (Carpenter and Brockington 1980; Fernando 1988; Cope 1989).

This is still a problem in Britain, as people from an African-Caribbean background, but not Asian, are more often admitted to psychiatric hospital, especially compulsory admissions, than white people (Coid *et al.* 2002a; Harrison 2002; Bhui *et al.* 2003). But this is more complicated than possible 'institutional racism' of the mental health services. Rather, it can be argued that this is the end-product of socioeconomic disadvantage, which is all pervasive in British society, both black and white. Indeed, people from social classes 4 and 5 have more in common with each other, irrespective of their ethnic background, in terms of their being over-represented in cohorts of 'socially excluded' people. It is true for poorer health, being more often in prison and psychiatric populations than their ethnic peers from classes 1 and 2, but belonging to the 'wrong' ethnic group appears to compound being in the 'wrong' social class, with its concomitant social disadvantage (Judge and Benzeval 1993; Audit Commission 1998; Pritchard and Butler 2000a,b; Coid *et al.* 2002b; Brugha *et al.* 2004; Bhui *et al.* 2005; Kahn *et al.* 2005; Thoits 2005).

A very important study exploring the psychiatric–criminal link gives us another perspective on this problem. Coid *et al.* (2002a,b) found a distinctive differential between ethnic groups in a national sample in British prisons. Based upon the total sample of prison populations, South Asians accounted for 33 per cent fewer male inmates than statistically expected, and 80 per cent fewer female inmates; white males and females accounted for 10 per cent fewer than expected, but the African-Caribbean prison populations were 5.4 and 5.9 times higher than expected (440 and 490 per cent more respectively)! Incidentally, the male and female inmate populations accounted for by 'other' ethnic British nationals were 54 per cent (males) and 2.3 times (females) more than expected. Table 7.1 presents the results.

However, it was noteworthy that unemployment figures were more than four times the national average among *all* prisoners, irrespective of ethnicity, with rates of 44 per cent for South Asians, 55 per cent for African-Caribbean people and 65 per cent for whites, reflecting the all-pervading negative impact of social class. The unemployed are at the bottom of the social class pile, as in effect they are excluded from it.

It might be argued that, like water to fish, class influence is so 'normal' we British do not notice it. Yet, ask a person visiting from overseas about 'social class' and their response may well surprise and be at odds with John Major's premise that 'we are all one class now', while Colin Powell's biography (1995) poses the question of where would he be if his father had emigrated to Southampton rather than New York – by inference not Britain's first black Chief of the General Staff. Paradoxically, while black and white prisoners had higher rates of early childhood problems, such as conduct disorders and being taken into care, than Asians, African-Caribbean prisoners had fewer adverse childhood backgrounds than white prisoners. Is this the 'social class' element showing?

Table 7.1 Representative British national sample of prisoners by ethnicity and gender (standardised admission rates)

Ethnicity	Male		Female	
	Expected	*Observed*	*Expected*	*Observed*
White	50,926	46,607 (–10%)	2,220	1,997 (–10%)
Black	1,052	5,680 (×5.4)	51	304 (×5.9)
South Asian	1,808	1,215 (–33%)	72	14 (–80%)
Other	520	803 (+54%)	22	50 (×2.3)

Source: Extrapolated from Coid *et al.* (2002a).

There were marked differences in the type of offences between the three groups, with more drug and violence against the person offences among African-Caribbean prisoners, who also had more previous convictions than the other two cohorts, with South Asians having considerably lower previous drug convictions than whites.

Unexpectedly, unlike earlier but much smaller studies (McGovern and Cope 1987), both male and female African-Caribbean prisoners had lower levels of mental health 'psychopathology' but, where there was mental disorder among the black prisoners, they had twice the rate of schizophrenia. This is strongly indicative of an ethnic prejudice in the compositions of our prisons. However, in view of the significantly higher rate of African-Caribbean prisoners being transferred from prison to psychiatric hospital, especially the forensic psychiatric services (Bhui *et al.* 1998; Coid *et al.* 2000), this may account for the lower 'psychiatric' profile of black prisoners in general prisons.

This overlap between 'criminality' and psychopathology shows one thing, the underlying all-pervasive cultural aspects of both ethnicity and social class. Yet, at the same time, there are differences.

The degree to which 'institutional racism' plays a part is, scientifically speaking, difficult to quantify, for how does one account for the lower Asian crime and psychiatric rates? In part, it has something to do with how disadvantaged families seek and gain help from the services, especially for young people (Audit Commission 1998). However, the ethnic/cultural issue is complicated, in part, by how people with problems are 'defined' and crucially define themselves.

Recent research has shown that, dependent upon their ethnicity, older people with depression attribute their problems differently. 'Whites' are more likely to consider some organic or reactive 'cause', whereas older African-Caribbean people more often attribute their problems to 'spiritual' distress, resulting in different pathways to help (Marwaha and Livingston 2002), while there are differing perceptions of the 'locus of control' between various ethnic groups (Wrightson and Wardle 1997). Moreover, the apparent variation in type of mental disorder among African-Caribbean people, namely relatively lower affective disorder problems and greater schizophrenic-type difficulties, may be linked not only to how people are assessed but to lifestyles (for example people who use cannabis long term). The

Swedish research is based upon lifetime medical registers, which permit researchers to track patterns of illness anonymously across families. People with first- and second-degree relatives with schizophrenia also have an increased susceptibility to developing schizophrenia. But there was a small but significant group of young men who developed schizophrenic-like disorders later, who had no relatives with schizophrenia, but who were long-term users of cannabis (Andreasson *et al.* 1990; Zammit *et al.* 2002). Moreover, in south-east London, there appears to have been an increase in schizophrenia over the past three decades, which may be associated, among a number of possible social factors, with a rise in the regular use of cannabis (Boydell *et al.* 2003).

This may be a factor in increasing the relative risk for schizophrenia-type disorder among young African-Caribbean cannabis-using men, as much as differing perceptions of schizophrenia in Britain (Cinnirella and Loewenthal 1999; Pote and Orrell 2002) or differential access to care (Bhui *et al.* 2003; Saxena *et al.* 2002) and/or differential impact of mental health legislation upon British African-Caribbeans (Eaton and Harrison 2000; Harrison 2002; Brugha *et al.* 2004). But it is also suggested that, within this complex of interacting factors, 'social class' may mediate against both those ending up in prison and those being compulsorily detained in hospital (Magnus and Mick 2000; Breslau *et al.* 2005).

The question remains, do the mental health services meet the needs of ethnic minority people and, if not, are they 'racist'?

The answer is that most public services do less well for ethnic minority people, which is also true for people in the lower socioeconomic groups. But what seems clear is that the mental health services are at the end of often life-long processes of discrimination that pervade British society and are a challenge to fully implementing the new Human Rights Act that came into force in 2000 (Rai-Atkins *et al.* 2002; Bindman *et al.* 2003).

This is not to exonerate either psychiatry or any of the services; rather, it is to place the situation in a different perspective. Moreover, British psychiatry, almost as much as British social work, has emphasised 'anti-discriminatory' practice, as British psychiatry has been at the forefront of major research dealing with the problem (McGovern and Cope 1987; Eaton and Harrison 2000; Coid *et al.* 2002a; Harrison 2002; Bhui *et al.* 2003; Brugha *et al.* 2004). Research published in the *British Journal of Psychiatry* for the Royal College of Psychiatry is impressive and contributes to making all aware of the discriminations within British society. Furthermore, it would be fair to argue that the *British Journal of Psychiatry* has a far greater empirical research orientation on discrimination than the *British Journal of Social Work*, which is far more 'experiential'. Governments can more easily ignore this, whereas hard data, giving facts and figures, are 'in their face', exemplified by the work of Coid, Bhui, Brugha and others from the field of psychiatry. It would be fair to say that the Royal College of Psychiatry has actively sought to confront these issues although, self-evidently, one experience of active discrimination is one too many (Thompson and Pritchard 1987). However, there are some encouraging signs. Based upon a recent study of women's suicidal behaviour, a very stigmatised activity in Asian communities, it was found that Asian women had significantly higher rates than indigenous Caucasian women. However, 17 per cent of the Asian women attributed 'racial harassment' as contributing to their suicidal behaviour. Clearly, 17 per cent is far too high, and how does it suggest an improvement? The biggest single factor attributed by these women to their distress was intrafamily stress, a far higher rate than white indigenous women. This was in part due to a clash of cultures, as the Asian women wanted a greater degree of personal choice than exists in the tradition of their culture of origin (Bhurga *et al.* 2003). Bearing in mind the high profile of ethnic issues and the 'temptation' to ascribe their stigmatised behaviour to external reasons, one cannot but conclude that this is an encouraging indicator of positive change. Indeed, bearing in mind Britain's colonial history and the recentness of 'empire', there is evidence to show that overt racial prejudice still involves a minority of whites, although sadly with a social class bias (Thompson and Pritchard 1987). While access to primary care for people from ethnic backgrounds has improved over the past decade, this is still less good for access to secondary health care (Saxena *et al.* 2002). There are no grounds for complacency, but we should avoid the temptation of castigating one sector of public service, rather than acknowledging that institutional racism is inherent in most societies, including our own.

This was true for institutional sexism, homophobia, regionalism and anti-traveller attitudes (Thompson and Pritchard 1987) but, compared with a decade or two decades ago, we have made progress. It is important for social workers to be 'up to date' not only about research, but also about the unfolding changes in our society, for things are better than they were.

In parenthesis, it may be that institutional ageism has yet to receive the recognition it deserves, but that may seem like special pleading on behalf of mature professionals.

However, we need to recognise that prejudice, including racial intolerance, is sadly found in every human society. Indeed, Indrah Singh (2003) said that he had experienced more racial prejudice in India than anywhere else in the world and sadly reminded us of the active discrimination occurring in Zimbabwe and Rwanda and the religious differences that can lead to violence in Nigeria and Sudan. Of course, the suppression of the Palestinian people by Israel, which has ignored UN resolutions for more than 30 years, graphically illustrates how a previously oppressed group can in turn become oppressors. This was classically seen with the Boers in South Africa, who were oppressed by the British and then imposed apartheid. This is a field in which none of us 'would 'scape whipping' and highlights the desperate need at societal, personal and professional levels to seek to implement the UN Declaration of Human Rights.

One area of persistent insensitivity in psychiatry needs to be mentioned, namely that some first-generation ethnic minority physicians' and psychiatrists' attitudes to their compatriots can sometimes leave much to be desired. Over the years, I have heard British-born Asian and Chinese physicians and students complain about their 'unreconstructed' colleagues' authoritarian attitudes not only against people of the same ethnic background, but also against 'low-class people', sometimes said with such insensitive disregard. While the 'class divide' is a long-known barrier to doctor–patient communication, unfortunately this can still be a particular problem. Indeed, it is a longstanding issue and, according to two eminent psychiatrists who were from minority backgrounds (Mahapatra and Hamilton 1974), the recruitment of physicians from the Indian subcontinent was a covert form of neocolonialism, luring Asian doctors to the West, denuding the continent of scarce trained personnel, which is admitted by the British Medical Association (BMA), and still occurs today. Moreover, using Asian doctors disproportionately to fill British vacancies in the less fashionable specialities or localities was another form of discrimination, in particular in the mental health and geriatric fields. The situation has clearly improved since the mid-1970s, but the need for sensitivity of language and cultural understanding remains for all professionals, irrespective of their own social, ethnic and cultural backgrounds. An ethnic minority practitioner's insensitive or judgemental attitude towards their indigenous working-class or compatriot patients is just as problematic as the white middle-class professional's insensitivity to clients from another ethnic or socioeconomic group. It is hoped that this acknowledgement of this longstanding problem will not be misunderstood, for it is noticeable that there is virtually no recent empirical research in this area.

Social class bias

Linked to this problem is the longstanding treatment bias against 'working-class' patients (Pallis and Stoffelmyer 1978). The middle-class mentally disordered person is far more likely to receive an integrated approach, namely appropriate psychotropic drugs and a 'talking' psychosocial therapy, than a person from the lower socioeconomic groups, and such trends still persist (McClelland and Crisp 2001; Mulvaney *et al.* 2001; Chew-Graham *et al.* 2002). Indeed, Magnus and Mick (2000) outline a position that has much merit when they argue that, instead of taking 'affirmative' action based upon 'race', as current in many US states, they suggest that social class should be the criterion for positive discrimination, as de facto this is what the Blair government is arguing for in British universities. The rationale is that there has been social progress, albeit still more is needed, but using ethnicity as the criterion ignores the fact that many ethnic minority families have become established middle-class people and, as such, are more advantaged than 'working-class' families.

Of course, this social class bias is not just a problem with psychiatry, but crosses the whole of medicine, e.g. cancer and asthma (Judge and Benzeval 1993; Duran-Tauleria *et al.* 1996; Herbert *et al.* 2002; Kahn *et al.* 2005). Most of the Royal Colleges, e.g. of General Practice, Medicine and Psychiatry, urge greater patient–physician partnership, which leads to better clinical and psychosocial outcomes when such relationships are established (Coulter 1999; Henwood 1998; Richards 1998; Pritchard *et al.* 2001, 2004b). However, compared with the earlier more rigid, authoritarian class discrimination identified by Pallis and Stoffelmyer (1978), there is evidence that matters have improved, although there are no grounds for complacency (Paykel 2001; Hawton *et al.* 2001; Mulvaney *et al.* 2001).

Pharmacology and the influence of the market

The advent of effective psychotropic drugs for mental disorder undoubtedly gave the public confidence to move from a predominantly 'custodial' care of people to 'care in the community' (Jones 1959). However, almost equal to the effectiveness of such drugs to contain and control both signs and symptoms, they have also been associated with extreme side-effects. Over the past 20 years or more, there have been undoubted reductions in the worst side-effects of the disabling kind, commonly seen in the 1960s and 1970s; yet, even with the most modern drugs, physicians and psychiatrists appear to be willing to tolerate their patients having what must feel like a high level of side-effects (Bazire 2001; Tohen *et al.* 2002). For example, in a most detailed comparative trial of a single anti-bipolar drug, compared with a combination of two drugs, the following side-effects were noted without comment: 25–50 per cent somnolence, 10–30 per cent dry mouth, 10–20 per cent increased appetite, 10–20 per cent increased tremor, 5–10 per cent occasional dizziness, 15–20 per cent headache, etc. and, over a six-week period, weight gains of between 2 and 4.5 kilos (Tohen *et al.* 2002). The problem is that psychiatrists often fail to ask themselves what these side-affects mean to the patient, especially those that have an impact upon their gait and facial expressions, when often the drugs rather than the disorder make some people look odd. However, what is often forgotten by the critics is that 'placebo' treatments, i.e. giving a mock tablet that has no known therapeutic value, also create side-effects in as many as 10–15 per cent of people! As we shall see, there are undoubted benefits from appropriate psychopharmacology, in reality life saving, but the professionals become accustomed to the side-effects, forgetting the unique experience of each individual patient.

As early as 1994, an in-depth meta-analysis of review articles over a 20-year period found that, on balance, lower or moderate use of anti-psychotics was better for maintaining patients long term, not least because they had fewer side-effects and self-evidently were better tolerated (Bollini *et al.* 1994), although of course drug companies and their representatives prefer physicians to prescribe larger rather than smaller doses. Despite improvements, much more needs to be done (Grunze and Moller 2002; NICE 2002, 2005).

However, adverse reactions are not just a problem for psychiatry for, at the extreme, it has been found that 0.5 per cent of patients who die in hospital do so, in part, as a result of a 'medical event', very often an iatrogenic (doctor caused) adverse drug reaction (Kumar and Clarke 1994). This means that, of the 630,000 annual 'all-cause deaths' in the UK (WHO 2001–5), if we conservatively assume that only half died in hospital and 0.5 per cent of these deaths were iatrogenic, then these are equivalent to 3,150 deaths annually. In parenthesis, this places the extremes of social service failures in cases of 'child abuse' in a very different perspective. Moreover, it is known that 4 per cent of all patients on long-term use of anti-inflammatory drugs have serious iatrogenic diseases, and a quarter of these, i.e. 1 per cent of the total cohort, die. We must avoid double counting, but that is equivalent to a minimum of 1,000 deaths in the UK alone.

Of course, no-one intended these adverse reactions, and only some ethereal idealist would really argue for a medicine-free world, that is until they had one of the serious 'thousand natural shocks that flesh is heir to' (*Hamlet*). The problem lies, for medicine and psychiatry in particular, in the research underlying the new drugs. There is a clash between the need to keep research development costs to a minimum balanced against the likelihood of the level of profit, sound research methodology and patient benefit, and demands upon prescribers to maintain vigilance (Inman and Pearce 1993; D'Arcy 1998; Freemantle 1999; NICE 2002). This is a *cri de coeur* exemplified by such prestigious organisations as the American Enterprise Institute of Procter & Gamble (Calfee 2000; Li *et al.* 2001), who found that media speculation about a new 'wonder drug' makes the ethical practice of the development of new drugs fraught at every turn (Abraham 2002). Unfortunately, even organisations that, at first sight, are entirely 'patient focused', e.g. the National Institute for Health and Clinical Excellence (NICE), are not only concerned with the efficacy of the drug but also its cost-effectiveness to the health service. Thus, a drug may improve the quality of life of a person with long-term schizophrenia, or a degenerative disease, but it may actually add to the overall health costs that government-sponsored NICE is charged to avoid (D'Arcy 1998; Corre 2002; NICE 2002, 2005). Moreover, an earlier study on the introduction of new drugs did not appear to be related to 'medical need' but more to various characteristics of GP prescribing (Inman and Pearce 1993) and, while the researchers did not say so, the inference was the impact of various 'sales' techniques upon the GPs.

The strongest criticism of medicine is the inevitable but uneasy relationship between the medical profession and the drug industry, all of medicine, not just psychiatry. Although it is easy and romantic to yearn for a golden age when we did not 'rely on drugs', just you look at photographs of ordinary people in the interwar years or up to the 1950s when necessary drugs were in effect severely rationed by people's ability to pay. They look older, as they bore the impact of what today are considered minor diseases but, in those days, ravaged the person, with the accumulative impact of illness and inadequate treatment. But, the drive of the 'profit motive' in the multinational drug industry cannot be gainsaid. This was exemplified in a conversation with an eight-year-old and her father.

The family had a small shilling (five pence)-sized savings box for Lepra, a charity that fights leprosy in the Third World. On the side of the box were the words of the leper speaking to Jesus 'If thou wilt, thou canst make me clean'. The child asked her father what this meant. He explained that the man with leprosy understood the special power of Jesus and therefore he was pointing out to Jesus that, as he had the ability, if he had the will, he could cure him. 'Does that mean we can cure leprosy daddy?' 'Yes' replied the father, which is of course true with modern drugs. 'Then why don't we?' asked the eight-year-old, with such devastating moral as well as technical logic.

Such wisdom from a child reminds us that 'out of the mouth of babes and sucklings' comes truth. The recent outcry of 143 of the 144 members of the World Trade Organization, following US Vice President Dick Cheney's personal intervention to stop the WTO relaxing patent regulations to assist poorer countries to have access to life-saving drugs, is a particular bad example of capitalism overcoming human ethics (Elliott and Denny 2002a,b).

One of the most important elements of true professionalism is that the professional acts in the best interest of their client/patient/service user. Such an ethic is fundamental to the public service ethos. So, in general, British surgeons in the NHS operate less than their American counterparts who have a different funding system. This reflects the old adage, 'Are you doing this for me, Doctor, or am I doing it for you?' because implicit in the interaction between professional and client is the degree of competing vested interests. From the 1960s onwards, Szasz (1970) has continued to argue that the only nexus to be trusted is that of the market, of the buyer controlling the seller, so that the consumer has the power to take their custom elsewhere. But Szasz and his like have quietly ignored the public service ethos and its mutuality with the citizen. Richard Titmuss's classic *The Gift* explained that, in the USA, patients have to buy blood, resulting in blood predominantly coming from disadvantaged groups of people, with the greater likelihood of carrying a number of blood-borne diseases. Hence blood products from the USA have proved to be more problematic. This is still the case today, despite technical improvements. However, in Britain, the citizen gives the gift of life as they willingly donate their blood to complete strangers. Because we take this as a norm, we often fail to grasp the wonderful significance of such generosity. It could be argued that even here there is an element of 'vested interest' as the mutuality is assumed, so we all expect that our blood type will be available if and when we need it, and our taxes support the advertisement and blood collection service. But if one is in the 'private sector', one is subjected to different kinds of pressures. To appreciate the world before the NHS, we need to read the novels of A.J. Cronin, e.g. *The Citadel*, as young doctors fought to be recognised, mortgaged half their lives to pay for the practices they were buying into and, of course, the more one did for the patients, the greater the financial return. To do this, Cronin showed that they became desensitised to practice rather than medical necessities, once cynically described to me as 'relieving the stuffed purse syndrome' as the physician, be they surgeon, psychiatrist, etc., subtly accepted at best, or encouraged at worst, a dependency that required their ministrations.

This was exemplified in my early academic career.

After nearly 16 years in practice, I looked forward to my new lectureship, freed from the energy-sapping demands of clients. Fortunately, my old Professor, Max Hamilton, said, 'if you teach a practice you need to practice'. In effect, all lecturers did a minimum day and a half practice, which included seeing private patients one or two evenings a week. I was closing a particularly successful case and suggested one more session (feed) after a holiday break. I was surprised when the client queried its necessity, but she acquiesced readily enough after the mildest justification. On reflection, I realised that I was seeing her for my needs, i.e. an easy 50-minute hour after my holidays, rather than her needs. This was unacceptable so I informed colleagues that, while I would continue to take private referrals – there was a waiting list – in future, all fees would be donated to one of three charities. Sadly, to a man and woman, all my colleagues stopped referring patients. Fortunately, I was able to continue with pro bono work, which maintains that vital practice–research–teaching interaction, not least to remind the protected academic with a minimal caseload just how demanding and difficult practice is.

This latter aspect is one of the greatest strengths of medicine, especially in the NHS, that academic medics maintain a practice and senior medics are encouraged to continue a research interest, all of which is shared with students in an evidence-based practice education.

My private practice experience taught me the subtle dangers of having a financial interest in the treatment of one's clients. This is not to say that those in private practice are not completely honourable, and probably more able to resist temptation than I but, as with NICE (2002, 2005) there is a clash of interests between efficacy and cost, so too in private practice, and with the pharmaceutical industry. When, in 1998, I became a research professor in a medical school, I had a score or more of appointments from eager drug representatives wanting to enquire about my research interests and could they help with funding. When they learned that I could not prescribe, not one returned to pursue the various research ideas put forward.

Yet we must not be hypocritical. All of us in the human services field make our livings out of other people's misery, pain and suffering. It is a harsh realisation, but one that we should recognise and take seriously, for the corollary is that we are obliged to do our very best at all times and that we must put something back into the service for the benefit of our fellow citizens.

Yet the human dilemmas surrounding pharmaceutical drugs can be profound.

'Mr X' was an outstanding colleague, widely regarded and respected. He developed a terrible degenerative disease, with catastrophic impact both physically and psychologically. The media had hyped up a new 'wonder drug' for his condition, which inevitably was very expensive. When looking at the two research papers on which the media story was built, I was horrified to find that the 'outstanding success' described by the journalist, which had raised enormous expectations, was nothing of the sort, as life expectancy post diagnosis increased by between 3 and 6 months.

Mr X received the drug but, in all honesty, more as a psychological tonic than a pathology-halting treatment. After 11 months, he died with great dignity, but he said 'I feel I've been cheated, it (the drug) really did nothing for me, but gave me false hope'.

The great American social policy analyst J.K. Galbraith said 'every corner of the public psyche is canvassed by some of its most talented citizens to see if the desire for some merchandisable product can be cultivated' (quoted by Barker *et al.* 1998). Yet, as we shall see, psychotropic drugs are not only life-savers but enable many people to live good-quality lives, despite suffering from some of the major mental disorders.

However, 'vested' interests can emerge in unexpected places. While in the USA during their last presidential election, I was regaled by a group of colleagues who sneeringly spoke of the shortcomings of the NHS: 'typical of what you'd expect from socialised medicine'. Similar to everyone else, I assumed that US medicine would be 'superior' and explored the ultimate outcome measure of 'all cause' death rates and, because of the high profile, 'all cancer' deaths between the USA and England and Wales. To everyone's surprise, and to British delight, while both forms of death rates had fallen substantially between 1974 and 2000 for people aged 24–74, initially the US deaths were lower in the 1970s than the Anglo-Welsh but, by 2000, we had had a proportionally bigger mortality reduction in most of the age bands (15–24, 25–34, 35–44, etc.) for 'all cause' and 'all cancer' deaths (Pritchard and Galvin 2006). This seemed to be 'big news' with obvious political implications, because the comparison had not always been so good (Evans and Pritchard 2000). However, both the *British Medical Journal* and the *Lancet* turned the paper down, despite the 'good news' for the NHS. Medical colleagues cynically suggested that such 'good news' might imperil further funding that the NHS still needs, and that such an outcome from 7.6 per cent of GDP expenditure on health compared with the USA expenditure of 12.3 per cent could be used by politicians to slow down on their promises to have the British GDP expenditure on health match the old European Union average. Too far-fetched? On being shown that British child protection had substantially reduced child deaths far better than in most other countries (Pritchard and Butler 2003), a Director of Social Services said 'that's good but don't shout too loudly, it will imperil my budget if the elected members think they could cut it – sadly we need one tragedy a year to keep them anxious in order to preserve our budget'.

However, to return to the practical problem of drugs in psychiatry, the aim is to find the balance between effective levels of appropriate medication and managing or reducing side-effects that can be tolerated, as opposed to side-effects 'which are worse than my voices'. It is acknowledged that some people find the impact of the side-effects more intolerable than the disturbance brought about by their mental disorder (Millett 1991; Buchanan 1996).

Professor Jamison (1995) explored this dilemma within her own life as she learned to manage her recurrent bipolar affective disorder with a proper balance of mood stabilisers and psychosocial support.

View of psychiatric services

With regard to consumer studies in the field of psychiatry, the early ones were undertaken mainly from a medical sociological perspective (Pilgrim and Rogers 1998), and there is a degree of 'Pausanias' syndrome here (Pritchard 1999). Pausanias was a close friend of Alexander the (so-called) Great. Pausanias consulted the oracle to learn how he might become world famous. He was told to kill the most famous person of his day and therefore, when his name was mentioned, Pausanias would be remembered. So he slew Alexander's father King Phillip; thus, like all assassins, he gained the dubious fame of being associated with the deaths of famous people of their times, e.g. John Wilkes Booth–Abraham Lincoln, Lee Harvey Oswald–J.F. Kennedy and Earl Ray–Martin Luther King. As an aspiring discipline, sociology attacked medicine, which, if you do not have to deal directly with the impact of the socially disadvantaged, is easy to blame on those who do. Not that some of the sociological criticisms are not accurate; the question is the underlying cause, which evidence would suggest is largely the gap between what research tells us is optimal intervention versus a minimal feasible service response, as the thinly spread mental health services battle to offer a client-specific service.

Nonetheless, psychiatry is confronting the challenge, as it has been found that the quality of the relationship between psychiatrist and patient is positively linked to outcome, as is the involvement of the patient in treatment decisions (McCabe *et al.* 1999). Hence, there is a current European multicentre project under way that focuses upon the patient's quality of life (McCabe and Priebe 2002). This in itself will be a major boost in the psychiatrist–patient interaction in focusing upon the patient's agenda. This was found in 'high-tech' neurosurgery, where it was accepted that 60–80 per cent of post-discharge emergency-type patients, which are the majority in neurosurgery, would suffer from medium- to long-term post-traumatic stress symptoms (McKenna *et al.* 1989; Heelawell and Pentland 2001; Pritchard *et al.* 2001). However, it was found by focusing upon what patients and their carers needed in the community that these stress symptoms were drastically reduced, seen in annual savings of £171,000 following speedier return to work by patients and their carers (Pritchard *et al.* 2004b).

Two British publications are making a major impact upon psychiatric thinking about better communication with patients. Barnes (2000) identified some of the practical effects of stigma: 34 per cent of her respondents had lost their jobs because of their mental disorder, 47 per cent had been harassed in public, 26 per cent felt compelled to move house and 25 per cent had been turned down by insurance or finance companies. Hence, think very carefully before advising anyone to trust in the sympathy of a profit-making company. Not surprisingly from a social work perspective, what users valued most was their relationship with their case manager, especially when they felt listened to, helped with practical housing and benefits assistance and helped to deal with family relationships. Rose (2001), in a very systematic and focused study, drawing respondents from semi-rural and inner city mental health service areas, was able to identify key issues for service users. These included the quality of information given, the care delivery process, how clinical and mental health crises were dealt with, user involvement, issues of advocacy, records and how to make complaints and general satisfaction.

The most startling finding was the considerable difference between the semi-rural and inner city respondents' views, far greater dissatisfaction being expressed by the inner city clients. However, it should be noted that four centres were surveyed, and the differences between them strongly suggested that clients' responses to them reflected something of the quality of staff. Table 7.2 reflects a synopsis of Rose's findings, and the scores shown are 'satisfied' and 'dissatisfied', with 'neutral' excluded.

Crucially, Rose (2001) was able to determine what contributed to these overall levels of satisfaction. There were marked statistically significant differences when respondents had had good information with regard to mental health problems, side-effects, benefits, work and community resources. Moreover, satisfaction was greater if clients felt that their personal strengths had been recognised in their need assessment and, crucially, if they felt involved in their care plan and their medication dosage and whether or not they felt overmedicated.

Bearing in mind that these assessments were determined by specially trained previous service users, the actual levels of expressed dissatisfaction (clearly exceeded by clients who were satisfied) are encouraging, and again reflect the individual quality of the specific professional or unit, rather than the overall system, a feature found elsewhere with service users from probation, social services and education welfare (Ford *et al.* 1997; Pritchard *et al.* 1998; Pritchard and Williams 2001; Pritchard 2001).

There are vitally important messages in this excellent, albeit relatively small, study, none of which would come as a surprise to experienced psychiatric social

Table 7.2 Consumer views of mental health services

Professional	Semirural (%) (n = 36)		Inner city (%) (n = 106)	
	Satisfied	Dissatisfied	Satisfied	Dissatisfied
Key worker	70	0	18	8
Consultant psychiatrist	61	8	21	19
CPN	68	7	73	5
Social workers	N/A	N/A	58	20
General overall satisfaction	64		62	

workers who would see these elements as prerequisites in any effective intervention (Butler and Pritchard 1986).

Society scapegoats not only the 'out group' such as offenders, mentally disordered, unemployed people, etc., but also those who work with such people, and psychiatry, not dissimilar to social work, does not receive much sympathy. Social work should know more than most disciplines how fierce and unfair the media can be when presenting the tragic but truly rare death of a child as being 'typical' of British social work. The predominant amount of 'good social work' practice is never reported, as it is not news. Indeed, preparing for a consumer study of probation, one of our pilot respondents said, 'I suppose the lads will bad-mouth the service, but they and I know, when the chips are down, the only person you can rely on is your probation officer'. This was confirmed in the eventual study (Ford *et al.* 1997) and further confirmed by other unlikely clients of social workers, persistent truants, who highly valued their individual social worker, although they sometimes complained about the system and, even in the fraught area of child protection, parents come to value their social worker's ministrations (Pritchard *et al.* 1998; Pritchard 2001; Spratt and Callan 2003), but they, like clients of psychiatrists, valued the quality of relationship almost above anything else.

Control issues

A perennial issue associated with the mental health field is that of control and, of course, 'psychiatry' is the 'senior' discipline and has greater compulsory powers than any other discipline, as will be seen in Chapter 9. Classically, based upon longstanding ethical appreciation that 'insanity is punishment enough', in certain situations, an individual is not responsible for their actions while the 'balance of their mind is disturbed'. This stems in modern times from the McNaghten Rules, which allow the defence of insanity in a criminal trial. Indeed, since classical times, when Ajax, in the Trojan war, ran amok, it was recognised that he could not help himself, and he was restrained by his saddened comrades, although later, when allowed to wander unsupervised, he committed suicide.

At the extreme of personal human violence, murder, this is often followed by suicide (Coid 1983; Wild 1988; Walford *et al.* 1990; Pritchard and Bagley 2001). It is an uncomfortable realisation that, on occasions, severely mentally disordered people can be a risk not only predominantly to themselves but, on very rare occasions, to others. These are rare situations, but it is important to acknowledge the slight risk, not to add further stigma to mentally disordered people but, rather, by dealing effectively with those poorly handled problematic situations, by better determination of risk, to reduce some tragic outcomes, which helps the public to get a better balanced view of the stereotypical anxiety of the violent 'raging madman'. Extrapolating from the latest WHO figures in the UK, it is a very salutary fact that over 4,000 people killed themselves, of whom between 50 and 75 per cent were or had been suffering from a mental disorder (WHO 2001–5), whereas 515 UK people were homicide victims; hence, logic would suggest that the focus and emphasis we give to our police force to combat murder is disproportionate compared with the suicide fatalities linked to mental disorder. Hence, a careful and case-specific but effective form of control might be necessary to protect the mentally disordered from themselves. Of course, the personal tragedy of the total stranger who is involved, reflected in the Zito campaign, makes a powerfully emotional argument, essentially because it triggers the public's latent fear and prejudice; yet, being killed by a mentally disordered stranger is an event far rarer than being a big National Lottery winner. Of course, the Zito Trust argues for better and more effective services, quite right too. However, it is easy to get things out of perspective, even though, if it should happen to you or yours, it is a 100 per cent tragedy. Yet all are at considerable more risk from the motor car, or indeed, being killed by lightening, so we need to get our proportional sense of risk more rationally based.

You may remember Marcus Aurelius' words that 'insanity is punishment enough', but he went on 'At the same time the patient should be kept in close custody. . . not. . . by way of punishment, but as much as for his own and his neighbours' safety'. The emperor went on to ask about the de facto community care arrangements and whether those in charge had been remiss because 'The object of the keepers of the insane is not merely to stop them harming themselves but from destroying others and, if this happens, there is a case for blame upon any who were negligent.'

Marcus brings together the classic issue of controlling because we care, a theme we find in every branch of the human services, especially social work and especially in the mental health field. We remove children from their parents, not to punish, irrespective of how each may experience it, but because we care for the child and are concerned to protect the parents from the consequence of either their negligent incompetence or disturbed active abuse. In probation, we control and contain, in part because we recognise that, in the chain of social disadvantage, crime is sometimes almost a rational economic alternative, as society has failed to provide adequate opportunities to offset the family background, which was unable adequately to socialise the person. And in mental health, we may have to control because, amid the vortex of the mental disorder, in their fright and panic or in response to unbelievably powerful instructions, they damage themselves or, infrequently, others, usually those who are close to them, including mental health workers. Prins' (2005) classic further edition of *Deviants: Patients or Offenders?* has a title that itself highlights the linked dilemma.

However, since the 1959 Mental Health Act, critics have been concerned about the compulsory powers in mental health. They argued that it gave too much power to psychiatrists and not enough attention was paid to the patients' human rights (Gostin 2000), but such critics, and now readers will see the source of my irritation, came from the field of sociology and had seldom if ever dealt with the practicalities of psychiatric emergencies in the field. While stressing 'rights' is all very laudable, they often ignored that what we desperately needed were resources. Consequently, the current legislation, the 1983 Mental Health Act, gave great emphasis to 'rights' but failed to deliver the necessary resources. Now the pendulum has swung the other way, following one or two high-profile media cases, such as the case of Christopher Clunis, resulting in the tragic death of Jonathan Zito.

The issue is truly one of human rights, predominantly of the sufferers and their families and, to some extent, the mental health workers and the general public. Clearly, one disaster is one too many, but it is a question of balance, based upon evidence-based practice and even cautious predictions of risk.

In 1998, British citizens, traditionally described as 'subjects', were given a wonderful boost, which superseded precedent, convention and royal prerogatives, when the European Convention of Human Rights passed into law in the Human Rights Act, filling the hitherto unfilled gaps in the unwritten British Constitution. Truly British citizens, including those who suffer from a mental disorder, have never had better protection against an arbitrary state since the European Human Rights Act was incorporated into British law. It will require time for case law to develop, to enshrine these rights into public consciousness. However, according to Bindman *et al.* (2003), in the field of mental health legislation, despite a number of challenges from aggrieved citizens against compulsory detention or delays in mental health tribunals, in most cases, the courts have leaned on the side of the authorities. Thus, all the 'panic' may not be necessary, except for those of us with a longer professional memory and an understanding of history. The forthcoming Mental Health Act is yet again likely to focus on rights, principles and the rest, not desperately needed resources to fund integrated treatment adequately, especially for the long-term seriously mentally disordered, which are in danger of being overlooked.

With this thought in mind, let us explore further the foundation of a model of practice that is inclusive of all the sciences that underpin the art of modern mental health social work, a bio-psychosocial approach.

8 Mental health social work with people with mood disorders

Objectives: by the end of the chapter you should:

1 recognise unipolar mood disorder – depression;
2 have knowledge of bio-psychosocial treatments;
3 understand the limits and problems of drug treatments;
4 explore a social work assessment – BASIC IDDS;
5 understand the potential of cognitive behavioural therapy (CBT);
6 recognise bipolar mood disorder and understand its treatment – mania;
7 understand the centrality of the family in mental health social work.

Unipolar disorder – depression

> The name of the slough was Despond.
>   (John Bunyan 1628–88, *The Pilgrim's Progress*)

> All Hope Abandon, ye who enter here.
>   (Dante 1265–1321, *Inferno*)

> And that dismal cry rose slowly
> And sank slowly through the air,
> Full of spirit's melancholy
> And eternity's despair.
>   (Elizabeth Barrett Browning 1806–61, *The Dead Pan*)

> I am a worm and no man.
>   (David, Psalm 22 *c.* 1000–700 BC)

We have defined unipolar and bipolar mood disorders, i.e. 'depression', 'manic depression' and 'hypomania' as outlined in the ICD classification; what is required is an emotional understanding of the person's experience. Using the approach as a framework, it is well recognised that many people do not match the textbooks, and we need to consider both the 'form' and the 'content' of the syndrome in the reality of people's lives to understand what might be required to intervene positively. From the outset, mental disorders do not occur in isolation, affecting both the sufferer and how he/she experiences the world, and all involved with them, especially the family. Moreover, there is good evidence that there are often psychosocial stressors that can contribute to any of the mood disorders (Blakely *et al.* 2003; Kessing *et al.* 2003, 2004; Qin *et al.* 2003).

To have a sense of the quality of the emotions experienced, the above poets give us a sharp reminder of how, along the continuum of 'normality' from joy to unhappiness, mood disorders span the range from psychic pain to ecstasy.

In John Bunyan's *Pilgrim's Progress*, the 'Slough of Despond' is a virtual description of depression, as the person feels mired in an emotional bog, a quagmire of misery, while Dante's insight often quoted as 'abandon hope all ye who enter here' reminds us that depression is a psychic hell. Just consider what being without hope means. Trapped, at that moment in time seemingly forever, in a current unchanging misery, no wonder despair follows, echoing Barrett Browning's agonising cry as the person is consumed 'full of spirit's melancholy and eternity's despair'. An 'eternity of despair' is truly dreadful and, in the old Christian church, such a stance was considered sinful as it denied the power of God's grace; hence, in the Catholic and Orthodox faiths, suicide is still theologically a mortal sin.

The psalmist David highlights another soul-corroding aspect, the abject sense of worthlessness that often accompanies depression, when he says 'I am a worm and no man'; thus, we see the main elements of severe depression, an emotional and often physical slough, hopelessness, a sense of unchanging helplessness and an over-riding sense of lack of self-worth, described by the poet John Clare (1793–1864) as he lay dying in Nottingham Lunatic Asylum, 'here I sit amidst the shipwreck of my own self-esteem'. Nor surprisingly, therefore, depressive ideations can often lead to suicidal ideation.

Of course, for all of us, the difficulty in dealing with the concept of mood disorders, and depression in particular, is that they seem to blend and merge with normative reactions to 'the thousand natural shocks the flesh is heir to'.

Rihmer (1999) from Budapest has a delightful teaching aid to help grasp the range of the depressive spectrum and why in practice it is hard to determine what is normal and dysfunctional and what differentiates between 'major' and 'minor' depressions. Many clinicians speak of and identify minor depressions, as it were a depression that did not come to fruition: subclinical depressions (SCD) are sometimes associated with chronic illness, which demoralises the person; the recurrent brief depression (RBD) and major depression overwhelm the person's ability to function. By and large, people tend to suffer from one of these patterns of depressions, says Rihmer (1999), and cause confusion for professionals, leading to arguments about genetic and environmental aetiology. He suggests that we can understand the total phenomena if we consider the types of depression visually as separate parts of an 'elephant'!

The relatively mild dysthymic disorder of mood is the trunk, subclinical depression might be thought of as the elephant's tail, while mild depressive disorder is the elephant's ear. Getting more serious is the recurrent brief depression, which is the elephant's legs, and, finally, major depression is the elephant's body.

So, imagine if the therapist could not see and had to diagnosis, as it were, by touch. They would say of dysthymic disorder, this is trunk-shaped depression, whereas the therapist with the subclinically depressed client would say, 'oh no, the condition is thin and snake like'. 'No, no', says the therapist with the mild depressed client, 'it's a flat, thin membrane type of syndrome'; the recurrent form would be described as trunk like, while the therapist with the client with major depression would assert that the condition is broad, large and massive. And, of course, all would be right because they would be describing their client at a particular point in time and with a different manifestation of the depressive spectrum.

Moreover, the mood disorders are not stationary as there is a dynamic and vortex with depression of four interactive and reinforcing emotions, depression–guilt–despair–aggression.

Dynamics of depression

| Depression | ⇔ | Guilt |
| Aggression | ⇔ | Despair |

While depression and misery are predominant, the other undermining emotions follow and thus impact upon every aspect of the person's life and, here, Seligman's (1975) concept of 'learned helplessness' is still useful and has implications for intervention and treatment. From this sense of helplessness can come the dangerous emotion of 'hopelessness', where the person feels stuck in a situation that they feel either they cannot change or will get worse. Richard Bentall's concept of mental disorder gives us not necessarily an explanation but a sensitive understanding for, in depression, the person blames themselves for all that appears to be going wrong, for they are a 'worm and no man', they have 'abandoned hope' and their self-esteem is zero, as their sense of self shrinks; a 'collapse of ego' is another useful idea. What is undoubted is that a depressive mood disorder, depression, is psychically painful and, at the extreme, engenders a deep sense of profound misery, which we must never forget is associated with suicidal behaviour and is the major affect related to suicide (Harris and Barraclough 1998; Pritchard 1999).

Perhaps the most accurate of the poetic insights comes of course from Shakespeare when Hamlet says 'There is nothing either good or bad but thinking makes it so'; this is an understanding that our sense of misery is related to how the person believes things are. Thus, reflecting Bentall, they will attribute their misery to their particular situation. This has a profound implication for treatment as we shall discover, as the person feels what they think.

Their world is always grey and likely to get blacker, affecting how they get on with other people, how they function socially and psychologically and, irrespective of whether this is 'causal', their physiology is disturbed, with disturbance of sleep, appetite and weight. Indeed, many deeply depressed people actually look quite ill. Moreover, in a sense, 'depression is contagious', for not only can it demoralise close family members but the therapist must be careful if they are working with a series of depressed people on the same day, because it is very easy to 'absorb' their negative view of the world.

At the severe extreme, their misery is so overwhelming that they are inert, can be virtually comatosed and, if they can be prevailed upon to speak, may express themselves ever so slowly. Some people express markedly delusional ideas, and it may be difficult to differentiate their state from a schizophrenic-type breakdown, for example saying that they 'are dead' or that they 'have died'.

It is noteworthy that, for many people, a unipolar mood disorder, depression, occurs over time and, retrospectively, family and therapist may realise that there has been a steady deterioration over months. Conversely, some people, especially if they have had a previous depressive episode, may slide into depression quite rapidly within a week or even days. This has important implications for the 'content' side of the syndrome.

The 'content' refers to how the condition impacts upon the life of the sufferer but, of course, the depressive disorder is not occurring in a psychosocial vacuum as a depressive disorder can be triggered by a stress precipitant, as the impact of life events coincides with any familial predisposition to depression (Shepherd 1994; Gelder *et al.* 2001; Tennant 2002; Angst *et al.* 2003; Goodwin and Gotlieb 2003; Targosz *et al.* 2003).

This may appear to be common sense, but we have already seen how apparent 'reactive' events are mistaken as 'causal', as in the case of childhood autism.

Freud's view of depression was that it was a symbolic loss of a key relationship, and this seemed to fit with Bowlby's view of a disorder of attachment. This was extrapolated to be associated with childhood parental bereavement. However, as with much of Freud's theory, this was wrong and in fact was challenged by Dr John Birtchnell (1970), who was very favourable to an ego-dynamic perspective. Nevertheless, he demonstrated the fallacy of Freud's initial position on depression. To his and other people's surprise, when he examined early parental bereavement and sought a correlation with subsequent mental disorder, especially depression, he found no statistical association. As we shall see, this is but one of a number of Freudian theories that collapse when the rational light of empirical research is turned upon his metaphysic, as highlighted by that doughty iconoclast Richard Webster, who is not afraid to challenge accepted stereotypes (1995, 1998).

What Birtchnell did find, however, was that, if the person had been bereaved and they subsequently developed a depressive disorder, they were more severely depressed than non-bereaved mood-disordered people. Birtchnell (1981) did further work in this field and explored the possible bereavement link with subsequent suicide in women. Again there was no statistical link but the quality of early or current sustaining relationships was crucial, which makes it easy to mistake reaction to an event such as depression as causal. This has been confirmed in recent international research showing that childhood bereavement is not significantly a subsequent factor in adults with a mood disorder but, when the two go together, the symptoms are worse, while the mediating factors for adults and children are the quality of family and other key relationships (Hurd 1999; Luecken 2000; Huprich 2003; Takeuchi *et al.* 2003).

The importance of relationships in mental disorders emerged from a brilliant study by Agid *et al.* (1999) that compared groups of people with unipolar, bipolar and schizophrenic disorders in relation to 'early parental loss' (EPL) before age 17 and age- and gender-matched control subjects. While there were higher rates of all three mental disorders, compared with control subjects, it was always worse if EPL occurred before age 9 and more severe in all three if the EPL was due to permanent separation, rather than death. Interestingly, among the non-patient matched control subjects, those with EPL had worse psychosocial outcomes, namely more divorce and unemployment, etc. (Agid *et al.* 1999). It is also another pointer towards environmental triggers upon mental disorders with differing genetic predispositions.

In essence, the 'symptoms' and the experience of the mood disorder will be expressed through that person's life situation and interpersonal relationships. The interactive theme can be seen in the psychosocial cost to carers of the sufferer, as carers may themselves develop a so-called reactive depression (Chentsova-Dutton *et al.* 2002; Pritchard *et al.* 2001, 2004b).

Thus, the depressive mood permeates the family and the person's social relationships and, initially, if the person and/or their family do not understand the process that is happening, they may attribute the symptoms to all sorts of factors which lie in their particular situation. Hence, it is very easy for the family to slip into blaming the client or inferring malign motives and there can be the practical issues of the disorder undermining the person's employment prospects or their ability to meet family obligations, which are especially relevant when children are concerned. It is noteworthy that depressed parents can be problematic at every stage in the child's life if they do not receive the effective treatment and support that can be made available (Ghodsian *et al.* 1984; Shepherd 1994; Fombonne *et al.* 2001a,b; Cairney *et al.* 2003). Hence, part of the informed social worker's role, as with informed psychiatrists, is to look out for possible child protection–mental health issues.

Treatments – bio-psychosocial

Antidepressant drugs are the foundation of effective treatment for severe unipolar mood disorders (Zaretsky 2003). It is known from analysis of brain chemistry that certain types of neuroreceptor are dysfunctional in those with mood disorders although whether this a result or a cause of depression is unclear. In any event there is evidence that, when the depression lifts, neuroreceptor biochemistry returns to normal. Of course, this does not mean that non-drug treatment is not important.

Baldwin and Birtwhistle (2002) provide a relatively simple and accessible explanation of the biochemistry underlying the range of mood disorders, including mania and bipolar disorder (Figure 8.1).

At the end of a nerve cells are neuroreceptors, which form the pathway for communication between nerves and the brain, in effect the telephone wires between the 'sender' and 'receiver'. The point at which nerves meet each other is called the synapse, which is microscopic in size. In order to transmit signals from one

Antidepressant action:
antidepressant blocks neurotransmitter reuptake
both at the dendrites and at the axon

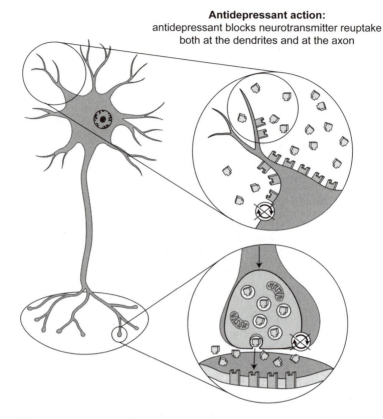

Figure 8.1 Downregulation of α_2 somatodendritic receptors by antidepressant drugs. Antagonism of α_2-autoreceptors increases the availability of noradrenaline at postsynaptic receptors.

nerve to another, there must be an electro-biochemical exchange between them, which is facilitated by chemicals called neurotransmitters. There is evidence that abnormalities in the level or function of serotonin (correctly called 5-hydroxy-tryptamine, or 5-HT), and two other transmitters, noradrenaline and dopamine, which appear to act on the central nervous system, are associated with depression and the disturbance of the person's mood.

Animal studies have shown that serotonin is associated with the sleep–wake cycle, appetite and sexual and aggressive behaviour, and it is suggested that depression is associated with a decrease in neurotransmission of 5-HT; many antidepressant drugs are thought to produce their therapeutic effects by acting on post-synaptic 5-HT receptors. Hence, the famous or infamous SSRI (selective serotonin reuptake inhibitors), the original Prozac, work by increasing 5-HT levels (Figures 8.1–8.4).

Depressive moods are also associated with increased levels of adrenocortico-tropic hormone (ACTH), which affects the levels of cortisol in blood; when a person is depressed, the cortisol levels rises. It has been suggested that, in some

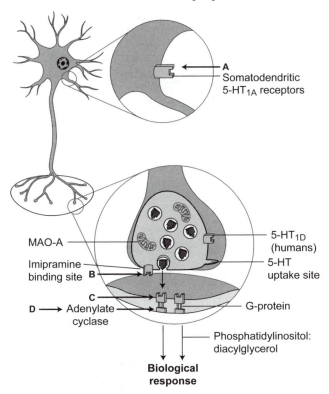

Figure 8.2 Possible neurobiochemical factors associated with depressed states. A, SSRIs and MAOIs desensitise the inhibitory 5-HT$_{1A}$ somatodendritic receptors; B, SSRIs and MAOIs desensitise the inhibitory autoreceptor on the presynaptic terminal. TCAs and SSRIs inhibit the reuptake of 5-HT into the nerve terminal after acute administration by binding to the serotonin transporter; C, postsynaptic serotonin receptors activated by increased serotonin in the synaptic cleft; D, information is translated from the receptor to the cell by second messenger systems.

patients, there is an enlargement of the adrenal glands but, again, whether this is causal, reactive or interactive is unclear.

The third class of biochemical neurotransmitter systems are the noradrenergic and dopaminergic systems. These are associated with maintaining arousal and drive in animals, but the former is as yet inconsistent in its pathological associations, while disturbance in normal levels of the dopaminergic cycle is linked to bipolar mood disorder and Parkinson's disease.

A simple way to grasp the implications of the contribution of these neurotransmitters to depression is to remember that unipolar affective disorder is, in effect, a syndrome of overlapping symptomatology, and the three different neurotransmitters probably affect the individual in a person-specific way. Thus, some symptoms will be expressed to a greater extent in some individuals than in others, and different drugs will have better or worse outcomes in different people; yes,

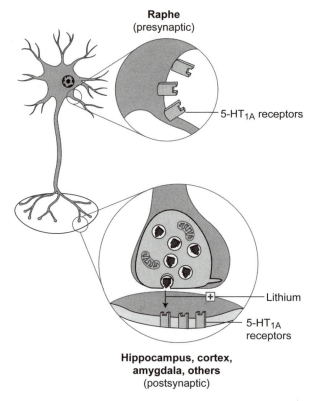

Figure 8.3 The neurobiochemistry of 5-HT$_{1A}$ receptors. 5-HT$_{1A}$ receptors may be somatodendritic or postsynaptic. Antidepressant drugs probably exert their action through effect at postsynaptic 5-HT$_{1A}$ receptors.

it is often a matter of trial and error before the best available drug for a specific person is identified.

The Prozac SSRI controversy

Modern antidepressant drugs affect neurotransmitters and, theoretically, as neutotransmitter levels return to normal, the patient's mood disorder improves. However, the controversy that surrounds the use of SSRIs is complex and, I suspect, is in part due to the patchy nature of current knowledge and, to be frank, possible vested interests both inside and outside the pharmaceutical industry.

The drug industry has not always been as scrupulous as it should have been, and as a result its reliability has been undermined. Consider the case of Dr Derek Healy. He was to take up a major psychology chair in Canada but was apparently 'black-balled' because he raised questions about the safety of SSRIs (Healy and Whittaker 2003). Healy claimed that some drug companies miscoded data on suicidal behaviour (Healy and Whittaker 2003) – in other words, they 'cheated'

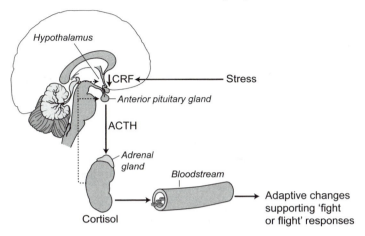

Figure 8.4 Adrenal gland function in terms of cortisol production. The hypothalamus–pituitary–adrenal axis may be disturbed in patients with chronic or resistant depression, with elevated cortisol levels and adrenal gland hypertrophy.

by either deliberately or through incompetence undercounting suicidal incidents possibly associated with SSRIs. A recent research meeting examined anti-acne drugs anecdotally said to be associated with an increased level of suicidal activity. The research funded by the drug manufacturer gave the drug a suspiciously high level of clearance (Jick *et al.* 2000). The study's cohort of patients not only failed to exhibit suicidal behaviour, but exhibited a significantly lower suicide rate than the national average; the study was, in effect, a 'whitewash', according to a meta-analysis by Hull and D'Arcy (2003). Anyone familiar with the suicidal behaviour field could not fail to note that the sample of Jick *et al.* (2000) consisted of a very distressed group of young people, with exceptionally serious acne, and yet the rate of so-called 'attempted suicide' (a term now jettisoned in favour of deliberate self-harm (DSH)) among the group was significantly lower than among the same age group in the general population (Hawton *et al.* 2003; Pritchard and Hansen 2005a). Thus, the authors misrepresented their data by not counting the probable DSH incidents; one almost might have said they were 'looking the other way'. Fortunately, not all drug trials are so seriously flawed.

The same Professor Healy undertook a meta-analysis of a series of 'gold standard' RCTs (randomised controlled trials) regarding the effectiveness of SSRIs and came to the conclusion that SSRIs reduced suicidal ideation in some people, but that there was an excess of DSH incidents in other people receiving active SSRI treatment compared with those treated placebos. Nonetheless, he did not damn SSRIs completely, but said that more precise research is needed to determine any benefits and risks (Healy and Whitaker 2003).

Various proponents of SSRIs have written papers, but we need to be careful as to their funding association (Wagstaff *et al.* 2002). A particularly valuable study, which shows how difficult it is to have very firm ideas on SSRIs, was undertaken by Kahn and Faros (2003), who focused upon actual suicides rather than episodes of 'attempted suicide'/DSH. Kahn and Faros (2003) analysed reports from the USA Food and Drug Administration (FDA) on controlled trials for modern anti-depressants, including SSRIs. Out of 48,277 patients involved in all the trials, 77 committed suicide, a rate of 0.16 per cent. Bearing in mind that we know these people were depressed, this was 14 times the general population rate (GPR) for US suicide, i.e. approximately 30,000 a year in a population of 276 million is about 0.011 per cent. So the Kahn team clearly had a more vulnerable cohort so one might have expected them to have a higher suicide rate, as in all probability these people were severely depressed. However, Kahn and Faros concluded that there was little difference between people treated with SSRIs, other antidepressants or placebo in these trials. So, is this a clean bill of health for SSRIs? I do not know, other than to say that the fact that there were no significant differences between the 'active' drug treatment and the passive 'placebo' drug-treated suicides must raise questions about the core sample and how quickly people are put on antidepressants.

A new study from Sweden on the presence of either SSRIs or other antidepressants in a database of 14,857 actual suicides, compared with control subjects, provides a good balance and a degree of support for SSRIs over traditional antidepressants (Isacsson *et al.* 2005). In brief, there were 3,411 detections of antidepressants in the suicide group compared with 1,538 in the control group. However, SSRIs had lower odds ratios of being associated with the suicidal cases than the other antidepressants. With regard to children, among 52 cases in people aged 15 or under, no SSRIs were found, whereas SSRIs gave a slightly lower risk in suicides of people aged 15–19. Thus, Isacsson concluded that, over the nine years, there was no support for the hypothesis that SSRIs were associated with an increased risk of suicide.

One of the advantages of SSRIs is that they apparently cause fewer and less severe side-effects, which has been assumed to make them somewhat safer than traditional tricyclic antidepressants. Yet this was not found to be the case in a RCT that compared the two drug types (Thompson *et al.* 2001a). Thus, clients, like practitioners, have to be helped to make their own judgement, based upon their own situation as to what medication suits them best.

This brief outline of the SSRI controversy has probably not helped you, as the evidence seems to justify 'sitting on the fence'. The problem is that a sucessful suicide, as well as each individual DSH event, is so highly idiosyncratic that I suspect that the RCTs have been too narrowly focused and, possibly, those crucial life-affecting psychosocial factors were not taken into consideration. In my opinion, anyone given only antidepressants, whether modern SSRIs or the older anti-depressant tricyclics, is being inadequately treated for, as we shall see, a combined approach involving both appropriate antidepressants and psychosocial support and care generally gives the best outcome. However, it is a worry that some of the undoubtedly positive effects of psychopharmacology are denied people because of this uncertainty, and some predominantly socially orientated practitioners might have a 'throw out the baby with the bath water' effect. Conversely, while SSRIs are increasingly used to treat dysthymia, the mild depressions (Wagstaff *et al.* 2002), in the USA, it was found that the outcome of SSRI treatment was no better outcome than that of psychotherapy (Williams *et al.* 2000). Of course, treatment with SSRIs would be much cheaper than psychotherapy and, recalling the Isacsson *et al.* (2005) study, have the advantage over traditional antidepressants of being associated with slightly lower suicide risk. The latter finding is supported by the British study by Martinez *et al.* (2005), although these authors acknowledge that there is a weak correlation with raised suicidal behaviour in people under 18 years of age.

In summary, it would be easier if there were unequivocal evidence about the outcome of antidepressants, SSRIs or the others, but life and research are not like that. Indeed, this analysis demonstrates the truth that we are always learning and that we are also at the edge of error and, whenever we move away from the straightforward type of physical diagnosis, e.g. pneumonia, appendicitis, and move into the field of the bio-psychosocial aspects of mental health, we find there is much we do not know. While only the best evidence is good enough for our clients, it is often just not there and we then have to make judgements on the best evidence available and how, if at all, it matches our client's situation.

Research, despite its limitations, is a far better guide than the fashionable but unverified theory; after all, medicine must have slain thousands when 'bleeding' was in vogue. Another example was Freud's initial insight that a proportion of mentally disordered women had been sexually abused by a male relative, often fathers, but he had to jettison the finding because of the professional outrage it caused, so instead he hypothesised that these women were fantasising (Webster 1998), whereas we know realise that there is a link between mental disorder in adulthood and abuse in childhood (Cheasty *et al.* 1998; Read and Argyle 1999; Hammersley *et al.* 2003; Holowka *et al.* 2003), albeit even here it is not entirely straightforward as, in the more careful well-defined studies, it is only the extreme type of abuse, emotional as well as sexual, that is associated with subsequent psychiatric disorder (Cheasty *et al.* 1998; Spataro *et al.* 2005). Care must be taken to deal with the reality of the person's situation, not add further stigma and guilt by overemphasising one particular aspect of contributory causes and assuming the presence of sexual abuse whenever a mental disorder appears (Pritchard 2004). Research will invariably create waves as the new data mean we need to relinquish older ideas in favour of better evidence-based knowledge.

> The old order changeth, yielding place to new. . .
> Lest one good custom should corrupt the world.
> (Tennyson, *The Passing of Arthur*)

Modern clinical psychiatry now accepts the benefit of 'combined treatment', that is antidepressants and a psychosocial input. There are many studies that show that a combined approach does better than placebo or a single approach of either drugs or some form of psychosocial therapy (Miklowitz *et al.* 2003a,b; Browne *et al.* 2000; Hirschfeld *et al.* 2002) not only for depression but also for obsessive–compulsive disorders (Biondi and Picardi 2005), alcohol problems (Wagner *et al.* 2004), depression and dementia (Bragin *et al.* 2005) and schizophrenia (Lenroot *et al.* 2003; Malm *et al.* 2003). Indeed, a combined approach is beginning to produce modest responses in that most difficult of all conditions, people with long-term substance abuse with co-morbidity with depression (Granholm *et al.* 2003; Drake *et al.* 2004; Gold *et al.* 2004), and here the social worker has an important role to play.

Miklowitz's team emphasise the importance of involving the patient's family in what is increasingly being called psycho-education for families, which is to explain the general progress of the syndrome and how it affects the person and its ramifications. Zaretsky (2003) argues that, although antidepressants are the foundation of treatment for the mood disordered, considerable improvement by psycho-education and specifically targeted adjunctive psychosocial interventions and that, overall, 'cognitive behaviour therapy' (CBT) is especially valuable in reducing relapses (more on CBT below).

The relative success of a combined approach provides further evidence of the benefits of the bio-psychosocial approach for example, building on Professor David Barker's work on the fetal origins of disease, Seifert (2000) showed that mood disorders will be impacted by the interaction of poverty, poor diet, depression and the need to deal with all these aspects to bring about improvement.

Taking this wider view, recent research on depression in children and adolescents is yielding some interesting results. In the past, we tended to dismiss the idea that children and adolescents develop proper mood disorders, because it was assumed that this was essentially reactive. This is no longer true for it is clear that some children, and especially adolescents, do develop a proper unipolar mood disorder, which, as in adults, benefits from a combined treatment approach (Waslick *et al.* 1999; Weisman *et al.* 2000; Compton *et al.* 2002). Hence the increase in the use of SSRIs for these disorders, but a European study is very sceptical abut the USA FDA board giving them approval, not least because of 'the lack of candidness of the pharmaceutical industry' (Trefferes and Rinne-Albers 2005).

One important feature that the experienced practitioner learns is that the lowest effective antidepressant dose should be given in order to minimise or even avoid the worst of the side-effects. Most people taking antidepressants will initially complain about a dry mouth and possibly a dry eye. Both can be tolerated when offset against the lifting of the miserable mood. But, as with all drugs, individual responses are highly idiosyncratic, and we must remember that 7–15 per cent of people have side-effects even with a placebo (Baldwin and Birtwhistle 2002). However, we must not make the mistake that some medical doctors do and see 'side-effects' as normal, as they can sometimes be very disabling, e.g. disturbance of vision, gaining weight, tremors and not least reducing sexual libido (Baldwin and Mayers 2003; Baldwin 2004), and recovering patients wryly complain that the loss of sexual drive is an underestimated 'cost' of recovering from their mental disorder. Hence the physician should be reminded to seek the optimal dose for their patients.

An important Cochrane systematic review on the older antidepressants, the tricyclics, found that responses were better with low dosages than on the so-called 'standard' dosage. It is thought that, because patients were maintained on the minimal level, they suffered fewer side-effects and, consequently, the drugs were better tolerated and taken for longer and more effectively, producing better longer-term outcomes (Furukawa *et al.* 2003). A disadvantage of the tricyclics, however, is that they can be fatal if taken in overdose and, in this regard, they are less 'fatally' safe than the newer SSRIs – the Prozac group of drugs – which is one of their attractions.

In the USA, an ongoing treatment project for adolescents with depression that emphasises an integrated approach, called Treatment for Adolescents with Depression Study (TADS 2003), is showing very promising results not only in treating the initial breakdown but in helping to reduce the further disorders in young and later adulthood (Weismann *et al.* 2000). The TADS study emphasises an integrated combined approach with the use of SSRI, CBT and family support, which produced far better results than a placebo or a unidimensional approach. It is expected that the clinical research team will be reporting over the next decade, and their work will certainly be well worth keeping up with. However, Compton *et al.* (2002) pointed out that most 'combined' treatments for depressed adolescents have been focused upon the treatment of depression, and there is less evidence to support such an approach when the situation is compounded by the adolescent being involved in substance misuse.

Problems with drugs?

A key issue related to mood disorders is the association with suicidal behaviour, both actual suicide and DSH, what used to be known as 'attempted suicide'. However, current research shows that suicide rates in women from most Western nations have fallen considerably over the past 25 years. This appears to be associated with improved psychiatry, community care, integrated combined therapy and, not least, the use of less dangerous antidepressants (Gelder *et al.* 2001; Pritchard and Hansen 2005b). However, one problem with drug studies is the vested interests, as we saw in our discussion on SSRIs. Moreover, I do not know of any studies that focus upon minimal dosages, as the vast majority of drug studies are funded by the drug industry. In the case of the mood disorders, this becomes problematic for, although antidepressants are undoubtedly life-saving in that they reduce the risk that depression will lead to to suicide, the older drugs were an easily accessible lethal method. Hence Prozac was the marketing man's dream – the apparent 'wonder drug', with relatively few side-effects – although they are less optimistic now (Wagstaff *et al.* 2002).

Many older drugs, especially the diazepams, which were often prescribed for depression in conjunction with anxiety, suffered from the problem that they resulted in dependency. Furthermore, many reduced the person's libido, which is also true of long-term use of anti-psychotic (schizophrenia) drugs, and were associated with weight gain, while the use of the modern SSRI with children and adolescents is now very questionable. Certainly, my own limited experience with the SSRIs has been related to young adult/student clients who had taken SSRIs for many months or even two or three years.

I want my life back – it was marvellous at first, I was worried about nothing, I was no longer depressed. But then I realised I was living in a dream world, literally I often felt I had no feelings – so I wanted to feel again, even if it was painful.

So, in effect, it is always a matter of judgement and, in principle, the lowest possible dose is best but always within the case-specific situation. There is evidence suggesting the maintenance of a person on the lowest level of an antidepressant for up to two years after the initial attack to minimise the risk of a further depressive episode (Furukawa *et al.* 2003), although this is an area of controversy (Angst *et al.* 2003). However, especially in the case of lithium and carbamazepine, there is good evidence that its long-term use does reduce the risk of relapse into depression (Wolf and Muller-Oerlinghausen 2002; Baethge *et al.* 2003). This includes the use of lithium for elderly patients (Wilkinson *et al.* 2002), although Klysner *et al.* (2003) also made the same argument for citalopram for elderly patients.

It is noteworthy that the modern use of lithium was revitalised when it was appreciated that, in much smaller doses than yesteryear, lithium as a long-term treatment for both unipolar and bipolar disorder was very good, and it is vastly cheaper than most antidepressants because it is a natural salt. Moreover, it has been claimed that 250 suicides a year are saved in Germany by the use of lithium as a prophylactic (Muller-Oerlinghausen *et al.* 2003). Again, the key is to find the best type of medication for the individual with the lowest dosage and lowest tolerable side-effects and, crucially, to ensure regular reviews to tackle any potential 'stress' factors and any accumulative side-effects. Ideally, what is needed are in-depth adequately funded and controlled long-term independent studies of combined integrated treatments, where the person might be free of their medication but, via regular in-depth reviews monthly, quarterly, six-monthly, test out as cost-effective as opposed to the psychosocial and fiscal cost of relapse and crisis. While research is crucial to answer some anxieties, when it comes to daily practice, only a person/family/situation-specific approach will be good enough to answer the question about this person at this time.

The 'last words' on problems with drugs will be left to Goodwin and Gotlieb (2003) in a brilliant and balanced review for the *Journal of Psychopharmacology*, which at first sight might be thought to be a 'drug'-orientated journal, but aims at the highest independent academic standards.

Goodwin and Gotlieb (2003) review the guidelines of the British Association of Psychopharmacology, which all should read, not least because it recognises that treatment is multimodal and crucially sees the patient and their family at the centre of all our concerns when they state:

establish and maintain a therapeutic alliance – communicate clearly and honestly what you think. Take the time to listen to what is bothering the patient . . . patients have social needs that merit assertive management.

(p. 171)

Classically, the basis of all research using drugs is to compare the outcome of patients 'blindly' receiving the active drug against patients who receive only the placebo, because it is known that simply having a drug can alter the patients' subjective feelings, to the extent that between 7 and 15 per cent of people receiving only a placebo drug develop mild side-effects (Baldwin and Birtwhistle 2002), such is the impact of the 'power and magic' of medicine. However, while medicine seems to want to go beyond 'placebo', they dismiss what would be better described as 'the self-reparative process'. Namely, when we inculcate hope for improvement in our clients, things improve; indeed, the place of 'the self-reparative process' should be a constant reminder that the quality of the rapport with one's client is of direct therapeutic benefit.

Areas of social work assessment

Social workers in this field are confronted with a range of theories, data and approaches, often with an overlap with the medico-psychiatric. My concern here is not so much with developing a 'care plan', but being concerned with the front-line therapist who is actually going to work with the client. How therefore can the social worker maintain their core psychosocial attributes, yet incorporate the necessary psychiatric information, without losing the essential individual client focus? The following practical approach is useful in every area of social work as it explores the modalities of people's lives ranging from their interpersonal relationships, their feelings, their social situation and crucially any 'biophysical' aspect of their situation. Thus, it can be utilised in any area of social work, which of course will have different areas emphasised, as well as in the mental health field. The mnemonic BASICID of Arnold A. Lazarus (1976) came from clinical psychology and has been modified for social work practice to become BASIC IDDS: Behaviour, Affect, Sensory, Imagery, Cognition, Inter-personal relationships, Drugs, Defences and Social factors.

A modality for practice assessment and intervention: BASIC IDDS

A.A. Lazarus eschewed explanatory theories as to the nature of a person's problem and focused instead upon what the person said the problem was. In part, this was to get away from the sterile debate between the Freudians and Behaviourists of the time, but also because he had an underlying theory that it was more effective to deal with the present 'complaint', i.e. what the client sought to change. The beauty of his 'multimodal' approach (1976) is its concentration upon the patients' concerns in the here and now and in a broad sense it belongs to the 'cognitive behavioural' school, as what the patient thinks and feels is important in both understanding the person's situation and offering treatment.

This is invaluable because, using the mnemonic BASIC IDDS, the therapist can immediately move from an assessment mode into a treatment intervention mode as, with their permission, they take notes of the difficulties as they see them, as well as check out under the various headings and explore any areas that they or we might have forgotten. Rather than describe the interactive elements, it will be easy to list them and demonstrate the problem and the appropriate bio-psychoso-cial social work intervention.

Lazarus argued that people express their problems in two broad modes: there is either 'too much or 'too little' of a behaviour or emotion.

The value of the BASIC IDDS system is that you can begin your interview easily and ask what is happening to the client (behaviour). How do they feel about this (affect), which is often linked to a feature that social workers often miss, how do they feel physically, have they any symptoms (sensory). You can then move on to how did they think about this (cognition) and, again, a little unusual for social workers, ask what idea they rehearse in their heads either to resolve the problem or to avoid it (imagery). This easily leads to how do they get on with people, especially key people in their world (interpersonal relations). Have they already started any treatment, medication or counselling, as either element may account for some of their behaviour and/or feelings (reaction to 'drugs'). Ask them how they usually deal with any painful material and, at the same time, observe their modes of defensive responses (defences). Perhaps the one unequivocally helpful aspect of Freudian psychology was that of 'defence mechanisms', which is how the person characteristically seeks to reduce any psychosocial stress/distress. Although Lazarus used neither 'defences' nor 'social' in his modality, it is self-evident that we need to understand their social position re employment/unemployment, do they live alone and what about their accommodation? Social factors, including housing issues, along with employment, community and amenities which are accessible to the client, are vital. We must never forget that we are as much social as physiological and psychological beings. Hence employment in particular is a major key to any person's social and psycho-physical health and identity.

The therapist does not have to stick rigidly to this order but, once you become accustomed to the format, you can move from any modality. So, for example, the client may start with social – no rent, threat of eviction – and this is where you start, even though it might quickly emerge that their problems follow on from a serious mood disorder.

Table 8.1 demonstrates the use of the BASIC IDDS system with regard to a middle-class person with a depressive mood disorder. It highlights the problems that the person is complaining about and shows the possible form of psychosocial intervention and, in this case, as an adjunct to antidepressants.

Cognitive behavioural therapy (CBT)

One of the most exciting and effective developments in the treatment of depression and other psychosocial conditions is that of CBT, first developed by Beck *et al.* (1979) and now backed by much modern and current empirical research (Kingdon and Turkington 2002; Clark *et al.* 2003; Gumley *et al.* 2003; Tarrier *et al.* 2004). It has a long and interesting history and has evolved since the early 1970s based upon the work of Aaron Beck, an American professor of psychiatry, who took the simple approach of asking himself the question, how does the client see, cognate the world? Are there gaps between the person's perception, beliefs and reality and what does the client need and wish to change? It reflected the Shakespearian insight of 'There is nothing either good or bad but thinking makes it so' or, as the classic philosopher Epictetus said of distressed and disturbed people, 'they are not so much disturbed by events as by the views they take of such events', which is the very essence of the CBT approach. Namely, it is the idiosyncratic response of the person to an event or a series of events that locks them into a patterned response so that things become ill as 'thinking makes it so'. In depression, some translate this as the half-empty glass syndrome, as the person translates everything around them in negatives and greys and downgrades themself, virtually undermining their own morale, spreading psychic panic in their own cognition, thoughts.

There is an interesting confirmation of Beck's concepts of depression, and therefore of CBT, in the work of Yeung *et al.* (2002), which was able to validate the depressive symptoms across cultures, Asians and white Americans in particular.

The approach grew out of the humanistic behaviour therapy movement, which saw an important part of human behaviour as 'learned', which of course has a crossover into the social, classically seen in educationally underachieving children, who have learned, been taught, not to have any educational aspirations. This concept was superbly used in social work by the late Professor Gerry Smale (1984) in his *Self-fulfilling: Self-defeating Strategies and Behavioural Change*, where he showed that the social worker's perception of their client, their belief in bringing about improvement and change, was an important factor in bringing such improvements about, and the need to improve the morale of the client and raise their expectations about themselves. Thus, if the social worker has optimism that they can bring relief and comfort into the lives of clients, they are more likely to do so. 'There is nothing good or bad but thinking makes it so' enhances the potential of the 'self-reparatory' process.

These forerunners of the CBT school had one thing in common, their core focus upon the person in distress and the importance of the therapeutic relationship. One variation of this is the work of Marion Linehan in what she describes as 'dialectic behaviour therapy' (Linehan 1993), where the 'dialectic' is the mutual engagement and dialogue between therapist and client to produce the basis for any treatment technique per se, that is the rapport or relationship. As we shall see, Linehan has worked as a psychologist with clients whom social workers would readily recognise, with what she categorises as 'borderline personality disorders': in effect, people with either life-long or since adolescence, personal and social problems, not least poor interpersonal relationship skills (Rizvi and Linehan 2001; Linehan *et al.* 2002; Welch and Linehan 2002).

CBT is available to social work, and a most succinct and brilliant paper on introducing social workers to CBT by Scott and Stradling (1991), though more than a decade old, is still worth consulting. They use a simple and effective example of Beck's idea of the development of the depressive reaction to an event, negative interpretation, reinforcing a further negative feedback, which can become fixed.

Table 8.1 Use of BASIC IDDS assessment in mood disorder

Area	Expressed problem	Possible bio-psychosocial responses
Behaviour	Avoids people Takes time off work	Counselling – possible 'assertive' Techniques – explore realistic expectations CBT and reframe Determine any activities with children
Affect	Low mood Constant misery, especially in the mornings Feels worthless Unaccountable guilt	Create therapeutic relationship Consider CBT Start appropriate antidepressants via referral to psychiatrist/ GP
Sensory	Feels tired Loss of appetite Loss of weight Tense headaches Fall in libido	Via relationship, highlight support available Monitor analgesics Teach relaxation techniques and biofeedback
Imagery	Often imagine themselves in self-defeating situations	Counselling, rehearsal techniques If images intrusive, teach thought-stopping techniques
Cognition	Finds thinking difficult Slow Feels worthless and a personal failure Guilty because they feel inadequate Suicidal ideas – 'there is no alternative – no hope'	CBT in conjunction with antidepressants Explore and identify areas for reframing 'Educate' person and family as to nature and process of unipolar disorder Consider consultation or referral to psychiatrist to deal with suicidal thinking

Interpersonal relations	Prior to problem – good circle of friends, good marital relationship and good parent Now finds children unmanageable 'Gone beyond rows' with partner Painful silences between patient and partner (you need to discover partner's views)	Counselling – consider family therapy/conjoint counselling with significant others if client agreeable Teach social skills if necessary Explore and check out relationships with children, especially if vulnerable
Drugs (treatment effect)	Has taken analgesics Increased use of alcohol First time sought psychological help	Liaise with doctors/nurse/psychiatrists Check out any source of prescribed and/or illegal drug Where necessary, liaise with permission with any other appropriate agency
Defences	Previously appeared a well-balanced and flexible person Now withdraws, some denial, tendency to self-blame and head off criticism	Counselling Remember defences are not to be confronted – explore extension and more flexible approach to dealing with psychic 'threats'/distress
Social	Graduate, middle class Situation threatens marriage, which could have major implications for accommodation	Check out financial and housing situation Are there potential stressors here? Check out, where necessary, benefit entitlements Liaise/advocate with other agencies

Real event – Husband comes home late, again.
Reactive thought – He's not interested in me, he's got another woman.
Emotional response – It's my fault, I'm unattractive, despair.
Reactive and reinforcing thought – I'm a bad wife.

The reality was her husband was late for reasons beyond his control, but she negatively interpreted this against herself, which can quickly build up a framework of self-deprecatory ideas.

Beck saw the depressive process as an interaction between a predisposition and life reinforcing events into a pathway leading to a depressive illness. This was not to deny a possible or probable underlying biogenetic tendency, but the 'illness'/disorder impacts on the experience in the person's life.

Early life experience → leads to dysfunctional assumptions about oneself and others → a critical life-shaping event → negative assumptions activated → (crucially a negative and automatic feedback is created) → negative automatic thoughts → symptoms of depression undermining – behaviour, motivation, affect, somatic and cognition → creating 'spirit's melancholy and eternity's despair' and, unless there is intervention to help the person reframe their cognition, they sink into a 'slough of despond'.

It is reiterated that this essentially psychological model is not at odds with the disturbance of neurotransmitter biochemical model, rather explaining how the person experiences the depressive cycle, as each model may be either a reaction or an interaction of both. Conversely, it can 'explain' a straightforward 'learned helpless' reaction depression. Thus, in some people, their life situations teach them to undervalue themselves, which may equally affect their biochemical reactions, whereas in others with an imbalanced biochemistry, they interpret the world negatively.

Scott and Stradling (1991) provide a nice example of two women at a coffee morning whose children are playing happily but noisily. Mother 1 is comfortable, secure in the knowledge that the children are not too intrusive or too boisterous, and aware that sometimes children do 'play up' in public, but she feels both children have not crossed an unacceptable line.

Mother 2, however, is quite distressed and getting more upset, as she sees the children's behaviour as close to riot and feels a total failure in her efforts to maintain what she feels is acceptable. The key difference between the scenarios is the difference in how the mothers perceive and evaluate the situation.

Thus, the 'distressed/depressive' mother feels that she cannot control the children and, as she cannot manage the situation, she is a 'bad person'.

This may stem from a general need to be seen to be in control, to be perfect, and such situations undermine her sense of self-esteem, which become associated with other perceived failures.

The event – children making a noise.
Automatic thought – I cannot control my children.
Automatic thought – because I have failed, I am a bad person.

Emotional response – despair, misery, inadequacy, depression
Automatic thought – I am no good and a weak person.
Emotional response – weak people are unloved, unvalued.
Automatic thought – I deserve to be unvalued.

This very neat normative outline from Scott and Stradling (1991) follows Beck's more detailed 'cognitive model of depression' (1976).

Early experience → formation of dysfunctional assumptions → critical incident/s → negative assumptions activated → negative automatic thoughts become locked into symptoms of depression as their 'content' and the 'form' of the condition merge. These then lead to and feed the five symptomatic areas of depression: behaviour, motivation, affect, cognition and somatic.

This last, the somatic, as we have seen, is often under-recognised by social workers and psychologists, but feeling miserable often changes people's bodily reactions, they develop somatic symptoms, including headaches, feeling faint, giddy, stomach pains and cramps, bowel disturbances, tremors, breathlessness, sweats and even palpitations. Indeed, one feature that often differentiates 'working-class' from 'middle-class' clients is that the former are inclined to describe their misery initially and often essentially in somatic terms. Not surprisingly, therefore, many people in the depressive loop find themselves treated for a range of physical symptoms that can confuse GP, expert and patient and their families (Lazarus 1976; Kingdon and Turkington 2002).

The process of CBT aims to influence the person's cognition about themself so that they can be helped to find an alternative explanation and to reframe their ideas. This is achieved by checking out the reality and accuracy of their perception. The key to the treatment is the modification of the dysfunctional attitudes, to break the cycle of negative automatic thoughts, assumptions and reduce and finally eradicate the learned, reinforced emotional response.

There is real benefit in colleagues from any discipline attending CBT training courses, although some may find that using CBT 'by following the manual' can restrict the benefits of the approach; although it is appreciated that for research purposes this may be recommended. Ideally, CBT is a relatively short form of intervention, two or three months; some even claim that 6 to 12 sessions are sufficient for some of the lesser psychosocial problems. A quite excellent 'textbook' that analyses typical cases is that from Kingdon and Turkington (2002), but they underplay the need for either renewed contact or accessibility should the stressors build up. Indeed, in parenthesis, it is feared that the CBT protagonist's emphasis upon relatively short-term therapy is to attract governmental support, rather than emphasising that it makes major impacts upon the person but the person often needs follow-up supportive treatment to prevent relapse and head off breakdown in the face of new psychosocial stressors.

A modified form of CBT has been found to be specifically useful in a range of conditions, not just with 'borderline personality disorder' (Linehan 1993; MacLeod *et al.* 1993; Bohus *et al.* 2000; Linehan *et al.* 2002), but also such things as post-traumatic stress disorders, generalised anxiety disorders and social anxiety disorders (Keller and Schuler 2002; Kingdon and Turkington 2002; Dugas *et al.* 2003; Ehlers *et al.* 2003). This makes sense, as the core aim is to help people reframe their lives in a highly individualistic way, bringing benefits of the technique, and crucially an engagement in a relationship with the practitioner. Moreover, as we shall see, CBT is increasingly used as an adjunct therapy for people suffering from the schizophrenias.

In the case of unipolar affective disorders, i.e. depression, CBT comes into its own as there is good evidence that it is more effective than other forms of 'psychotherapy' (Scott and Stradling 1991), it helps prevent relapse (Cahill *et al.* 2003) and, in a range of studies, has been found to reduce depressive symptomatology, improve self-esteem and social functioning, give patients a better understanding of their condition and general improvement in quality of life (Page and Hooke 2002; Jane-Llopis *et al.* 2003; Cahill *et al.* 2003; Merrill *et al.* 2003; Miranda *et al.* 2003).

But from the misery of depression, we now turn to the opposite side of the coin of mood disorders, bipolar disorder, often described as manic-depressive disorder. As with the depressive mood disorders, socioeconomic or psychosocial stressors can be associated with the onset of a manic attack (Kessing *et al.* 2004).

Mania

> O wonderful, wonderful and most wonderful and yet again wonderful and after that out of all whooping.
>
> > (*As You Like It*, 3:2, Shakespeare 1564–1616)

> To see the World in a Grain of Sand
> And a Heaven in a Wild Flower,
> Hold Infinity in the palm of your hand
> And Eternity in an hour.
> > (William Blake 1757–1827, *Auguries of Innocence*)

With regard to mania, Tudor physicians sometimes described mood disorders as 'ecstasies' (to be out of mind), as they recognised that some 'moonstruck' people ranged from profound despair to excited ecstasy. A useful concept from Freudian psychology is that, while depression is a collapse and shrinking of the ego, in mania there is an incredible expansion of the ego, as their sense of their self-esteem explodes into 'O wonderful, wonderful and most wonderful and yet again wonderful and after that out of all whooping' (Celia, *As You Like It*), in this case the 'madness of love'.

The person who is manic is so elated that one almost cannot help but share the intense excitement of the mania, as all their senses seem to expand, inflate and anything and everything is possible.

Sometimes, the person's excitement, with their accelerated thoughts, is in the words of Keats 'touched with fire', which is the title of Professor Jamison's book on the association of bipolar disorder, manic depression, with the poets (Jamison 1996). Moreover, such is the speed of thought, the truly psychedelic perspective of the mania, that they may be misdiagnosed as being psychotic as their intense poetic insight reveals in the words of the great mystic poet William Blake (1757–1827) 'To see the World in a Grain of Sand, and Heaven in a Wild Flower, hold Infinity in the palm of your hand and Eternity in an hour', whose ecstasy demanded that he write in 'capital' letters – the very opposite of an 'eternity of despair'.

But we should not be misled by this poetic ecstasy for, in such prolonged states, people's lives are disrupted as they and others have dysfunctional reactions to the manic situation. Moreover, for most people who suffer from a bipolar disorder, there is a degree and phase of depression either before or after the dominant manic attack, which is an added dimension to their stress. However, Professor Jamison felt as both a person and a professional, the bipolar nature of her mood disorder made the depressive phase 'bearable and worthwhile' (1995). But we must not make the mistake of assuming that because there is poetic or creative force that sometimes accompanies genius, that this is not a disorder which requires intervention, although some evolutionary psychologists suggest that the extremes of mental disorder, especially bipolar and the schizophrenias, may have had some benefit to humankind, even though it may have been at great cost to the individual (Pinker 1998; Warner 2000). However, recent studies of the morbidity of bipolar disorders show that, without adequate preventative treatment, between 30 and 60 per cent of people will have either a subsequent depressive or manic disruptive episode within the next year, with considerable costs to the individual (Angst *et al.* 2003; Post *et al.* 2003). Furthermore, these 'costs' can include the family of those around the disturbed person, as the disorder disrupts their ability to relate appropriately to others and their social circumstances.

'Mr White' was ordinarily an ideal family man, competent professional, pillar of the local church and good neighbour. However, over the past 20 years, he had four episodes of bipolar disorder. The first, at the age of 20, started as a hypomanic attack. Although, initially, he had enormous energy and was highly productive he gradually became a total nuisance to his colleagues as he could not contain himself. The family still shudder at the memory of his expressed erotic ideas about nubile young women neighbours, 'my, "Joan", you're a pert little thing, do you know your breasts yearn to be sucked' and other such and even more explicit remarks. His behaviour was totally misunderstood and, on two occasions, this involved violence as he misinterpreted other people's response to him. After the episode subsided into melancholia, he began to express suicidal ideas as he was horrified at his own behaviour.

Fortunately for Mr White and his family, after the second attack, later subsequent episodes were recognised by his family, and they were able to gain early treatment, and the successive breakdowns were not as severe as the first two. This is not uncommon, and this may be why many colleagues may not have seen a 'pure' manic attack, with all its extremes, because intervention occurs early, as suffers are encouraged to have prophylactic (preventative) treatment.

The seriousness of the disorder is that, as with unipolar disorder, bipolar disorder carriers a risk of suicide, especially as with depression, the manic-depressive disorder is recurrent and persistent; therefore, effective treatment is not only life enhancing but also life saving (Maris *et al.* 1992; Pritchard 1999; Kleindienst and Griel 2003).

Bio-psychosocial treatment

The first line of treatment for bipolar disorder is pharmacological. The mania needs to be brought under control as quickly as possible, not least because, by minimising any social disruption, we minimise any subsequent social consequences and/or stigma. The problem with mania is that it fits the 'popular' vision of madness, Milton's 'demoniac frenzy', which can trigger all the latent cultural anxieties surrounding mental disorder. Modern evidence-based psychiatry recommends a group of drugs known as 'mood stabilisers', although in the recent past virtually any and every major tranquilliser was used. A key drug is lithium, which is effective in many cases quite quickly but, more importantly, as a preventative medium- or long-term prophylaxis. It is claimed by the pharmaceutical industry that more recently introduced mood stabilisers, such as clonazepam and olanzapine, work more quickly than lithium (Rendall *et al.* 2003; Curtin and Schulz 2004). This may be true; however, it is also the case that lithium at currently adminstered doses is both highly effective (Kleindienst and Griel 2003) and, being a natural salt and way past patent rights, very much cheaper. But, as always with pharmacological treatments, the therapist should always go for the drug that best suits the individual patient, with minimal tolerable side-effects.

With regard to long-term preventative treatment, the balance of evidence seems to come down on the side of lithium, albeit sometimes in combination with other mood stabilisers (Fawcett 2003; Kleindienst and Griel 2003).

In the last decade or so, for some bipolar patients, anticonvulsant medication seems to be the type of drug of choice, e.g. sodium valproate, which is more often used for treating the brain disorder epilepsy (Wang *et al.* 2003). This suggests that, for some people suffering from bipolar disorder, it may be that the problem lies in imperfectly co-ordinated electro-neurotransmitters or may be another manifestation of epilepsy, a disease known to humankind for thousands of years (Julius Caesar is known to have suffered from epilepsy), but still not fully understood.

In parenthesis, the effective treatment of epilepsy is one of the unsung successes of Western medicine. Before the Second World War, there were thousands of people held in our old psychiatric hospitals because of their epilepsy, whereas now, the vast majority of sufferers lead totally normal lives, having the benefit of long-term anti-epileptic (anticonvulsant) drugs.

As with all mood disorders, there do appear to be psychosocial stressors that precipitate an attack, with the corresponding risk of subsequent dysfunctional life-disrupting episodes (Angst *et al.* 2003). Therefore, apart from the pharmacological evidence, there is increasing evidence of the benefit of an integrated combined bio-psychosocial approach, especially when it is specific and targeted (Zaretsky 2003). CBT, for example, helps the person understand and control their condition, not least in assisting in compliance with the prophylaxis, and in addition with psycho-education for both the person and their families, i.e. explaining the process of the condition and its effect to the client (Colom *et al.* 2003; Miklowitz *et al.* 2003a,b; Zaretsky 2003). This is exactly the sphere in which social work skills are especially appropriate, as it involves the development of a therapeutic relationship with the sufferer and their family. By explaining what is known about bipolar disorder, we form an alliance with patients and family, demystifying and crucially avoiding blame. The greatest criticism of the anti-psychiatric movement was that it shifted the 'blame' for the disruption from the person to their families and pseudocorrelations were made between parents who had 'eaten sour grapes and [set] the children's teeth. . . on edge' when, again and again, the families' negative response was reactive not causal.

This brings us to a feature that pervades the whole of mental health social work and for any and every disorder, namely the centrality of the family.

The centrality of the family

It may seem a cliché but nothing is more important to the client than their family. How they impact on and react to their family, and the absence of a family, exposes the person to 'isolation', which reduces the person's ability to cope within the community. Time and again, when we look at the treatment of the mentally disordered and other psychosocial problems, while treatment, therapist and agency are important, it is the family upon whom the majority of people rely and from whom they receive the most consistent and long-term support (Leffley and Johnson 1990; Bassuk *et al.* 2002; Enoch and Goldman 2002; Fry and Barker 2002; Teichman *et al.* 2003). Indeed, even in modern Britain and the major Western countries, via the transport and communications networks, families are still the main source of support and, in this sense, the 'extended family' persists. This is seen in the absence of families in cultures with stronger 'extended family traditions', such as Asian and Catholic countries, where, against expectations, suicide rates are relatively far higher than in 'secular' Britain. This is apparently because, in countries such as Italy, Spain, China and Hong Kong for example, the extended family is supreme, but among elderly people who are either childless or unmarried suicide rates are proportionally far higher than in the UK because their services depend so much on the extended family (Lau and Pritchard 2001; Pritchard and Baldwin 2002; Pritchard and Hansen 2005b). The overlap of mental disorder and homelessness (see below) also highlights the core role of the family;

even when there is conflict, the most consistent support to the 'homeless' person is still the family. Indeed, it is when the ties with the family break down that homelessness occurs but, for many, this is a relatively temporary situation, as the family offers some subsequent support (Pritchard and Clooney 1994; Scott 1993; Barker 2001; Social Exclusion Unit 1998a,b; Eynan *et al.* 2002; Ash *et al.* 2003). This means we need to take seriously the burden of the family of bipolar patients for, without strengthening and supporting a 'family alliance', the danger of relapse of the person increases significantly (Reinares and Vieta 2004). Consequently, one general rule of thumb for the mental health social worker is to support family links when we can and, if there is a continuing source of conflict, then aim to minimise it, aiming to aid the restoration of at least minimal good relations between the client and their family. However, it must be appreciated that living with a mentally disordered person puts an enormous strain, emotional, social and often financial, upon the family (Banks 1998; Henwood 1998; Phillips *et al.* 2002; Falloon 2003). Hence, where appropriate, we need to offer them as much support as possible, which will invariably be of value to the primary client.

'John' was 35, from a professional family. One way in which he coped with his mixed mood disorder was through substance abuse. There were periods of intense conflict with his parents, especially his father, who sometimes felt that John's manic phases, which caused considerable social disruption, were deliberately designed to offend his parents' middle-class sensibilities. At one level, it would have been easy to identify totally with John, especially in his earlier years. 'Just think Mr P what it's like to have a taxi man wake you up at 3 a.m. in the morning demanding his money, while John tells the whole neighbourhood that he's back with his "rejecting parents".' This happened not just once but was almost a quarterly occurrence over a number of years as, after a family crisis, John would leave home until the next breakdown, when he would return in one extreme state of his mood disorder, compounded by his 'self-medication' of substance abuse because he refused the prophylactic treatment offered.

Parenthood is the most rewarding, demanding and taxing role we have. The perfect parent, like the perfect child, has yet to be born. The danger for the social worker is to overidentify with one side or the other, rather like Mind and the National Schizophrenia Fellowship. The former invariably advocates on the side of the patients, de facto against the parents, while the NSF is sympathetic to the strains placed upon the families. The research evidence takes the part of the parents as they, along with the client, carry the psychosocial burden in every area of breakdown, be it psychosocial or physical (Pritchard *et al.* 2001, 2004a,b); indeed, this is why a single word definition of good parenthood would be 'altruistic'.

Psycho-education is an increasingly used concept that concerns the direct involvement of the family in the 'treatment alliance' with the patient (Leffley and Johnson 1990; Miklowitz *et al.* 2003a,b), which focuses upon helping family and patient to understand something of the natural history of the condition (Colom *et al.* 2003; Miklowitz *et al.* 2003a,b; Miklowitz 2004). The aim is to demystify and destigmatise the situation by sharing modern knowledge of what we understand of the condition. Crucially, when sensitively handled, it can help both patient and family to understand something of the risk of stressors increasing the risk of relapse, and therefore avoid them, or get earlier invention to ward off a breakdown. This should be done collaboratively, especially if there has been a firm psychiatric diagnosis, although it is crucial that the various members of the community mental health team are speaking with one voice and all know of the decision to inform patient and family. In the past, there was a tendency to avoid giving a diagnosis, for many reasons, but mainly not wishing to demoralise those involved. It is now recognised that leaving people in the dark that their relative suffers from 'nerves' is both patronising and unhelpful. People are generally much more able to cope with quite serious situations, medical and social, if they are informed and aware (Henwood 1998; Rowlands 1998; Pritchard *et al.* 2001, 2004a,b).

The family's importance to the person with a mental disorder, be it mood disorder or schizophrenia, cannot be overstated, and the concept of 'expressed emotion', i.e. critical, hostile comments from family members, has long been known to be associated with breakdown (Leffy and Vaughan 1998), not causal per se, but influential in the person's situation.

This is a key area of work for the social worker in supporting and/or helping to 'interpret' the patient's situation via 'psycho-education' (Craighead and Miklowitz 2000; Miklowitz *et al.* 2003a,b; Kim and Miklowitz 2004). Understanding the family system and their psycho-socioeconomic antecedents is central, and the 'integrated treatment' approach, which includes family therapy, CBT and appropriate pharmacology, utilises wherever possible the family as 'allies' and, within a project called 'systemic treatment enhancement programme' (STEP) propounded by Professor Miklowitz, results are superior to usual treatment outcomes (Morris *et al.* 2005). Of particular importance is the improvement in morale of both the person and their family, reversing the potential vicious cycle of 'expressed emotion', where confused, disappointed, hurt, frightened family members do not understand the vulnerability of their relative.

The role of the family 'carer' is at last being recognised by government and the medical profession (Banks 1998; Henwood 1998; Rowlands 1998), and it has been shown that psychosocial support to the carer, as well as the patient, makes a great difference, improving quality of life for both and saving money for both families and the general economy (Pritchard *et al.* 2001, 2004a,b). Hence, Leffley and Johnson (1990) have rightly urged us to seek a 'family alliance in the treatment of the mentally ill'. Not only is the value of such an approach evidence based, it is, on reflection, what most people would want for themselves, to maintain optimal relations with their family so that they too can support and/or be mutually supported by their family.

9 Mental health social work with people with schizophrenia

Objectives: by the end of the chapter you should:

1 recognise the range and types of the schizophrenias;
2 understand the impact of the syndrome upon all involved;
3 know of the extreme risks associated with schizophrenia;
4 understand the rationale and the limits of psychotropic drug treatment;
5 understand the rationale of the bio-psychosocial approach to intervention;
6 be better prepared to work with people with schizophrenia;
7 consider 'controversial' treatments for severe mental disorder.

> Canst thou not minister to a mind diseased . . .
> Raze out the written troubles of the brain,
> And with some sweet oblivious anti-dote
> Cleanse the stuffed bosom of that perilous stuff
> Which weighs upon the heart?
>
> (*Macbeth*, 5:3)

Impact of psychosis: a psychosocial vortex

The more experience one has of working with vulnerable and troubled people, the greater the danger that we become familiar and desensitised to the impact of their condition. We are all familiar with the surgeon who cracks jokes amidst the gore, the 'patter' we might receive from the oncologist as we are his/her fifth cancer patient of the day, as he/she needs to be 'detached', but this professional approach can become depersonalising, belittling and inadvertently stigmatising – as with medical doctors, so too with social workers. We need to remain sensitive to the enormity of the impact that both schizophrenia and its diagnosis can have upon the client and their family.

Their thought processes are disturbed and disturbing, with misattribution so that the person may fear that they have been taken over by aliens, or in their confusion their communication with their loved ones becomes misunderstood and sometimes frightening. As all share the cultural stigma against mental disorder, the initial insight that many people have that something is going wrong can in itself be a bitter experience as they fear 'I am not in my right mind', that they are going mad.

Imagine our thoughts no longer in our control, if we begin to hear voices in our heads that do not belong to us, that accuse us of terrible things, or belittle us, mocking our most intimate anxieties – if these hallucinations also affect our other senses, smell and touch, then is it surprising that we behave in a highly disturbed way?

Yet here's the rub, while we all, to a greater or lesser degree, have some idea what it is like to be depressed or excited, the experience of schizophrenia usually lies outside the normal range of people's experience. The nearest we ever come to this is in confused dreams or under the influence of psychedelic drugs.

Indeed, schizophrenia is so outside our usual experience that the greatest student of human nature, Shakespeare, had to counterfeit the emotional experience and gave us stereotypes of 'moonstruck madness' from the observer's point of view, rather than the sufferer's perception. In *King Lear*, the legitimate son Edgar is in hiding pretending to be mad:

> I will . . . take the basest and most poorest shape
> . . . in contempt of man
> Brought near to beast; my face I'll grime with filth,
> . . . with presented nakedness outface
> The winds . . .
> The country gives me proof and precedent
> Of Bedlam beggars, who with roaring voices
> Strike in their numbed and mortified bare arms
> Pins, wooden pricks . . .
> Sometime with lunatick bans, sometime with prayers
> Enforce their charity . . .
> Poor Tom, Poor Tom's a cold.
>
> (2:2)

Yet, despite Shakespeare's efforts, he does not authentically reach the qualitative nature of the psychological vortex that attends people in the midst of an acute attack. Perhaps the most effective literary descriptions of a psychotic attack come from Franz Kafka's *Metamorphosis* and *The Trial*. In *Metamorphosis*, we read of a man who has taken to his bed for a vague uncertain reason as slowly he turns into a wood louse. Kafka creates the most eerie and chilling atmosphere, as the narrator convinces, as he is convinced, that he is truly turning into a scaly wood louse. But the man appears simply to accept his transformation as he gets further and further from reality.

In Kafka's *The Trial*, however, we enter the world of the paranoid. The narrator visits a large building and almost imperceptibly his visit begins to have sinister overtones as he experiences people around him condemning and judging him. He 'knows' he is accused, but he cannot determine either charge or offence for which he is now standing trial, as he and the reader are dragged into this vague half-dream world of threat and insinuation. Kafka's genius is that he gets close to the slippage between a person's hold on reality and them moving into a world of different and incomprehensible meaning. For example, 'Michael', a 38-year-old man, described his third episode of schizophrenia, which he himself later described as 'Kafkaesque, which of course reflected the content of his life.

> I felt uneasy. I thought was I getting ill again, did I really need to get any more tablets, but they did my head in, have made me fat and made my mouth so sour that I couldn't speak properly. . . . I noticed he was looking at me. I tried to ignore him and walked on but he was following me. I was not looking for sex, the tablets had ruined that, but he seemed to know that I was gay. To my relief, he walked around the next corner but I still didn't trust him, was he just a look-out . . . (days had passed).
>
> I tried to stay in the house but I was getting very anxious, I could feel as much as hear the voice beginning again, a whisper, I had to get out . . .
>
> I hurried by them, they were laughing and one said to the others, 'he's gay, a queer and he'll get AIDS'. I tried to tell myself that this wasn't happening, that I was just anxious, but it was . . . I started to run but coming the other way were two men pretending to be joggers, I panicked and ran into the park but they followed me and as I ran into the bushes I heard them call out to each other . . . Everything was threatening and I knew I was in danger, I thought I was going to wet myself and then I heard them say 'why don't you kill yourself, you're a dirty queer, you're going to get AIDS, why don't you kill yourself and save you the trouble'. Their words were in my head, I couldn't get my breath, I felt I was going to faint. I knew I was in deadly danger as either they would finish me, or I might finish myself. I was terrified.

'Michael' had never come to terms with his sexual orientation and continued to feel guilty about it and, in his previous attacks, the hallucinatory voices centred around his low self-esteem and his sexuality and his fear of contracting AIDS. He was in reality remarkably continent, having only had three lovers in the whole of his life, and only once had he ever had a casual sexual contact, more than ten years before. However, this almost became an obsession for him as he feared that this contact might have infected him. We hear from Michael the pattern and 'form' of the disturbed thoughts, followed by emotions and then 'content'-specific hallucinations following. He contacted his social worker, who was able to provide an emotionally secure situation so that he could get psychiatric treatment, based upon a trusting relationship. Although 'Michael' insisted that he was at risk of assault, that 'they' were out to get him, he accepted psychopharmacological treatment given by injection and, within a week, the worst of the persecutory and dangerous suicidal ideas had abated.

But consider, if you felt you were being followed, spied upon, urged to kill yourself by strangers or worse, voices in your head, you too would feel anxious and fearful. For while there is a period when the person suspects they are ill, especially if they have had previous episodes, the experience becomes real and overwhelms the earlier insight, with all the subsequent normal emotional response to the perceived threat.

Here is the paradox, the 'concept of normality', in that the person (a) makes every effort to maintain a psychologically normal response to their early disruptive feelings and (b) has normal reactions to the content of the disorder so that, being convinced of the threat, they react as anyone would – flight, predominantly, or if especially threatened, but more rarely, fight. One needs an active act of imagination to understand what the sufferer must be going through and of course 'no man is an island'; the client's content will involve and inevitably effect their family and those around them. Again, their response to the first episode will be very normal; initially, they will seek to make sense of what is happening and, as yet, not appreciating the nature of the disorder, will respond emotionally to the person's behaviour and attribution. Very quickly, each can blame/accuse the other of being unreasonable and, of course, as it begins to dawn upon the family that their relative is ill, this itself must be a dreadful and fearful experience – for after all 'madness', being 'loony', happens to other people, not themselves. Dependent upon the relationship of the sufferer, if they are the parent, imagine what the child must feel to hear from their parent bizarre and perhaps overly intimate anxieties; if they are the young adult, imagine what their parents and grandparents or siblings may feel as the young life, which promised so much, begins to unravel before their eyes.

'Michael's' situation of course was fairly typical of a paranoid schizophrenic illness and is fairly obviously extreme and disrupted. Table 9.1 offers a breakdown of the key assessment points and how to understand his specific problems and the necessary intervention following the BASIC IDDS model.

'Nicholas', aged 19, was at the other end of the spectrum. Here, we have to rely upon his mother as our informant as 'Nicholas' was withdrawn and taciturn, finding his experience beyond words.

> We didn't realise anything was wrong for some time. 'Nick' had done well in his GCSEs and we were very proud of him and hopeful. After his exams, he had his first serious girlfriend and this lasted nearly six months and, at first, we put down his moods, his lethargy, his irritability, to 'young love' not going smoothly. He started dropping his friends and again when we learned he'd finished with 'Anne', or rather she had finished with him, we thought it was typical adolescent depression, and of course he wouldn't speak to us about it and we didn't press him. We

Table 9.1 BASIC IDDS. Assessment of paranoid schizophrenia – 'Michael'

Problem	Intervention
Behaviour	
Agitation	Counselling, restart atypicals
Withdrawal	Arrange later CBT
	Family support and psycho-education
Effect	
Anxiety	Counselling and support
Fear	CBT to reframe beliefs system
Suspicious	
Sensory	
Hears voices	Counselling regarding diet and exercise
Distressed by side-effects	Discuss with psychiatrist later moderate dosage
Loss of libido	
Weight gain	
Interpersonal relations	
Avoids people	Family therapy and psycho-education
Quarrels with family	Social workers acts as 'bridge' between client and family – interpret feelings to deal with high expressed emotion
Cognition	
Low self-esteem	CBT allied to long-term counselling support
Fears for his life	Reframe deluded ideas
Fears he has HIV	
Imagery	
He 'sees' people looking at him	Teach 'imagery'-stopping techniques to help manage
He 'feels/imagines' people are around the corner 'waiting' for him	hallucinations
Drugs/treatment	
Side-effects precipitated him stopping his atypical anti-psychotics	Liaise with psychiatrists and GP
	Include 'Michael' in discussions regarding restored atypicals
Defences	
Avoidance	CBT and supportive counselling
Displacement of affect	
Social	
Underemployed	Recognise frustrations of being underemployed
Unemployed	Below capacity. Explore employment (sheltered) possibilities
Isolated	Encourage joining appropriate interest group (e.g. church, art/history groups, gym, etc.)

then found that he was missing school and, as both my husband and I went out before him, we were shocked to find that over three months he'd hardly been in college at all. He slept in late and, at the other end, kept his computer on till the early hours. He started getting interested in transcendental meditation and New Age kind of things. Previously, he would tell us what was going on his life, but he became more withdrawn and taciturn and, finally, we became alarmed when his best friend came around to see him and Nick simply went upstairs and wouldn't talk to him. His friend alerted us to the fact that, for nearly six months, Nick had become more and more withdrawn, dropped out of everything and 'sorry to say he's become a bit weird, not like himself at all'. His friend denied that Nick was into drugs, although admitted that a year before they had both tried cannabis, more a mutual dare, than any real interest and had not continued with the experiment. This was a wake-up call for us, for we suddenly realised that, over the past 12 months, Nick had been growing away from us and everyone, and that he virtually never initiated a conversation, that he had become dirty in his personal habits and that he'd lost something of himself.

Before, he'd been a bright, outgoing lad but now, why now you'd think he was mentally handicapped; we were distraught with worry and really panicked when Nick's grandfather told us that Nick reminded him of his late brother who had ended up in a mental hospital just after the war.

When trying to communicate with Nick, one appreciated his mother's description and something of their frustration as, when he did respond, it was often in a rather childish, fatuous way, sadly typical of 'simple' schizophrenia. Hence, it is understandable how the early nineteenth-century psychiatrist described this form of the disorder as 'dementia praecox', dementia of the young, as like Nick, such sufferers seem to regress and lose psychosocial developmental skills – in effect, they became emotionally and socially retarded. Sadly, this form of schizophrenia seems to be more disruptive of the developing personality, as the patient regresses into an earlier developmental stage and presents classic passive symptoms of lethargy, low mood, poor arousal, withdrawal, poor personal attention and psychosocial isolation.

Dual diagnosis: schizophrenia and substance abuse

Another type of situation, which has increased over the years, is the person with schizophrenia and an involvement in substance misuse, especially cannabis, rather than the so-called hard drugs such as cocaine, LSD, etc. (Margolese *et al.*

2004). The potential problem association of a cannabis link with schizophrenia came from an early Scandinavian study (Andreasson *et al.* 1990), which analysed the Swedish Psychiatric Register. They identified young national servicemen who later developed schizophrenia. They belonged to one of two groups, those with first-degree relatives with schizophrenia or heavy and prolonged cannabis users, a theme confirmed in later research (Zammit *et al.* 2002). This aroused a degree of dissent, in part because cannabis is a drug increasingly used socially and it undermines the argument for decriminalisation of the 'softer drugs'. This is not the place to argue for or against but to report recent research that shows quite clearly that prolonged cannabis use increases the risk to the person of having a schizophrenic breakdown (Smit *et al.* 2003; Arendt and Munk-Jorgensen 2004; Berger 2004).

A study from Australia is especially useful as it spans a 25-year period, from 1975 to 2000; in effect, it charts the general increased use of cannabis in Western societies. It was found that only 8 per cent of people with schizophrenia were also substance abusers, mainly cannabis, but this rose to 26 per cent of all patients (Wallace *et al.* 2004). In addition, these dual diagnosis patients, i.e. schizophrenia and substance disorder, a term psychiatrists are using increasingly, were significantly more often involved in subsequent criminal behaviour, including violence, 68 per cent compared with 12 per cent of non-dual diagnosis people.

An important element in the cannabis–schizophrenia interaction is that cannabis users, particularly when starting young, were substantially more likely to develop schizophrenia with more negative symptoms. Furthermore, the breakdown occurred earlier, a mean of 6.9 years earlier than in people who developed schizophrenia but had no history of substance abuse (Green *et al.* 2004; Veen *et al.* 2004).

Of course, it may be that people who are going to develop schizophrenia are more likely to start using cannabis earlier, but a study from the Netherlands found that this 'self-medication' hypothesis had not been proved (Smit *et al.* 2003). Of course, smoking is far more deadly than cannabis and is associated with the fivefold increase in malignant disease in young women in Britain (Pritchard and Evans 1997), but as usual with any social situation, drugs and/or alcohol complicate matters and often make things worse (Eckert *et al.* 2002; Gossop *et al.* 2002; Ash *et al.* 2003). It may not be welcome news, but the level of new research focusing upon cannabis begins to suggest that, as smoking is to cancer, cannabis may be to schizophrenia, as well as being its own 'cancer risk', while the possible therapeutic use is still unclear and of course not 'street available' (Kalant 2004; Hall and Currow 2005). While the schizophrenic condition, with its genetic endowment, needs psychosocial stressors to be triggered, it may be that cannabis enhances the minimal genetic element. Although there is little doubt that, compared with 25 years ago, cannabis is more readily available and used 'socially', this may be a feature in the reported increase in the incidence of schizophrenia in south-east London (Boydell *et al.* 2003).

It is not being claimed that cannabis 'causes' schizophrenia, but it is clear that its use makes people more vulnerable to mental disorder, especially schizophrenia.

'Duncan' was a very bright African-Caribbean teenager who aroused some opposition because he was active in equal rights activities. He passed his 'A' levels a year early and decided upon a gap year, against the wishes of his teacher father. During this time, his use of cannabis increased, which caused his parents considerable alarm, as his mother, a nurse, knew of the association with mental disorder, and a paternal uncle had had a number of schizophrenia-like illnesses.

Duncan's university career was broken up by periods of significant failure to produce work on time and some minor violent episodes, where Duncan may have been as much a sinner as sinned against. After an academically successful first year, he was a virtual absentee in the second and needed to repeat the year. He had a schizophrenia-like episode at the beginning of his repeat year and had a medical suspension. He was treated with anti-psychotic drugs and only with much persuasion was he helped to return to university. He had great difficulty in completing his year, but he was strongly supported by other students, though there were bouts of quite acute paranoia. He explained 'It's my mantra, this is out of harmony with the world, which can detect the evil forces, if I can get my mantra on an even keel all will be well' but 'don't you go on about the spliffs, I need them to keep me calm', as Duncan oscillated between reasonable appreciation of the reality of his situation and periods of depressed mood and great suspicion: 'It's not that all white people are racists, I sometimes think they are.' He would charm with self-deprecatory humour 'I'm probably not an easy guy to be with', but later might refuse to come for a counselling support session. Duncan, with support, completed his degree to the genuine pleasure of all who knew him but sadly, after returning home, he resumed his cannabis and, following a family row, Duncan left home and spent some time homeless; we learned from his distraught parents that he was the victim of a particularly nasty violent attack because he was black, mentally disordered and homeless.

The case of Duncan reminds us that the person with schizophrenia is often not the only victim, but distressed and loving parents, who are often unfairly blamed (Skinner and Cleese 1994) and too easily blame themselves. Moreover, the consequences can be socially devastating, not least with its association with homelessness and being the victims of violence (Eckert *et al.* 2002; Ash *et al.* 2003; Walsh *et al.* 2003), whilst also having a lower life expectancy and not just because of suicide (Harris and Barraclough 1998).

So, how do we intervene and assist the person with schizophrenia and their family?

A bio-psychosocial approach to treating schizophrenia

When considering working with people with schizophrenia, nowhere is the bio-psychosocial approach more appropriate. For example, while there is a clear indication of a genetic predisposition to schizophrenia in many people, like most conditions, it awaits an environmental 'trigger' from a range of stressors to push the person over the edge (Leff 1992). Consequently, in treating the person with schizophrenia, we need to take into account the totality of the person's situation, not just their interpersonal relationships, family and friends, but also cultural factors, including ethnicity, social class and the economic situation, as well as the necessary psychopharmacological approach. This is succinctly summed up by Warner (2000: 106) when he says:

> From the womb to the workplace, the environment shapes schizophrenia. The physical world and human society control how many people will develop the illness and how its course will run. Biological factors are particularly important in establishing the predisposition to the illness; psychological factors such as the reaction to stress, can trigger the onset; and sociological factors, like the domestic environment or stigma, influence its course and outcome.

However, this integrated approach nonetheless means that the front line of treatment is the anti-psychotics to help control the disturbed bio-psychosocial functioning, which assists the person to respond appropriately to those around them.

Psychopharmacology

The advent of anti-psychotic drugs, classically Largactil (chlorpromazine), allowed us to free the previously confined mentally disordered person as the anti-psychotics reduced their symptoms and also gave the public confidence that we could pursue the 'care in the community' policies (Jones 1959; House of Commons 2000). The drugs were seen to calm people and made them more able to respond to others. The fact that we never matched resources to care in the community, nor the fact that government gets very anxious about any high-profile cases, which makes them sound more oppressive than they wish to be, does not alter the fact that the vast majority of people with schizophrenia do not need to be in hospital for most of the time.

The problem with the older drugs, now called 'typical' anti-psychotics, the neuroleptics, such as chlorpromazine, thioridazine, haloperidol and fluphenazine, is that, although all were an improvement on the earlier treatments, the side-effects are often considerable: in particular, what are known as extra-pyramidal symptoms, which occur over time in many patients, e.g. Parkinson's disease-like symptoms, awkward stiff gait, rigidity, facial tics, shaking, mask-like face and dystonic reactions, experienced as restlessness, anxiety, agitation, insomnia, described as akathisia (Tandon and Jibson 2003), which can be quite frightening for both the patient and their family. Moreover, we should not forget that both antidepressant and anti-psychotic drugs can produce sexual difficulties and loss of libido as a particular distressing side-effect (Baldwin and Mayers 2003; Baldwin 2004).

While these 'typical' anti-psychotics were very good at reasonably speedily reducing the acute symptoms of schizophrenia, their side-effects were such as to undermine the client's desire to take the medication. And not maintaining the anti-psychotic drugs was associated with earlier and more frequent relapse. Moreover, it is especially important to start anti-psychotic treatment as soon as possible to reduce the impact of the disease; the typicals, with their occasionally quite early severe side-effects, led to treatment breakdown (NICE 2002; Tandon and Jibson 2003).

The so-called newer 'first-line atypical' anti-psychotic drugs, i.e. basic first type of pharmacological treatment, with which the vast majority of clients with schizo-phrenia will be treated today, are risperidone, olanzapine, quetiapine, amisulpride and, in the USA, ziprasidone. Different drugs seem to suit different people, and the physician will often need to find the medication that is best for that individual, although probably 70 per cent of people with schizophrenia are treated with either risperidone or olanzapine. The key benefit of these 'first-line atypicals' is that all these drugs have considerably fewer or less severe side-effects; therefore, they are more tolerable to people, with the additional benefit that they are more likely to use the drug appropriately and not stop treatment (NICE 2002; Tandon and Jibson 2003).

Clozapine is another atypical used for people who have not benefited from the above atypicals, so called 'treatment-resistant' schizophrenia (see below), but it must be used with great care as it can cause serious, but usually reversible, blood disorders, such as reducing the person's white cell count. Nonetheless, under strict and careful monitoring, clozapine can relieve the suffering from the extreme dis-tress of their schizophrenia, and therefore is within the treatment armoury.

As mentioned earlier, drug trials are difficult to evaluate, especially when sup-ported by the pharmacological industry, and I will eschew an exploration of the dozens of papers making claims for one drug over another but turn to the National Institute for Health and Clinical Excellence (NICE) for its overview, but bear in mind that it is equally concerned with efficacy and economics.

There is general agreement that the first-line treatment for schizophrenia is an anti-psychotic (atypical preferred) drug, but its choice should be based upon a discussion between the physician and the client who should explore costs, in terms of side-effects, and benefits (NICE 2000). This is to achieve three distinct treatment goals (Tandon and Jibson 2003):

1   bring active symptoms under control (not least remembering the association of psychosis and suicidal ideation; Pritchard 1999; Harkvy-Friedman *et al.* 2003);
2   assist the person to re-establish normal functioning;
3   implement a maintenance phase aimed at preventing relapse.

NICE also agrees that there is little to choose between the four main atypicals used in Britain, amisulpride, olanzapine, risperidone and quetiapine, and therefore the decision in each case should rest upon the least intrusive side-effects. They also urge that the lowest clinically effective dosage should be used as there is evidence that the greater the dose the more likely are side-effects, especially the EPS although, in Tandon and Jibson's meta-analysis (2003), quetiapine was found to be better than the others, and possibly less of a problem for weight gain.

The worry with the various RCTs, as reported by NICE (2002) and Tandon and Jibson (2003), is how relatively short a period these trials last, usually around 6–8 weeks, some even as short as four weeks. Yet these drugs are often prescribed for months, and in low doses as prophylactic (preventative) even for years. One other point of warning is that, while some physicians might prescribe two of the atypicals together, typicals and atypicals should never be used concurrently, so we need to ensure that our client is aware of the dangers of inadvertently mixing them up.

What all authorities agree on, however, is that, although the person-appropriate medication is necessary in the treatment of schizophrenia, it

> should be initiated as a comprehensive package of care that addresses the individual's clinical, emotional and social needs. The clinician responsible for treatment and key worker should monitor both therapeutic progress and tolerability of the drug on an ongoing basis.
>
> (NICE 2002: 2, p. 97)

One unusual medication that has attracted interest is that of polyunsaturated fatty acid supplements, e.g. cod liver oil of the omega-3 EFA type, readily purchased from any health food shop. The media ran a couple of stories, and some serious studies looked at the effect in terms of people with schizophrenic behaviour and possible anti-psychotic properties. Joy *et al.* (2004) undertook the typically rigorous Cochrane review and concluded that, while some claims were overoptimistic, omega-3 EFA given as a single supplement and in addition to anti-psychotic drugs was of some benefit. There is, therefore, probably a reasonable case for suggesting that people with schizophrenia take one capsule a day – thus avoiding any suggestion of overuse – not least because it has other beneficial properties with regard to helping to combat cardiovascular disease, and as many people with schizophrenia have less good lifestyles, in particular they are often heavy smokers. Thus, omega-3 EFA can be recommended as a general contribution to improving the person's diet. Of course, they are relatively inexpensive and in small doses are virtually free from side-effects.

One final word on psychopharmacology. Most drug studies are a combination of tests against another drug and/or a placebo, i.e. does drug X perform statistically significantly better than the placebo, which is a compound without any known chemical benefit. The reason for this is that, in many medical conditions, not just in mental health, about 10–15 per cent of patients given a placebo 'improve' over a short time.

Why is this? Medicine seemingly accepts this as a normal response, not recognising that the placebo effect might be better described as the 'self-reparative' process. In effect, the doctor/shaman has 'appealed' to the person's optimism and 'belief' in the 'priest/physician/expert', thus inculcating hope and optimism. I remind trainee psychiatrist and medical undergraduates of this 'self-reparatory' power and urge them to maximise it in the service of their patients. This is not fanciful, for a recent Cochrane database systematic review (probably the most rigorous type of in-depth review of many research studies in the form of a meta-analysis) showed that, when comparing placebo 'treatment' with no treatment, there were definite statistical gains using placebos in some areas of the person's life (Hrobjartsson and Gotzsche 2003). This human phenomenon can be utilised within that central therapeutic vehicle, the client–social worker relationship, for whenever the 'self-reparatory process' is invoked, the person's mood improves; this is another aspect of the positive elements within cognitive behaviour therapy (CBT).

Psychosocial approach to working with a person with schizophrenia

The textbooks make great mention of the frequent emotional withdrawal of people with schizophrenia, which can be marked in an acute attack. However, we should not make the mistake of thinking, 'the person's not at home'. Rather, they are defensively withdrawing either because of their difficulty or because they are preoccupied with their inner world, but this is a normal reaction to an abnormal situation, and the importance of establishing a rapport cannot be overstated. This was dramatically demonstrated to me when I returned to the back wards of a hospital where I had had a student placement more than 15 years earlier.

George was part of a project to reintroduce speech to people with 'mute' schizophrenia; most had not spoken for a decade or more (Barker *et al.* 1998). His had been a particular severe case of catatonic withdrawal, and I had felt especially sorry for him and on occasions had spoken to him, of course without getting any answer or emotional response. Years later, when I visited the project, George greeted me, recalling the time when I had been there. This was very moving and also a salutary reminder that even the most withdrawn person does not lose their humanity.

Hence the importance, which even the most pharmacological orientated authorities acknowledge, of an integrated approach, which includes the psychosocial in order to meet the full needs of the person and their family, at whose centre is the therapeutic relationship (Baldwin and Birtwhistle 2002; NICE 2002; Goodwin and Gotlieb 2003; Tandon and Jibson 2003; Zaretsky 2003). This demands that we pay particular attention to establishing a therapeutic rapport with the person. This can be difficult because, in some people, the schizophrenic syndrome gets in the way and demands the greatest care and attention on our part. Nonetheless, as with all professions working with people, it is the professional's responsibility to communicate with the client. This demands that we are aware of our own body language, the style and pace of our speech, and the need to ensure that we do not either under- or overstimulate the person. We use appropriate vocabulary, and especially with this condition, try to avoid using similes or metaphors, as sometimes the persons almost thinks 'concretely' and literally, so one does not ask 'are you feeling brassed off' or comment on the weather that it's 'raining cats and dogs', as this may well confuse, as they see neither 'brass' nor 'cats and dogs'. Hence, we follow the person, remembering that a quiet calm voice is invariably the best, crucially paying attention to the pace of our speech as sometimes the other person has difficulty in comprehending or taking in what we are saying. Calm, patient communication, with a willingness to have silences, avoiding the impression of rush, and wherever possible respond to the person's normality. For example, in fraught situations, one waits for a quiet period and makes the enquiry 'is it possible to have a cup of tea'. Indeed, in those emergency situations where one is unsure what is happening, if one behaves as a social visitor and asks for tea, in a normal response the person under stress reacts appropriately to a request from a guest, which calms the situation down.

Yet because a person is suffering from schizophrenia, this does not always mean that they are unable to communicate; indeed some people can be quite voluble, to the extent that one may consider whether they are suffering from a schizoaffective disorder, which seems to combine elements of schizophrenia with one end of the mood disorder.

In terms of treatment, the drug treatment is the same as for schizophrenia, although possibly with a mood stabiliser added (NICE 2002; Goodwin 2003; Tandon and Jibson 2003) but most important is that we respond to the affect the person is presenting. Typically, such a person may have a set of well-defined ideas, which may initially sound quite reasonable, if a little esoteric, but as they unfold, one emotionally realises that there is a psychotic element to their ideation. If we engage with them, initially we might feel a little confused as to who has the greater grasp upon reality – always an interesting philosophical point but we won't pursue it. These ideas often centre around philosophical or scientific ideas, especially astronomy, astrology or religious topics, which appear to the lay person to be a little 'cranky', but allowing the person to continue, one begins to appreciate there is a loss of hold upon reality.

'Matthew' was a former flatmate of a post-graduate student of mine, with a previous history of admission to psychiatric hospital. When well, he was an interesting, intelligent man, with a real sense of humour and with a good degree of insight, and, with encouragement, he would continue his maintenance resperidone. However, he would then stop his medication and over some months his 'hobby' of astronomy would become an obsession, and he would send the most detailed essays arguing that the planets were being influenced by other than gravitational forces, along with some mathematical formulae as 'proofs'. The first four pages sounded impressive but one learned not to accept his telephone call, which could well last an hour and was impossible to end politely. But one could not help be flattered that he thought you important enough to communicate his great secret, along with copies of letters to Tony Blair, Margaret Thatcher and Bill Clinton. He would remain in this slightly raised affective state for months, quite incapable of working, and needed a degree of supervision because he tended to neglect himself for his 'studies'. But he never failed to be polite and pleasant, if a little persistent and obsessional. He would then appear to be mildly depressed and then willing to consider returning to his medication, when with great politeness, and one sometimes wondered whether he was laughing at us, he might write or ring to explain that the planets were not being influenced by other than gravitational forces, but strongly advised one to destroy his earlier communication 'just in case the CIA were on to us'.

What 'Matthew' reminds us is that people are not like the textbooks and, despite it seeming a cliché, one really must respond to each person in their individual circumstances and how their version of schizophrenia is presented. Moreover, we should always consider the person's strengths, not just their apparent weaknesses and problems. It is amazing the fortitude and resilience that people show in lives which, to an outsider, have little joy in them. Yet the person battles on, and we should always be certain that our intervention adds to their psychosocial resources, not undermines them. The psychosocial elements of our work with people with schizophrenia are highlighted in Table 9.2.

With regard to the psychological, all the usual core counselling skills are required, plus the extra sensitivity needed to communicate with someone whose own communication 'receptor/transmission' may be disrupted. In respect to social factors, employment and accommodation are crucial issues (Platt 1984; Pritchard 1988; Social Exclusion Unit 1998a; Eynan *et al.* 2002; Park 2002; Blakely *et al.* 2003; Desai *et al.* 2003). Indeed, Warner (2000) points out that the absence or

Table 9.2 Key psychosocial issues affected by schizophrenia

Psychological	*Social networks*
Perceptual and cognitive disturbances	Income maintenance
Communication problems	Employment
'Personality' strengths and weaknesses	Housing/accommodation
Self-esteem	Cultural/ethnic
Interpersonal relationships	Amenities/neighbourhood
Children and their needs	Services – voluntary and statutory
	Schools and child provision

inadequacy of either not only is a barrier to recovery and reintegration, but adds to the alienation and stigmatisation that often accompany schizophrenia.

One perennial problem is how do we deal with the client's overt expression of their hallucinations and/or delusions? Do we 'humour' them and pretend that we are going along with their reality of the voices, or strange smells and/or a sense of being touched; by responding as if we share their beliefs that they are possessed by aliens, communists, God, the devil, etc.?

There are two general 'rules' to be recommended: first and foremost, the social worker should always give acknowledgement of the reality of the emotion that is likely to be associated with either the hallucination or the delusion, especially the latter, if the person seeks to discuss how they should respond to the voice and/or ideas. Their emotional reaction is undoubtedly real. If they are fearful 'that they are being watched by aliens', this is a perfectly reasonable reaction and, in that sense, normal.

Secondly, wherever possible, without directly challenging the delusion, nor inadvertently reinforcing it, quietly and gently express sympathy but say you have a different perspective. They may come back and ask 'do you think I'm imagining it, do you think I'm mad?' Again, avoiding the confrontation, bearing in mind the likelihood of a degree of insight/half-appreciation that something is wrong, the answer is to reiterate your sympathy at the reality of their distress but raise the question that they may well be responding to various stressors, which can make matters confusing.

'Michael', in his acute stage, said 'they've killed all the gays and they are coming for me next'. It would not have been helpful to pretend this was true and then argue for going to hospital as a place of refuge, because 'Michael' may very well have been unsure about his delusion. And his comment, while expressing an emotional truth, may also have been testing out the reality of his experience. The reply was 'that must be terrifying. I can see why you seem so frightened. But I don't see it like that but, if that is what you think, it must be very distressing.' The key is not to argue, or challenge, but offer an alternative view of reality, while at the same time giving full recognition to his feelings. Of course, there is never an always and always a never and, in those rare circumstances in which the person is so agitated that an alternative view may incite aggression, one may have to compromise, but whenever possible, don't, unless there seems to be absolutely no alternative.

Sometimes with people who are suffering from dementia, one is perhaps more likely to respond in harmony with their ideation but, again, avoid it if possible.

'Mary' was 88 years old, an intelligent, kind and loving woman, whose late-onset Alzheimer's was destroying her cognition and sense of reality. She was agitated that she had to go and find her dog, which was outside whining because it was dark and cold: 'Snowy hates the winter and being outside'. I commented that she was showing great concern for Snowy but perhaps she was experiencing an old memory, as Snowy died peacefully some years before, and therefore she did not need to go out. 'Oh dear, am I getting mixed up again?' 'Yes, but we all do sometimes, shall we have a cup of tea?' And she, the lady to the last, responded with dignity and grace and asked what kind would I like. Later, as her condition got worse, with some degree of cerebral irritation, she became very agitated and one would have to say 'You stay here, I will go and check' and then, on your return, seek to divert her from the idea that was distressing her.

At the other end of the spectrum, we always need to consider whether the person with a severe mental disorder has children or not. If so, what is happening to them and how is the situation impacting upon them? There is clear evidence of an important psychiatric–child protection interface (Falkov 1996; Pritchard and Bagley 2001; Pritchard 2004), which will be discussed in detail in the appropriate chapter.

There are three major research-supported psychosocial approaches that are often of benefit to people with schizophrenia and their families

Psychosocial treatment packages

Family management – high expression of emotion

It is now accepted that the family are an important source of support to most people with a severe mental disorder (Miklowitz *et al.* 2003a,b), and that the unsupported 'blaming' of families (Skinner and Cleese 1994), rather than recognising the mutuality of their distress, should frankly be a thing of the past. We ought not to mix up the imperfections of interpersonal relations that can occur in most families, as a primary cause of the mental disorder; the family should not become an area of stress, rather than support. Yet again and again, the last bastion of continued sustained support comes from the family, despite the considerable stress upon the family having a member who has schizophrenia and, unless case-specifically contraindicated, we should seek to sustain and maximise that support (Reinares and Vieta 2004). In our effort to understand and empathise with the person with schizophrenia, it is easy to forget just how demanding and stressful it can be living with a person with schizophrenia (Falloon 2003).

'Walter' was a 38-year-old man, six feet tall, very overweight, compounded by poor diet and heavy smoking. He lived with middle-class parents in their seventies, both of whom were slightly built and now beginning to be physically frail. Over a 20-year period, when things 'got especially bad', the parents would seek help in managing Walter, who physically, emotionally and financially dominated them. Walter had been an intelligent youth, but his first schizophrenic episode in his late teens had severely disrupted his development and potential. He had not worked since this breakdown, and the nature of his disorder was such that he reminded one of the large adolescent sparrow bullying his fraught, overworked parents. The parents tolerated a great deal, 'we love him, he's ours, he doesn't really mean it' and, after a particularly bad session, he might express remorse but would assert 'its not my fault, I'm ill'.

Ordinarily, Walter stayed in bed until lunchtime, occupied himself with esoteric books, later the internet, and had an elaborate form of rituals to keep 'the voices at bay'. He intermittently took his anti-psychotic medication, which meant that life was sometimes tolerable, but limited for them all – the parents' social life had been virtually ruined by the intransigence of Walter. On a number of occasions, there were exacerbations of his schizophrenia, which would be very alarming for him and his parents, as he shouted back at his voices, broke furniture, insisted that his parents share his rituals so that they were not allowed to enter some rooms, could only walk in certain paths in others and could only sit on certain chairs. If thwarted, he had been known to strike his parents. While his behaviour might seem like that of a spoilt adolescent, he was clearly under the influence of severe delusions, and the social worker's role, as the key worker in this situation, was to negotiate with Walter and his parents, to persuade him to recommence his medication and then to do some CBT exercises, which helped Walter cope better with his voices and, at the same time, helped his parents to handle their understandable ambivalence better. Walter's life was undoubtedly a tragedy with the damage the schizophrenia had caused, but his parents also suffered, as latterly there was concern that Walter might physically harm them. Yet any suggestion of admission was resisted by these heroic parents because, despite everything, 'with your help, we can and should manage. He's our son, we love him.'

Such an example is not uncommon and reflects something of the stress endured by the family and the person with schizophrenia. Falloon (1985) recognised this and, in a series of brilliant studies, highlighted something of the family dynamics/interactions that occurred in families who had a member with schizophrenia (Malm *et al.* 2003). In brief, Falloon found that there were two broad responses to the crisis situation in how the families dealt with their emotions. In 'high expressed emotion' (HEE) families, who, compared with 'low expressed emotion' families, were found to be overcritical, undermining, rejecting or overinvolved, leading to greater relapse on the part of the sufferer. Crucially, Fallon and colleagues and others found that via family therapy this HEE could be reduced, with subsequent benefits to the family member (Falloon and Pedersen 1985; Falloon 1998; Phillips *et al.* 2002). However, Pharoah *et al.* (2003), typically in a Cochrane review, was very cautious, but found that there were some positive outcomes. By and large, a family management or family therapy approach did encourage compliance with medication, reduced the frequency or relapse of symptoms and improved levels of expressed emotion in families, to the emotional well-being of all involved. However, the reviewers were uncertain as to the specific mechanisms and, although a promising approach, they concluded that more research is needed, although already completed trials should inform practice. Hence, it should become part of an integrated armoury of psychosocial intervention with people with schizophrenia (Malm *et al.* 2003; Miklowitz *et al.* 2003a,b).

Psycho-education

In the past, we were so afraid of the stigma of the diagnosis that sometimes people might be involved with the mental health service for years, but never be given a diagnosis, or 'label' or explanation of what was wrong. We tended to use euphemisms rather than explain the nature and process of the problem, be it a severe mood disorder or schizophrenia, and often spoke about 'nervous breakdown' but without any adequate explanation of the process and outcome (Miklowitz *et al.* 2003a,b). Today, however, we recognise the need for a treatment alliance with client and family and between the professionals and the people involved; in conjunction with the psychiatrist, the key worker might well be charged to explain the situation. Crucially, this should help the patient and the family to arrive at some decisions about medication. Over the last decade, 'educating patient and family' about schizophrenia and the other severe mental disorders has become common practice, and it helps to demystify and destigmatise the situation. Especially important is when we can tackle the almost inevitable 'blaming game'. If only the parents had been more/less strict, if only they had given more/less, etc., then he/she would not have had their breakdown. If only he/she had not left home/stayed at home, had more/fewer friends, then the breakdown might not have occurred. Psycho-education, in effect, brings together the family management approach to schizophrenia with appropriate family therapy, but most of all informs both client and their family, enabling them to make better decisions about their treatment and their lives.

Pekkala and Merinder (2002) did the usual careful Cochrane database systematic review and, while they were sometimes critical of too extreme claims, they came to the conclusion that psycho-educational approaches were a useful part of the total treatment programme. Moreover, the intervention was relatively brief and inexpensive, and there should be further research efforts to identify specific outcomes. Indeed, as already mentioned, Miklowitz *et al.* (2003a,b,) did just this and found that, in conjunction with psychopharmacology, the psycho-education approach, involving crisis intervention sessions if necessary, improved the situation and was also very effective in bipolar management, improving the use of the medication and family and client morale.

An interesting variation on this approach has been reported by Dyke and colleagues (2003), who have used a group therapy approach, bringing a number of families together for weekly group sessions, which seems to have had some better results than treatment as usual or a single approach to psycho-education.

Cognitive behaviour therapy

Undoubtedly the biggest advance in psychosocial intervention with people with schizophrenia has come from cognitive behavioural therapy (CBT) (Barraclough *et al.* 2001; Kingdon and Turkington 2002; Tarrier *et al.* 2004). However, it must be stressed that this is usually considered appropriate in conjunction with psychopharmacology, not least to minimise the disruption caused by the symptoms, therefore helping the person to be better able to communicate. The CBT approach is outlined in Chapter 8 on mood disorders, for which it was initially designed. But Kingdon and Turkington (2002) have been making great strides with CBT and, hearing personally of patients' experiences with CBT, one cannot but be impressed. It is reiterated, however, that CBT sometimes sells itself short as it tries to emphasise what a brief and therefore cheap intervention it is. It is ideal for the early onset of an episode, but the person needs longer term support, crucially for the practitioner to be available if needed. There is evidence that people knowing they can get help, for example at the end of a telephone, often cope with the crisis better and, in fact, often don't contact the professionals because they are willing to attempt to ride out the crisis (Morgan *et al.* 1993; Pritchard *et al.* 2004a–c). However, we have to remember that the schizophrenia can be dysfunctional, which apparently accounts for the negative findings on social skills training alone (Pilling *et al.* 2002). A most promising approach was carried out by two US social workers on the 'Soteria project' whose aim was maximum combined psychosocial support and minimal use of medication. Over a two-year period, Bolar and Mosher (2003) found marked improvement on a number of measures, relapse, better social function, work and reduced but more compliant use of medication. The benefits are self-evident, not least from reduced side-effects.

Perhaps the most ambitious use of CBT and schizophrenia was by Barraclough and colleagues (2001), who took on that most difficult group of people who have both substance abuse problems and schizophrenia. The key seemed to be the use of motivational interviewing to engage the person into their own medium- and long-term care. Over a 12-month period, the combined CBT and motivational interviewing group did very much better on improved social functioning, reduced symptoms and considerably lowered substance misuse.

If people with mental disorders were more like surgical patients, with a well-defined problem, with known natural history and outcome, then perhaps we might mirror the surgeon's 'technology', though without a psychosocial approach surgical patients do less well (Pritchard *et al.* 2004a–c). But life is messy and made more complex when the person's functioning is disrupted by the bio-psychosocial disorder we call schizophrenia. The question therefore is can schizophrenia be cured?

Perhaps the question of 'cure' can be answered by the poet: 'Call no man happy till he be dead' says Solon, but this is not being miserable, just careful and avoiding hubris. Professor Max Hamilton, a doyen of British psychiatry, used to say 'medicine seldom cures, improves often but should comfort always', so too with social work and psychiatry when working with people with schizophrenia. The textbooks suggest that approximately 30 per cent of people never have a second episode, another 30 per cent have other episodes but without too many dysfunctional effects, while about a further third of people have protracted damaged lives. Yet the evidence is that this last group can be helped more than this dismal figure suggests, while the wisest thing Sigmund Freud ever said was 'work binds people to reality', so we should always consider the psychosocial benefits of being involved in employment. Furthermore, we must consider as part of a wider psychosocial approach to schizophrenia, and relevant to any mental disorder, issues of day care and housing.

Day care and housing support

Catty *et al.* (2001), in the usual excellent Cochrane review on the value of day care, report many studies with positive outcomes. Giving a structured day to the unemployed person with schizophrenia also gives a degree of 'relief' for the supporting families. The reviewers, as always, are cautious, not least because there were few RCTs of day care versus no day care, but this should be seen as part of the armoury of intervention to assist both the person and their family.

With regard to the person's accommodation, Rebecca Pritchard, former Service Director of Centrepoint, explores issues of housing and mental disorder in Chapter 13. But it is a timely reminder when considering psychosocial intervention for schizophrenia not to forget housing issues. A Cochrane review by Chilvers *et al.* (2002) is very positive about the part assisted housing support can play, but cautions against the potential inadvertent risk of making the person 'dependent' upon professionals. This is an important consideration in a condition that can make a major impact upon their lives. Therefore, we cannot think in terms of 'cure' of schizophrenia, rather improvement and prevention of further breakdown or, where the stressors have overwhelmed the person, an active preventative approach to reduce these stressors. This is not a counsel of despair for just a brief recall of 20 or 30 years ago shows us just how much the situation has improved when an integrated bio-psychosocial model of intervention is used. This leads us to consider what psychiatrists perhaps with unfortunate language call 'treatment-resistant schizophrenia' and the problems that can follow from this.

'Treatment-resistant' schizophrenia and threat of violence

It is suggested that between 5 and 20 per cent of people with schizophrenia do not respond to the anti-psychotic medication (Kane 1996). Such people have the unfortunate designation of 'treatment resistant', whereas we should be describing such situations as treatment failure or limits of treatment, as the term may inadvertently contribute to the further stigmatisation of the mentally disordered.

The Royal College of Psychiatrists explored this problem in a special supplement of the *British Journal of Psychiatry*. It makes sad reading; although it has to be admitted that anti-psychotic medication is the first-line treatment for people with schizophrenia, it showed a marked lack of imagination in its overfocus upon alternative uses of drugs, rather than what Kuipers (1996) was recommending, de facto dealing with the underlying problems.

Kane (1996) highlighted five factors that led, either singly or in combination, to 'refractoriness' (another unfortunate term) to treatment.

1   The drug used is not effective.
2   The impact of adverse effects of the drug used.
3   Non-compliance by the patient of the prescribed drug and/or dosage.
4   Presence of co-morbid conditions, especially substance misuse.
5   Patients who fail to keep up the maintenance phase of treatment, i.e. after initial quite large dosages, small maintenance doses appear to become inadequate.

However, realistically, it has to be recognised that people with schizophrenia, especially those with paranoid schizoid delusions, can be very disturbed and disturbing and, unless and until we can assist the person to manage their life, this behaviour can undermine their future ability to live a normal life again. The last thing we want is the person in the middle of an acute attack of schizophrenia to be so disruptive that they shatter any psychosocial supports they may have and, of course, violence, actual or perceived, is the most disturbing and stigmatising element of all.

Why are people violent, including people with schizophrenia? Essentially for four reasons: (a) they experience threat; (b) they fear they cannot control the situation; (c) pre-emptive or defensive strike; and (d) social stressors, which are often the underlying mechanism in interpersonal violence (Zink and Sill 2004). For the person with schizophrenia with their highly sensitive but impaired perception, it is easy to misinterpret another's reaction to you. Of course, command hallucinations tell the person to strike for some 'psychotic' reason e.g. 'he's the devil, kill him and save the world – this is death, kill them and bring everlasting life to the world'. Yet, in my experience, whenever there has been violence, it is mainly because either I or other people have mishandled the situation, namely we have been insensitive to the person's distress, or we have rushed things, or we have our own macho agenda; male workers are culturally less good at ignoring the 'masculine challenge', to which our boyhood teaches us to react actively. The key, however, in dealing with potentially violent situations is to know the history of the person, for the individual with schizophrenia is, like any other citizen, far more likely to be aggressive if they have a previous history of aggression.

When previous aggression is added to possible paranoid delusions, this is the case in which one takes every precaution and one should not be alone with such a person without an adequate alarm system. Forearmed is forewarned, provided we don't, by our anxious, fearful, subtle aggressive posture, feed in to their anxiety, fear and pre-emptive aggression (Special Hospitals' Treatment Resistant Research Group 1996).

Controversial treatments for people with mental disorders

It is acknowledged that there are treatments still used for mentally disordered people, not just schizophrenia, which merit a brief review. Perhaps the most controversial treatment in psychiatry, mainly associated with mood disorder, but sometimes used for people with schizophrenia, is electroconvulsive therapy (ECT).

Tharyan and Adams (2002), in a brilliant Cochrane review, found few or no benefits for ECT for people with schizophrenia, and it was not as effective as anti-psychotic drugs. Even the claimed short-term benefits of ECT over drugs to bring about symptom reduction was very short-lived. Thus, based upon Tharyan and Adams (2002), there appears to be little evidence for the efficacy of ECT for schizophrenia. However, the converse is true for people with severe mood disorders; when antidepressants don't work, ECT can be life saving in that it reduces the risk of suicide (Sharma 2001; Van der Wurff *et al.* 2003).

Psychosurgery

Two conditions in which psychosurgery might be considered as a last resort and, associated with depression, are people with long-term Parkinson's disease and obsessive–compulsive disorder (OCD) (Montoya *et al.* 2002), which needs to be briefly reviewed, although many feel it is a doubtful treatment regime (Pilgrim and Rogers 1998).

If ECT was not controversial enough, then psychosurgery, with its shades of *A Clockwork Orange* and *One Flew Over the Cuckoo's Nest*, in the words of Aristophanes 'takes the biscuit'. In part, this stemmed from undoubted crude, if not punitive, use of psychosurgery. Classically, these were leucotomies, in which neurosurgeons, at the behest of the psychiatrist, trephined through the frontal lobes of mentally disordered patients considered 'intractable', possibly dangerous to themselves and others, especially staff, and/or it was done as a treatment of last resort. I well remember knowing patients who had received a leucotomy in the 1940s and 1950s, but their 'frontal' disinhibited, sad and pathetic behaviour was almost as much to do with the hideous institutionalisation of those days as the surgery. Worse, at the beginning of my career, leucotomies were still being done, anecdotally, at the behest of 'disciplinary' staff on very dubious grounds. Invariably, the treatment in those dark days was done at the request of someone

as a 'last resort' to help. Or the worst example I saw, was as a de facto disciplinary procedure against Mr Z who, after being threatened with the treatment, was
so mishandled and provoked that his attack on the staff justified his leucotomy.
Today, neither would Mr Z be a long-term patient, nor would the hospital regime
be so oppressive and staff and patients so institutionalised that such behaviour or
treatments would occur.

In parenthesis, when ill-informed people, without experience of the impact of
those old 'Bins', urge that we abandon 'care in the community' and go back to the
'asylums of the good old days', they know little of what they are talking about.
They have not thought through the problem associated with 'cul-de-sac' and the
'corruption of care' (Martin 1984), which bred staff such as Ken Kesey's 'Big
Nurse' in *One Flew Over the Cuckoo's Nest* who, in Orwellian language, used
the words of care and compassion as a form of psychosocial control and often
malignant psychological manipulation. Kesey is a great read; social work students
are asked to 'make a case' for 'Big Nurse' while psychiatry students are asked to
read it and ask themselves if it is familiar in any way.

Yet 'here's the rub': while any treatment is absolute, i.e. irreversible – once
brain tissue is severed or removed, at the present state of knowledge it cannot
be restored – there are major ethical issues in its use. But, and there is always a
but, in some very restricted situations, there may be a justifiable case for psychosurgery, based of course upon evidence that it is more effective than alternative
treatments.

Stereotactic psychosurgery is used outside the mental health field in severe
cases of epilepsy and the severe late stage of Parkinson's disease, with claims of
up 50 per cent improvement, and it is worthwhile considering as a minority of such
people also have an accompanying mental disorder (Carr *et al.* 2003; Molinuevo
et al. 2003; Weintraub *et al.* 2003). The main benefits arise from reduction in
tremors and rigidity, thus improving the person's quality of life (Vitek *et al.* 2003),
although not everyone is convinced. Sometimes the overall benefits are not as
long-lasting as the patient hopes and, if there are minor adverse affects, this may
make the procedure 'not worth it' (Short *et al.* 2003). However, what all agree
on is that such patients have to be carefully selected so, on the one hand, these
people are at the extreme of OCD and therefore have been 'harder to treat' but,
on the other, it is a great benefit to some. When it works, it can be a most moving
experience for staff and patient.

Today, 'psychosurgery' for psychiatric conditions in Britain only occurs for
severe and intractable OCD, and is only allowed after very careful selection and
all other treatments have failed. 'Informed consent' is taken very seriously, and
permission to proceed is given only after the most stringent checks. However,
there are claims of good improvements in about 40–60 per cent of patients with
mild or no adverse neurological or cognitive outcomes (Montoya *et al.* 2002;
Gabriels *et al.* 2003; Kim *et al.* 2003).

At the 'extreme', psychosurgery was given to five people who had a history of
severe self-mutilation, associated with OCD or schizoaffective disorder. In very
carefully selected cases, minimal limbic unilateral leucotomy was found to be

very effective in four of the five people (Price *et al.* 2001). Small numbers but 100 per cent for four out of the five people and their families.

We need to maintain an open mind, for certainly I have seen one or two OCD patients over the years whose lives have been positively transformed by stere-otactic surgery, but the doubts must remain. The issue is the irreversible nature of the treatment and the need for psychiatrists in particular to remain open minded for, on two occasions in the 1960s and 1970s, the psychiatrist's, rather than the neurosurgeon's, enthusiasms for 'high-tech' medicine led to patients undergoing psychosurgery for perhaps mixed motives. That possibly could not happen today but what is clear is that there is much we do not understand in this area. For example, neurosurgery is not an uncommon treatment for intractable unstable epilepsy and, of course, such epilepsy can lead to death. A study from Japan on 226 patients with unstable epilepsy showed that, over a period of 15 years, 28 per cent of these patients also had psychiatric disorders, mainly mood disorders but some neurotic–behavioural disorders. After primary neurosurgery for the epilepsy, 22 out of 61 patients were free of their psychiatric symptoms up to two years after surgery, but these patients' psychiatric symptoms appeared to be linked to seizures. Thirty-nine patients continued to suffer from mental disorder, mainly of the neurotic–behaviourally disordered type, eight of whom got worse (Inoue and Mihara 2001). It is difficult to draw any firm conclusions and, therefore, certainly with OCD, until our psychosocial and pharmacological treatments improve, in extreme irresolvable cases, then perhaps, maybe, psychosurgery can be an option; certainly if, with careful explanation and selection, etc., the person wishes to be considered for such a treatment. Moreover it is known that there is an enormously important role post-surgery for a counsellor/specialist nurse, for much of the associated psychosocial distress following major neurosurgery is substantially reducible and much is preventable (Pritchard *et al.* 2004a,b).

Long-term psychotherapy

It will be considered 'controversial' to suggest that psychotherapy may be considered to be a controversial treatment but, in the continued pursuit of social justice and evidence-based practice, the key question of effectiveness places long-term psychotherapy in the controversial category. Furedi's (2003) book speaks of 'The curse of the talking cure', and the strength of his argument comes from (a) the reluctance or inability of the long-term psychotherapies, especially those of an ego-dynamic orientation, to establish an evidence-based practice and (b) the association with the problem of the vested interest of the therapist when fees are related to the extent of the therapy. It is the exact opposite of Szasz's position that one can only 'trust' the professional if as it were he/she is controlled by the market – the 'cash nexus'. In a very detailed Cochrane systematic review looking at studies exploring the use of an ego-dynamic or psychoanalytical approach for either schizophrenia or severe mental illness, Malmberg and Fenton (2001) found no evidence that these approaches were superior to other treatment methods. In most cases, the approach was less effective, and being time-consuming, was generally more expensive. The term 'worried well' is sometimes used to describe the kind of person who enters long-term 'psychotherapy', who subjectively may well feel benefits. So be it and this must be a 'good thing'. However, in terms of schizophrenia and other severe dysfunctional mental disorders, it seems that the psychoanalytic type of treatments are of questionable value. Moreover, in view of the century of psychoanalytic treatments, one might have thought that there would be a substantial body of empirical evidence that not only does psychoanalysis resolve these problems but it would be as good if not superior to an integrated bio-psychosocial approach. But there is no such evidence. For the anxiety, social phobias, etc., people, if they can afford it, may receive benefit from the approach, but it is not a treatment recommended for the serious mental disorders (Malmberg and Fenton 2001).

In parenthesis, I was not always so sceptical about the ego-dynamic approach, and still find the concept of defence mechanisms invaluable. In the early 1970s, examining the 'Family dynamics of school phobics' an 'oedipal pattern of mother–son and father–daughter alliances' was identified (Pritchard and Ward 1974), but later it was appreciated that there was a far simpler and probably more accurate explanation for why, within a warring family, mothers and sons are in opposition to the father, the discontented husband. This of course was in the days before divorce was made relatively easy for the average family (1971); prior to that, families had little choice but to live on in state of emotional siege and, although modern divorce has its casualties (Hetherington 2005), in the 1970s very often the children were the battleground between warring parents. Now, here is the paradox, the great Hans Eysenck wrote a paper on the outcome of psychotherapy (1953). The paper was written in German and, although he was initially cautious in his comments, he later began to refer to his 'research' without any qualifications and damned psychoanalysis out of hand (1964). Many people who had never read Eysenck's original work cited it as proof that ego-dynamic treatments did not work. He was challenged by Durressen and Jorswieck (1962), again in a German paper, about his faulty methodology and his bias in his conclusions of an early meta-analysis. A colleague and I translated the Durressen and Jorswieck paper into English in 1976, but the *British Journal of Social Work* felt the issue was somewhat dated and 'historical' (translation available on request from the author). Eysenck's methodology was hugely flawed, yet this paper is often cited by the anti-psychoanalytic 'lobby'. However, as the long promised empirical comparative outcomes studies have not emerged from this approach, one might conclude that Eysenck was right for the wrong reasons.

It must be remembered that these are not 'academic' trivia, for one of the 'complications' of schizophrenia and the other mental disorders is that they can lead to the fatal outcome of suicide, a topic that will be explored in some depth.

Part III
The emergency perspectives

10 Mental health social work with 'suicidal' people

Objectives: by the end of the chapter you should:

1 understand the multiple factors contributing to suicide;
2 recognise the difference between suicidal and 'deliberate self-harm' (DSH) behaviour;
3 be able to make judgements about risk;
4 be aware of the potential distortion of misunderstanding ethnic factors in the suicidal behaviour;
5 be better prepared to work with DSH 'survivors' and the families of people bereaved by suicide.

What do people feel like when they are contemplating suicide? The following poets tell us.

> To be, or not to be – that is the question:
> Whether 'tis nobler in the mind to suffer
> The slings and arrows of outrageous fortune,
> Or to take arms against a sea of troubles,
> And by opposing end them? . . .
> For who would bear the whips and scorns of time,
> The oppressor's wrong, the proud man's contumely,
> The pangs of despised love, . . .
> The insolence of office, . . .
> When he himself might his quietus make
> With a bare bodkin?
>
> (*Hamlet*, 3.1)

> Oh it was pitiful!
> Near a whole city full,
> Home she had none. . .
> Mad from life's history,
> Glad to death's mystery,
> Swift to be hurled. Anywhere, anywhere
> Out of the world!
>
> (Thomas Hood 1799–1845, *The Bridge of Sighs*)

Hamlet's famous soliloquy in which he debates whether or not to commit suicide in response to a 'sea of troubles' illustrates a core theme underlying most suicidal behaviour, the desire to free oneself from overwhelming stresses. Shakespeare, always psychologically authentic, describes the emotional reasons that lead Hamlet to consider making 'his quietus'. Suicide is essentially a reaction to either internal psychical or extrapsychical pressures. Hamlet went on to rehearse the moral dilemma of his time, when suicide was a 'cardinal sin' and perpetrators would be consigned to hell. This is still the case in theological terms with the Orthodox and Catholic churches, although the strength of such religious anathema varies in different countries (Neeleman *et al.* 1997; Pritchard 1999; Pritchard and Baldwin 2000; Lau and Pritchard 2001). This can still lead to someone who has committed suicide being buried outside 'holy ground', e.g. in Greece. Although the Bible makes no specific moral comment about suicide, suicide is condemned in the Koran and remains a virtual taboo in Islam and is even more stigmatised in Islamic countries than in traditional Christian countries (Pritchard and Amunullah 2006).

Hamlet's position is highly personal, however, as in his 'psychological perturbation' (Schneidmann 1985), he confronts his torment alone, as he assumes no-one else had any responsibility. Yet less than 50 years later, John Donne could write 'Any man's death diminishes me because I am involved in Mankind; and therefore never send to know for whom the bell tolls; it tolls for thee.'

This acknowledges the range of social factors, and Thomas Hood's view of suicide is highly social, as he contemplates the plight of a homeless young woman's desperate response to her 'life's history' being ignored by a whole city. His compassion for the victim is only matched by his castigation of the rest of us, who pass by and do nothing to alleviate her misery. Hood's approach was before Durkheim's great insight that suicide, the most personal of actions, was nevertheless influenced by social factors. Durkheim's classic seminal sociological text *Le Suicide* (1868) demonstrated something we now take as self-evident, namely that changes in death rates are indicative of social changes for better or worse. For example, declines in European infant mortality came through better pre- and antenatal care, and currently in the UK the rate is six per thousand, whereas in Sierra Leone the rate is 116 per thousand (WHO 2001–5), a good example of how mortality rates reflect societal conditions.

Modern attitudes to suicide vary, although cultures are still strongly influenced by their relatively recent past, so that, even after 70 years of assertive secular government, the former Soviet Union countries' attitudes to suicide still reflect the earlier traditions of Islamic and Russian Orthodox faiths (Wasserman *et al.* 1994). Yet students in modern secular Britain have often initially asserted that they believe in the possibility of 'rational suicide', invariably citing terminal illness and old age as epitomising such a logical course of action.

Practice teaches otherwise. I had thought that suicide could be a rational act until former clients raised serious questions, which undermined my previous sense of certainty.

'Mr X' (62 years) was a rich, highly educated and independent man. He took the greatest care to kill himself because of four 'natural shocks that flesh is heir to'. He had terminal cancer, and had been given less than six months to live; his son had bankrupted the family business and was in prison; his daughter had been killed in a road accident; and his wife had left him because she could not cope with these disasters. By an amazing fluke, he was discovered and, with barely minutes to spare, he was resuscitated. On gaining consciousness, he was furious and asserted his human right to do with his life as he wished. The professor of psychiatry told him that 'anybody who tries to kill themselves is, in my book, mentally ill and my job is to treat the mentally ill'. A furious row ensued but, threatened with being 'sectioned' under the 1959 Mental Health Act (MHA), Mr X was bullied into been seen by one of the professor's 'nice young men'. I was mortified by such imposition of treatment but, after an equally stormy altercation, the professor insisted that I act as directed under the MHA and offer Mr X treatment. I did so largely in the hope of protecting Mr X from any further indignity. Mr X, being an honourable man, took his antidepressants as agreed and as an act of kindness agreed that I should work with him. This led to Mr X being discharged sooner than expected, and I continued to maintain supportive contact with him, in part to protect him from any further professional imposition.

Some months later, the professor shared with me a letter written to both of us:

Dear Professor Hamilton and Colin,

The pain is well controlled and they have revived their estimates and I've probably got another two or three months. Thank you both very much, life is very precious, I must have been 'mad'.

Mr X died three months to the day later and the professor and I attended his funeral. I was wiser and humbled as Mr X had come to terms with his losses and, with great gallantry, contentedly enjoyed his last weeks of life.

The second lesson to make one pause was the case of Mr Z (56 years), who was also in a terminal state with a very atypical but rapid dementia.

'Mr Z' had changed, within a space of eight months, from being a kind, caring, loving husband who was a pillar of the community to becoming an obscene parody of his former self, unkempt, aggressive, unruly, cognitively deteriorating at a remarkable rate, as he made sexual overtures to any adjacent female. We feared for the physical safety of his slightly built wife, facing this severely psychologically disabled truculent prop-forward-sized man as, after being frustrated over trivia, he had beaten her – totally out of character.

The 30-year-old marriage, which had been the epitome of devotion, was now a living hell as, on the one hand, Mr Z defied any firm diagnosis but continued to deteriorate psychologically and physically and, on the other, had becoming a frightening bully for both family and staff.

'Mrs Z' refused our offer to admit him, and we began to plan a compulsory admission against the wishes of Mrs Z because we feared for her safety. Our only 'comfort' was that, at this rate of deterioration, he was not expected to live more than a few months.

In a window of opportunity of being unattended, Mr Z took a massive overdose and was comatosed. At midnight, the family faced me with the emergency decision of calling for an ambulance for the apparently dying man, who had hastened his end in an apparent islet of sanity, according to a scrawled note, to save his wife from the violent man he had become.

Very reluctantly, for I thought I was putting the wife through further trauma, I called the ambulance. Mr Z was successfully resuscitated, although I learned that Mrs Z felt like Kent in *King Lear*, who would have said 'let him pass! He hates him that would upon the rack of this rough world stretch him out longer.'

Mr Z made a full physical recovery, but it was clear that some of the family, and perhaps colleagues, felt I really was 'stretching him out longer'.

Because of the nature of Mr Z's brain disease, there were three different university professors who were very interested in the forthcoming post-mortem – a psychiatrist, a neurologist and an endocrinologist, as well the psychiatric social worker – as there were some interesting diagnostic prognostications to be confirmed.

After some months, it became apparent that, against all expectations, Mr Z had stopped deteriorating; indeed, after about three months, he began to improve. Within six months, he exhibited clear cognitive improvements and, within a year, Mr Z had reverted to the kind, considerate, loving family man that he had been previously. While there was a degree of residual slight disinhibition, so that he was quietly jovial, rather than his previous shy gentle self, he made a full recovery. He did not return to work, taking early retirement, and then went on to complete an Open University degree, fulfilling a lifetime ambition.

The irony of this situation was that Mr Z outlived two of those university professors, while this practitioner had learned a very important lesson. We must always give our client another chance for, as Hamlet said: 'There are more things in heaven and earth, Horatio, than are dreamt of in your philosophy.' Sometimes we are not only wrong, we do not know sufficient about the particular individual to make such de facto 'total' judgements, for we 'experts' can get it wrong.

In a research project, I came across the case of a 68-year-old widow, comatosed following a major subarachnoid haemorrhage (SAH), which is a special type of stroke (Pritchard et al. 2001). 'Mrs Y' was very seriously ill, with a massive bleed, and she was being nursed in a non-specialist general hospital as there were major bed pressures on the regional neurological unit, and it was thought that, even using the 'intensive care' ambulance, she was not fit to be moved. The neurologist, genuinely thinking of the best for patient and family after three weeks of no apparent improvement, suggested closing down the life-support machines. The family, i.e. sons and daughters, were outraged and insisted that she continue to be treated.

Nine months later, Mrs Y completed my questionnaire about her experience of an SAH!

We now know that, with appropriate and timely help, even large SAH bleed patients can and do make a very good recovery with major or total psychosocial recovery (Pritchard et al. 2004b). Yet this lady, in many a well-meaning professional's view, had no life that was worth preserving and in effect at that time was expendable.

We need to be extremely careful not to judge other people's situations as if they were our own for, in all probability, many people under 40 years old might think that a seriously ill person of 68 years with cancer might very well be better cared for with minimal or no intrusive treatment. But not if you are the 68-year-old!

The problem is that there is evidence that people with apparently terminal disease such as some cancers and quite elderly people, 85 years plus, only express the wish to die when the pain is poorly controlled and/or they feel neglected, excluded and rejected (Draper and Anstey 1996; Duckworth and McBride 1996; Linden and Barnow 1997; Agbayewa et al. 1998). A significant number of people with malignant disease become depressed, not so much reactively, but a co-morbid clinical depression, which responds positively to antidepressant treatment (Bottomley 1998; Berard 2001; Jones 2001).

Some of the poets have mused sentimentally over death:

> I have been half in love with easeful death,
> Called him soft names in many a mused rhyme . . .
> Now more than ever seems it rich to die,
> To cease upon the midnight with no pain.
> (Keats 1795–1821, *Ode to a Nightingale*)

Wordsworth paints an almost sentimental picture of the death of Chatterton, a young poet:

> I thought of Chatterton the marvellous boy,
> The sleepless soul that perished in his pride. . .
> We poets in our youth begin in gladness
> But thereof comes in the end despondency and madness.
> (*Resolution and Independence*)

Hence, some students of English may feel that death is sanitised and self-inflicted death acceptable. Yet the reality of death is often foul. The impulsive young homeless person who ingests the caustic fluid; the young man, desperate with unrequited love and in a semi-drunken frenzy, wishes to hurt and be hurt 'to show her', dies in front of the hurtling lorry; the rejected young mother whose refuge is in alcohol mixes it with sleeping tablets and dies in her own vomit; the homeless vagrant, whose now decomposed body confounds the mystery of how he died; while the desperate businessman, in a moment of frenzy, thinks the soft waters of the river will ease his pain, as he jumps 60 feet and dies not of drowning but of multiple fractures.

The message must be that we always offer the person in distress another chance. True, I have lost clients from suicide, more anon, and sometimes felt a sad acceptance that at last they are at some sort of peace, but realised that they died mainly because our treatment for their madness was just not good enough. If we eased up on the fight against death, where would be the stimulus, the spur, to reach out to another person in despair which, at the present state of knowledge, we cannot ease, to continue our research to seek to give them the help they need?

There are always dangers in drawing historical precedents out of context, but Nazi Germany was quite happy to 'accept' suicide as a form of 'natural health cleansing' as 'inferior people slaughtered themselves', thus improving the 'purity of the race' (Retterstol 1993). Not that anyone today would countenance such a perspective.

Problems of definition and extent of the problem

But what is suicide and, nationally, just how big a problem is it? In British law, it is a legal definition rather than a diagnosis and is determined by a coroner rather than a physician, although many coroners are medically trained. Like a crime, there need to be two established facts, the *actus reus* (guilty act – the killing) and the *mens rea* (guilty intent). Thus, while it is often relatively easy to determine that the person killed themselves, the question also has to be decided, did they intend to do so?

'Suicides' therefore end up in one of two WHO mortality categories, 'suicide' where the coroner's court decides it was an intended self-killing, or 'other violent deaths', which contains undetermined deaths as well as 'open verdicts'. As suicide still carries a degree of stigma in most Western countries, and completely so in the vast majority of Islamic countries, it is believed that most countries suicide rates are probably under-reported. In part, this occurs because coroners often seek to ameliorate the family's bereavement if there are any doubts (Kolmos and Bach 1987; Maris *et al.* 1992). This may explain why suicide rates vary so greatly between countries; Table 10.1 lists the latest figures available for five continents.

Traditionally, the highest male rates have been in Finland and Hungary, currently 323 per million (p.m.) and 445 p.m. respectively (WHO 2001–5). Although the rate in Japan, at 365 p.m., has historically always been high, it fell throughout the 1970s and 1980s, but has returned to previous highs following recent economic difficulties in the country (Aihara and Iki 2002).

However, more countries are now reporting to the WHO and the highest male rate was in Russia at 693 p.m. and Belarus at 603 p.m., perhaps reflecting the turmoil over the past decade.

The lowest male rates have traditionally been in Greece, Portugal and Spain followed by England and Wales. However, since the two Iberian countries rid themselves of dictatorial regimes and with more honest reporting, they have shown rises year on year since the change. Greece is still the lowest at 53 p.m. men and 9 p.m. women, with England and Wales at 98 p.m. and 28 p.m.

For general interest, the 'cultural' issue of how countries report suicide is seen in Table 10.1 where for example 'Catholic' Mexico report rates of 63 and 13 p.m. for men and women, but more 'honest' Chile reports 182 p.m. and 30 p.m. for women. In parenthesis, the probability of internal variations in reporting suicide is seen in the fact that, apart from Greece (53 p.m.), a Greek Orthodox country, and 'Catholic' Mexico at 63 p.m., all other Catholic countries have higher suicide rates than 'Protestant' secular England and Wales. However, in the 1970s, 'Catholic' Ireland, Italy and Spain used to report lower male rates than the Anglo-Welsh, but their current disclosure seems to reflect changing attitudes to suicide in the more traditional countries (Cantor *et al.* 1997; De Leo *et al.* 1997).

The Islamic taboo on suicide is seen in the figures for Egypt, 1 p.m. and 0 p.m. (36 and 13 cases only), and Kuwait, but the former Soviet Islamic countries give the game away, showing that suicide crosses all cultural boundaries as Islamic Kazakhstan has rates of 502 p.m. and 88 p.m., and Uzbekistan has rates

Table 10.1 World suicide rates (per million) by gender, 2002 (C, mainly Catholic country; O, Orthodox; I, Islamic)

Country and year[a]	Males	Females	Male–female ratio
Australia (2001)	201	53	3.79
Belarus O (2001)	603	93	6.48
Austria C	305	87	3.51
Belgium C (1997)	312	114	2.74
Bulgaria O	256	83	3.08
Canada (2000)	184	52	3.54
Chile C (2001)	182	30	6.07
Czech Republic C	245	61	4.02
Denmark (1999)	214	74	2.89
Egypt I (2000)	1 (36)	0 (13)	2.77
England and Wales	98	28	3.50
Finland	323	102	3.17
France C (2000)	279	95	2.94
Germany (2001)	204	70	2.91
Greece O (2001)	53	9	5.89
Hong Kong (PRC) (2000)	161	101	1.59
Hungary C	455	122	3.73
Ireland C (2001)	214	41	5.22
Italy C (2001)	111	33	3.36
Japan	352	128	2.75
Kazakhstan I (2001)	502	88	5.70
Kyrgyzstan I (2001)	191	41	4.78
Korea (Republic)	247	112	2.21
Kuwait (2000)	16	16	1.00
Mexico C (2001)	63	13	4.85
Netherlands (2003)	127	59	2.15
New Zealand (2000)	198	42	4.71
Norway (2001)	184	60	3.07
Poland C	266	50	5.32
Portugal C	189	49	3.86
Romania C	239	47	5.09
Russia Federation O	693	119	5.82
Scotland	197	59	3.34
Singapore (2001)	115	69	1.67
Spain C (2001)	122	37	3.30
Sweden	189	81	2.33
Switzerland (2000)	278	108	2.57
Ukraine O	407	84	5.56
UK	108 (3,124)	31 (942)	3.48
USA (2000)	171	40	4.28
Uzbekistan I (2000)	118	38	3.11

Source: WHO (2005).

Notes
Brazil and China currently unavailable.
a   All 2002 unless stated otherwise.

higher than the Anglo-Welsh at 118 p.m. for men and 38 p.m. for women. This strongly implies that suicide is a reality in Islamic societies but it is hidden, and this has practical implications when working with Islamic families (Pritchard and Amunullah 2006).

Before we congratulate ourselves on the low numbers of suicides in England and Wales, it should be noted that 3,124 men and 942 women killed themselves in the UK (2002), which exceeds the tragic 9/11 toll of 3,074 innocent victims. Moreover, we must remember that these figures represent individual tragedies of lives snuffed out. Furthermore, the toll of suicide does not just stop with the deceased, but the relatives left behind are locked into an irresolvable guilt at 'what went wrong'; Edwin Schneidmann (1985) has suggested that, for every single suicide, there will be as many as ten seriously grieving and affected people, which gives a further twist to the bald figures.

However, there is one other awkward fact about defining and counting suicides. Not all people who intended to die, died in the incident and, sadly, not all people who actually died definitely wanted to die, which in a sense was an 'accident'. This is often related to an impulsive act under stress, and the person, especially the younger person, did not appreciate the lethality of the method used. In part, this is one reason why medical doctors, dentists, nurses and farmers in Britain have a disproportionately high suicide rate because they have easier access to more lethal means; occupation matters (Koskinen *et al.* 2002)!

Nonetheless, it can be said with confidence that the levels of reported suicide in most countries are an underestimate rather than the reverse and, in the USA, with its easy access to firearms, there were more than 10 times as many suicide deaths as deaths on 9/11, 32,000+ to 3,074 (Pritchard and Wallace 2006); indeed, for every major Western country, suicide remains a major public health problem and now exceeds road deaths for at least the last five years (Pritchard 2002).

An important practical issue in a multicultural society is that different religious and cultural groups have different attitudes to suicide (Neeleman *et al.* 1997). This may account for Greece having the lowest reported self-killing in the West, as in rural areas suspected suicides are still buried outside 'hallowed' ground (Madianou and Economou 1994) – shades of the 'churlish priest' attitude to Hamlet's Ophelia: 'her death was doubtful'. Though to be fair, suicide was still a criminal indictable offence in Britain up to 1961 and, of course, assisting someone to die is still a criminal offence. Nevertheless, old ideas still persist and, when working with Islamic families, one has to be especially sensitive, lest inadvertently one causes offence; yet if working with a translator, it is vitally important that they understand the nature of your questions, not to condemn but rather to save someone from the extreme consequences of either severe depression or an episode of schizophrenia.

Supervising a student's mental health caseload, the social worker was doubly keen to eschew any of the remotest trace of racism and concentrated upon 30-year-old 'Ali's' experience of racial intolerance. On more careful questioning, however, it transpired that Ali had successfully integrated into British society following his family's expulsion from Kenya. He had a successful education and held a good job for a number of years. But, similar to his mother, he had developed a depressive illness, which went unrecognised, as did the fact that his elder brother had probably died from suicide. Careful liaison with the family and the GP resulted in Ali accepting antidepressants, with very positive results.

This is not an uncommon error for while, self-evidently, institutional racism exists, it can blind us to other problems experienced by people from a culture different from our own.

'Mr XX' was a successful Asian businessman, respected and revered in his community and by his business associates. When he began to express ideas of persecution, it was far too easy not to think through what he was presenting. His unrecognised and undiagnosed schizophrenia had terrible consequences. In response to command delusions, he sought to protect his family from the coming end of the world and, after killing his wife and children, killed himself.

Membership of an ethnic minority is not a safeguard against mental disorder; indeed, recent research on female attempted suicide found that racial intolerance as a cause of the women's deliberate self-harm was far less important than intrafamily or interpersonal relationship problems (Brugha *et al.* 1997). A simple perusal of Table 10.1 shows that cultural factors are far more complex and that we should rid ourselves of a number of stereotypes, e.g. that Sweden has a particularly high suicide rate, whereas in fact it has always been considerably higher than that of England and Wales but, since the mid-1970s, Sweden's rate has been generally falling, while our rate has fluctuated, in part with unemployment rates, and is still higher than the earlier rate, especially for young male adults (Pritchard 1988, 1992b,d; Pritchard and Hansen 2005a), as shown in Table 10.2. (Note the differences between the 1970s and the average of 2000–2 rates, especially for the younger males aged 15–34 in England and Wales.)

Interestingly, Japan's recent rate is up almost a third on what their male rate was in the 1970s and 1980s, a very good indicator of the Durkheimian thesis of social change influencing mortality rates, dramatically seen in the astronomical rates of the Russian Federation, Belarus and Ukraine.

Table 10.2 Three-year average annual suicide rates by age and gender in England and Wales, 1974–6 versus 2000–2 (numbers and rates per million)

	Age (years)								
	15–24	25–34	35–44	45–54	55–64	65–74	75+	All ages
Men								
1974–6								
Number	203	358	326	474	409	359	150	2,280
Rate	63	112	120	152	156	178	197	96
2000–2								
Number	246	569	571	471	294	195	192	2,541
Rates	77	150	148	138	107	95	132	99
1974–2002 ratio of rates	1.22	1.34	1.23	0.91	0.69	0.53	0.67	1.03
Women								
1974–6								
Number	97	169	202	348	320	323	159	1,619
Rate	30	51	72	111	113	128	95	64
2000–2								
Numbers	68	136	173	140	104	97	132	850
Rates	22	35	45	40	39	42	53	32
1974–2002 ratio of rates	0.73	0.69	0.63	0.36	0.35	0.33	0.56	0.50

Main factors associated with suicide

It must be stressed that suicide is multicausal and, when we come to individual cases, we sometimes can find no apparent reason for the death – hence we are generalising.

In the West, and we must stress we are mainly focusing on research from Westernised countries, the biggest single factor is gender (Beautrais *et al.* 2003; WHO 2001–5). The suicide rate is lower among females than among males, ranging in the West from 1:2.15 in the Netherlands to 1:5.82 in the Russian Federation; the UK female–male ratio is 1:4.28. Interestingly, this male bias in suicide is almost completely reversed in the People's Republic of China (Pritchard 1996a). Nonetheless, for practitioners in all the other countries, including Catholic and Islamic, we need to remember this male bias.

Next is age. Tables 10.2 and 10.3, showing suicide rates by age and gender in England and Wales, illustrate a general pattern of suicide in the West, namely that suicide rates usually rise in each successive decade, are lowest in adolescents and young adult males (15–24) and usually highest in elderly males (75+) (Duckworth and McBride 1996; Pritchard and Baldwin 2000, 2002; Lau and Pritchard 2001; WHO 2001–5). However, the trouble with research is that new data mean a rewriting of the textbooks and, recently, suicides among the elderly, especially women, have fallen dramatically, expecially in Britain, so that today the highest rate of suicide is among 50- to 64-year-olds (Pritchard and Hansen 2005b).

Thus, we see that the suicide rates have fallen substantially among both elderly men and women, whereas those among the male 'youth and young adults' group (15–34 years) have risen significantly, and suicide rates among women of all age ranges have fallen. Why this is is unknown, but one speculates that it may reflect something of the improved morale of women following their improved emancipation since the early 1960s. However, as can be seen in Table 10.3, this phenomenon of increased suicide rates among young men and reduced suicide rates among young women is found throughout most Western countries.

However, as has already been said, suicide rates follow changes in society, and one link is unemployment, which is associated with suicidal behaviour (Platt 1984; Pritchard 1988, 1992b,d; Agerbo *et al.* 2003; Blakely *et al.* 2003; Qin *et al.* 2003). Table 10.3 covers the period before the oil crisis of 1973, i.e. when Arab states began to charge an economic cost for their oil, rather than perpetuate the former colonial system, which was associated with sudden and massive rises in unemployment in the West. Although it should be reiterated that unemployment is itself associated with 'confounding' features of more mental disorder and membership of an ethnic minority, and the chronic socioeconomically disadvantaged (Hunt *et al.* 2003; Qin *et al.* 2003).

After gender and age come a series of associations that overlap and compound the risk for individuals in the various categories.

Most important, some would say the next most important, is mental disorder. Study after study shows that suicide can often be the extreme consequence of mental disorder (Appleby *et al.* 1999; Harris and Barraclough 1998; Cavanagh *et al.* 2003), the mood disorders, severe depression rather than anxiety disorders

(Chioqueta and Stiles 2003; Waern *et al.* 2003). This is always made worse by the co-morbidity of alcohol or drugs misuse (Conner *et al.* 2003; Hawton *et al.* 2003), followed by schizophrenia (Bentall 2003; Potkin *et al.* 2003), which is perhaps not surprising as a recent study found that as many as 22 of 100 people with firm ICD diagnoses of schizophrenia experienced 'command hallucinations for suicide' (Harkvy-Friedman *et al.* 2003). If we include the 'personality disorders', adolescents diagnosed as personality-disordered, who developed depression in adulthood, died at twice the rate of non-diagnosed young people (Johnson *et al.* 1999). If we include the substance misusers in the category of mental disorder, then the assumption of some policy-makers that 90 per cent of all suicides are related to mental disorder gets very close (Department of Health 2002). However, I think this is an overestimate, for there are some social factors that predominate and then precipitate a reactive depression, which are initially social rather than a psychiatric illness. This is yet another indication of the overlap and interaction between the so-called medical and social models.

There are some very helpful results from Sweden where health registration methods were used to explore suicides over a 20-year period (1949–69) yielding 8,396 people (Runeson and Asberg 2003). Bearing in mind the heavy weighting of depression, which does not have a strong genetic component, as well as of the schizophrenias, which do, the findings regarding subsequent suicide of first-degree relatives are very informative (Freedman *et al.* 2001; Carter *et al.* 2002; Jones *et al.* 2002). Since 1969, 9.4 per cent of all family relatives died from suicide compared with 4.6 per cent of non-family members. Compared with the current Swedish male suicide rate of 197 per million (p.m.), the controls are very similar at 207 p.m., whereas the familial suicides are 433 p.m., more than twice the 'expected' rate. It highlights the futility of the nature versus nurture argument but unequivocally gives further weight to the interaction of bio-psychosocial factors.

As already indicated, substance abuse, both drugs and alcohol, is also associated with suicide (Jones *et al.* 2002; Conner *et al.* 2003; Hawton *et al.* 2003) but next, in approximate descending order of association, is criminality, as there are disproportionally more suicides among offenders, men and women, than the general population (Pritchard *et al.* 1997b; Towl 1999; Pritchard and Butler 2000b; Coffey *et al.* 2003; Howard *et al.* 2003; Sattar 2003). Amazing in the twenty-first century, however, is the considerable degree of overlap between mental disorder and crime and substance misuse in these cohorts. In effect, they are people with multiple problems, very often stretching back into their childhood and another aspect of the psychiatric–child protection interface (Lyon *et al.* 1996; Pritchard and Butler 2000a,b; Howard *et al.* 2003). One worrying aspect is that many of these offenders, the majority of whom are quite young, under 35, often had some contact with a range of services but seemingly failed to engage with them, which is an essential prerequisite for effective intervention (Ford *et al.* 1997; Pritchard *et al.* 1998). It transpires that typically more of these young adults die within 4 weeks of leaving prison, either from a straight suicide, often an overdose, or from a drug-related death (Jones *et al.* 2002; Bird and Hutchinson 2003).

Table 10.3 Changing youth and young adult suicide rates (per million) by gender, 1973–5 versus 1995–7

Country	GPSR		15–24 years		GPSR versus 15–24, ratio of ratios		25–34 years		GPSR versus 25–34, ratio of ratios	
	Male	Female	Male	Female	Male	Female	Male	Female	Male	Female
Australia										
1973–5	156	75	159	45			167	84		
1999–2001	204	52	213	55			341	76		
Ratio	1.31	0.69	1.42	1.22	1.08	1.77	2.04	0.90	1.56	1.30
Canada										
1973–5	181	70	241	49			232	95		
1998–2000	197	53	214	51			245	57		
Ratio	1.08	0.76	0.89	1.04	0.82	1.37	1.06	0.60	0.98	0.79
England/Wales										
1973–75	93	62	58	29			106	51		
2000–2	100	28	76	19			149	36		
Ratio	1.08	0.45	1.31	0.66	1.21	1.47	1.41	0.71	1.31	1.58
France										
1973–5	227	88	115	48			176	69		
1998–2000	285	94	125	35			260	76		
Ratio	1.26	1.07	0.60	0.73	0.87	0.68	1.48	1.10	1.17	1.03
Germany										
1973–5	276	147	204	74			288	115		
2000–2	203	71	123	29			170	42		
Ratio	0.73	0.48	0.60	0.39	0.82	0.81	0.59	0.37	0.81	0.77

Italy										
1973–5	77	34	31	22			59	30		
1999–2001	111	34	67	16			101	25		
Ratio	1.4	1.00	2.16	0.73	1.50	0.73	1.71	0.76	1.19	0.76
Japan										
1973–5	195	148	195	133			232	151		
2000–2	345	130	150	67			259	111		
Ratio	1.77	0.88	0.77	0.50	0.44	0.57	1.12	0.74	0.63	0.84
Netherlands										
1973–5	105	73	78	26			86	75		
2000–2	129	60	83	27			143	52		
Ratio	1.22	0.82	1.06	1.04	0.87	1.27	1.66	0.69	1.36	0.84
Spain										
1973–5	60	22	19	10			38	12		
1999–2001	126	39	72	13			115	27		
Ratio	2.10	1.77	3.79	1.30	1.80	0.73	3.03	2.25	1.44	1.27
USA										
1973–5	182	66	171	46			233	84		
1998–2000	178	42	176	31			216	43		
Ratio	0.98	0.64	1.03	0.67	1.05	1.05	0.93	0.52	0.95	0.81

Note
GPSR, general population suicide rate.

There are other features, listed below, which in effect have the common theme of creating a stressful situation for the individual and, depending upon their personal circumstances, their biophysical endowment and their psychosocial resources, they are at increased risk of suicide.

Physical illness, either the apparently terminal or long-term chronic, or the impact of an HIV diagnosis, are self-evident and deceptively 'make sense'. However, it must never be forgotten that the vast majority of people in such circumstances do not engage in suicidal behaviour.

The interactive element in suicide is again seen in the raised risk of being homeless (Scott 1993; Bughra 1996; Baker 1997; Eynan *et al.* 2002) and/or living alone, i.e. being isolated (Lipman *et al.* 2001; MacDonald *et al.* 2001; Cairney *et al.* 2003). On reflection it is self-evident that if a person is alone, in the throes of a mood disorder, unsupported, feeling rejected, neglect and there is no-one around to show any care, in desperation, they are more likely to die and a relatively less lethal method, such as drugs, with no-one to intervene is more likely to end fatally. Linked to this theme of isolation is the sequel of divorce/separation, which makes men more vulnerable to suicidal behaviour; again this reflects the emotional crisis that can surround key relationships and/or a troubled situation. Nor should we forget the impact of discharge from an institution, for despite prison being an almost unimaginably terrible place for any human being, as one 'lifer' inmate told us:

> you can get used to anything. It takes about three years, the first year is a mixture of confusion, fear and depression, oh god, especially the depression. That's why you shouldn't let people kill themselves then. It might be different afterwards if they've a really long sentence, death might be preferable.

Bearing in mind the level of frank mental disorder in our prisons, ranging from 10 to 30 per cent, one wonders how psychiatrically depressed the above informant was. Yet leaving the secure structure of prison can be very disorientating, and discharges can end in binge drinking and drugs, sometimes ending fatally (Jones *et al.* 2002; Bride and Real 2003).

There is much more to say about the child protection–psychiatric interface (see Chapter 11) but increasingly it is recognised that victims of child sex abuse are significantly over-represented in psychiatric caseloads and may exhibit suicidal behaviour as adults (Hawton *et al.* 1985; Bagley and Ramsay 1997; Pritchard and King 2004). These issues will be explored more fully, but the link between child neglect and abuse and subsequent psychiatric disorder is the next big practice breakthrough, which will both improve services, i.e. help to break the cycle of abuse, and reduce subsequent mental health problems (Falkov 1996; Pritchard and Stroud 1999; Stroud 2001; Pritchard 2004).

Unemployment

On undertaking a Department of Health (DoH) project to examine drug use among south coast teenagers in 1985, I did not find what the DoH 'politicians' wanted/ expected and reported that the key issue was relative poverty; for some reason, I never heard from the DoH again. However, to try to get a handle on the extent of the seriousness of drug misuse among teenagers, one indicator of the seriousness of such behaviour would be the extreme consequence, namely a death. Examining the local health region and district authority mortality statistics, they had very low numbers. Self-evidently, one youth dying of illegal drugs is one youth too many, but policies are assumed to be about degrees of risk, which underpins the concept of public health. Turning to the British mortality statistics, the WHO confirmed the low death rate over a 20-year period i.e. 1972–84, and to place this in context, this was compared with suicide rates, which recalling from my student days male suicide was about 95 per million. While the early 1970s rate was around 95 p.m., by the mid-1980s it had almost doubled. This was a stark example of the link between suicide and unemployment. A seminal paper by Professor Stephen Platt (1984) had drawn attention to this phenomenon, but the politicians of the day had criticised it because it was too clinically based and not representative of the national situation. By examining changing patterns of national suicide rates with that of unemployment, it was shown that there was a link between national suicide and unemployment rates (Pritchard 1988), which was further demonstrated throughout the Western world (Pritchard 1990, 1992c,d, 1994). Moreover we were able to predict this interactive effect in the later 1990s recession (Pritchard 1994), although there are specific age and gender issues. Namely, it is the youth and young adults who bear the greatest burden of unemployment and also of suicide compared with other age groups (Pritchard 1996b; ILO 2000) a feature that persists today, seen in the raised 'youth and young adult' (15–34 years) rates in most Western countries (Pritchard and Hansen 2005a). This is demonstrated in Table 10.3, which shows the general population suicide rate (GPSR) for the early 1970s and then for the latest year data are available, mainly up to 1999 (WHO 2001–5). The suicide rates for youth (15–24) and young adults (25–34) are shown separately, and in six of the ten largest Western nations, the index of change of young male suicide has worsened significantly compared with the GPSR over the period. It is striking that, despite rates for England and Wales being down close to their early 1970s level, youth (15–24) rates are still 64 per cent and young adults (25–34) 59 per cent higher than in the earlier period. Indeed, increases in the Anglo-Welsh younger male rates are among the worst in the West and, although Italy and Spain are far worse, this may be because of the changes in attitudes to reporting suicide in Latin countries (Cantor *et al.* 1997; De Leo *et al.* 1997). Whereas the Australian rises look valid as they use the British system as do the New Zealanders, youth in both countries suffered especially badly in the early 1990s recession (Pritchard 1992d).

Interestingly, the young male situation is not mirrored in young female suicide rates, which may be linked to the different methods employed by young women. Men are classically much more violent against themselves, and most suicides among men involve hanging, drowning, slashing and jumping, and occasionally shooting or carbon monoxide inhalation from car exhausts; in contrast women mainly use drug overdoses, which has actively been made more difficult over the past decade by moving away from potentially lethal overdosing on antidepressants.

Mental health social work is very demanding, and nothing is more fraught than work with people who are at risk from suicide – that is if we know they are at risk. The late Professor Schneidmann had a very unusual concept that helps to utilise the research knowledge in a client-specific assessment. He used the term 'psychological perturbation'. This consisted essentially of a cognitive set of ideas and feeling.

First, psychic pain or distress; second, psychological restriction – there does not appear to be any alternative; and, third, penchant for action.

This is very useful as it highlights the state of mind of the person, irrespective of the contributory risk factors. It reminds us to consider this client at this moment in time in their specific situation. But, of course, the therapist, social worker, psychologist, etc. needs to be able to establish a meaningful relationship with the person to understand their state of mind for, in most cultures, we do not tell 'strangers' about our distress; in most cultures, the active thought of suicide is unacceptable, so people will hide their serious suicidal ideation. This is why, within the suicide statistics, one meets in the Coroner's courts an entirely unexpected and seemingly purposeless but clear-cut suicide, as the person experienced their psychological perturbation alone and tragically had a penchant for action. The mental health practitioner has to be something of a detective and always be aware of the possibility of suicide, although this does not always work to plan.

I was seeing 'Mr Brown' monthly for a recurrent depression after helping him through his divorce. His depression seemed relatively mild because, for the last decade, he had only lost a few weeks off work, though as he worked mainly by himself, despite his undoubted anxiety and feelings of misery, he could just about cope.

He lived quite close and, as I was going into town with my infant daughter to meet my wife and baby daughter, Mr Brown was there. I felt 'waylaid'. He was very polite but insisted that he needed to see me. I was not pleased but agreed that I could step inside his home but only for ten minutes and promised him that I would bring his next appointment forward to the following Monday morning, thinking I was using the classic structuring response to an overdemanding client. He saw my predicament, a 2-year-old etc., and then apologised profusely, telling me just how much he had appreciated my care and concern over past 18 months and that few people, least of all in his own family, had ever taken so much trouble with him. I stopped thinking, pleased with the compliment, and reassured him we would meet on Monday. As the day progressed, I began to feel that Mr Brown's remarks were almost like a valedictory address and, after discussing the situation with my wife, I returned to Mr Brown in the early evening. There was no answer, his garage door was locked and he seemed not to be at home. It was too late; he had taken all his antidepressants, at a time when they were far more lethal than those prescribed today, and his suicide note, which among other things exonerated me, was no comfort. With hindsight, I should have referred him to the emergency duty team, but then with hindsight we would always be perfect.

Two themes that always seem to exist in the suicide dilemma are a current sense of depression, which often hides a sense of aggression, but is turned against the self, with a sense of rejection. This rejection is two-way. The victim often feels rejected by those and society around them, 'the whole city' was nearby but did nothing, said Thomas Hood, and here is the paradox, we the 'survivors' feel rejected by the suicide – we or our society were so unimportant that they left us – suicide is 'the ultimate rejection'. How this affects the families of suicides will be dealt with later, but few of us can remain neutral when faced with such a stark reality.

The list of contributory factors is long (Table 10.4), and yet a key issue has yet to be discussed, namely 'attempted suicide', which is the problem to which we now turn.

Deliberate self-harm – 'attempted suicide'

Suicide is one piece of behaviour, which in fact is markedly different from 'attempted suicide'. There are crucial differentiating factors, which have profound practical implications. Unfortunately, it does not make practice less difficult, but highlights the need for client-specific judgements to be made, as a previous 'attempted suicide' is a major indicator of risk of actual suicide, although the majority of 'attempted suicides' do not die, although in a lifetime, after one 'attempt', 20 per cent of such people eventually die from suicide (Maris *et al.* 1992).

One important technical matter is that the term 'attempted suicide' is seldom used because it assumes a desired destination, i.e. death. In the 1970s, the term 'parasuicide' was used, but this too seemed to infer a destination or an unfulfilled desired end. For accuracy, and avoiding any 'assumptions' about the person's state of mind, the official and more useful term is 'deliberate self-harm' (DSH). The person has been hurt, it was done by themselves and appeared deliberate, i.e. it was not an accident. As will become clear, while there is an overlap with suicide per se, there are major differences associated with DSH and suicide, but DSH itself is a risk factor in eventual suicide.

The key differences from suicide are that DSH is predominantly a female activity, rather than male, and is done proportionally more by young people, not older, which is the reverse of suicide. It is invariably reactive, whereas suicide can be the result of 'hidden' command delusions, as well as other internal and external psychological stressors. DSH, especially among children and adoles-

Table 10.4 List of factors associated with suicide (not mutually exclusive); psychosocial autopsy (%)

Depression (mainly severe but could be impulsive and reactive)	90
Crucial – a previous deliberate self-harm episode (plus any of the above)	70
Schizophrenia – both acute and chronic	40
Male sex	80
Age – rate increases by decade (being under 30 and female 'protects')	60
Substance abuse (especially if multiple – overlaps with personality disorders)	40
Personality disorder (especially after violent event, either victim or perpetrator)	30
Criminality (range of offenders – overlaps with personality disorders and substance abuse)	25
Physical illness (especially if inadequate support or pain relief)	15
New HIV infections (especially at time of diagnosis)	15
Gay and lesbian youth ('coming out' period still fraught)	15
Access to lethal method (crucial in impulsive actions – guns, high buildings – age linked)	10
Victims of child sexual abuse (CSA) as adults (controversial – see text –males more so)	10
Unemployed (especially the under-35s)	15
Homelessness	15
Isolated living	15
Recent divorce/separation (especially if male)	10
Discharged from long-term institutional care (children's home, prison, etc.)	10
Other high emotional situations (victim of violence, traumatic relationship, unrequited love, frustrated anger)	10
Male child sex abusers (see text on research comparing CSA and mental disorder; suggested CSA four times rate of mentally disordered?)	10

cents, might be thought to be flight from a stressful situation, rather than a flight to death, although DSH among children and adolescents, as well as young adults, is associated with all the 'usual psychosocial suspects' of child neglect and abuse, substance misuse in particular, high emotional tension and especially being the victim of violence, if they are female, or the perpetrator of violence if they are male (Pritchard 1992c; Bagley and Ramsey 1997; Kung *et al.* 2002; Bergen *et al.* 2003; Spirito and Overholser 2003).

A seminal study by Platt *et al.* (1992) explored DSH in 15 different European cities by age and gender; unfortunately, they did not include a British city. It confirmed the marked female and young bias in DSH, but also noted that some cities in the same country had markedly different DSH rates. Utilising Platt *et al.*'s figures, comparing the DSH rates with the national suicide rates and taking the countries closest to the Anglo-Welsh suicide rate, Table 10.5 highlights the different interaction between DSH and suicides (Pritchard 1999).

Overall, average male DSH to suicide was 5:1 and female 19:1. If, however, we take the Dutch city of Leiden figures as closest to British ones, the ratios come down to 4:1 for males and 14:1 for female DSH to suicides. What is striking is

Table 10.5 Comparison of DSH by city with national suicide rates (per million)

City, country and gender	Age (years)					All ages
	15–24	*25–34*	*35–44*	*45–54*	*55+*	
Men						
Padua (Italy)						
DSH	690	1,010	450	430	460	610
Suicide	51	99	92	135	286	112
Ratio	13.5:1	10.2:1	4.9:1	3.2:1	1.6:1	5.5:1
Leiden (Netherlands)						
DSH	720	750	620	530	190	570
Suicide	89	154	156	173	233	130
Ratio	8.1:1	4.9:1	4.0:1	3.1:1	0.8:1	4.4:1
Guipuzcoa (Spain)						
DSH	1,160	650	660	360	400	670
Suicide	84	106	102	149	297	116
Ratio	13.8:1	6.1:1	6.5:1	2.4:1	1.4:1	5.8:1
Average DSH–suicide ratio	11.8:1	7.1:1	5:1:1	2.9:1	1.3:1	5.3:1
Women						
Padua (Italy)						
DSH	1,260	1,450	780	870	480	910
Suicide	16	32	35	51	82	41
Ratio	78.8:1	45.3:1	22.3:1	17.1:1	5.9:1	22.2:1
Leiden (Netherlands)						
DSH	1,120	1,100	1,630	1,420	390	1,050
Suicide	44	72	75	138	125	75
Ratio	25.5:1	15.4:1	21.7:1	10.3:1	3.2:1	14.0:1
Guipuzcoa (Spain)						
DSH	1,120	1,800	770	600	190	850
Suicide	19	26	23	46	95	39
Ratio	59.0:1	69.2:1	33.5:1	13.0:1	2.0:1	21.8:1
Average DSH–suicide ratio	54.4:1	43.3:1	26.1:1	13.5:1	3.7:1	19.3:1

the extent of DSH among 15- to 34-year-olds in comparison with actual suicide, especially in young women, 8:1 for young men and 25:1 for young women.

However, age and gender, while especially important in determining subsequent risk after DSH, require a case-specific analysis to seek to determine whether an obvious predisposing or precipitant cause lay behind the DSH. For example, the presence of a mental disorder gives far greater weight to a DSH, for almost 30 per cent of people who experience more than one episode of schizophrenia are involved in DSH (Harkvy-Friedman *et al.* 2003) and, of course, an initial

DSH makes a second DSH more likely and a third DSH is often fatal. In a recent study, 50 per cent of people who died from suicide had one or more previous DSH incidents (Langlois and Morrison 2002), but self-evidently 50 per cent of people who died had no known prior DHS. Not easy!

Clearly, in exploring the interface and overlap of DSH with suicide, we are trying to get some idea of risk of fatality. On the other hand, despite the irritation that can be caused by some people, especially the under thirties, who seem to be involved in frequent DSH especially of an apparently mild non-lethal nature, it should be remembered that, whether or not this is a 'gesture' or 'attention' seeking' or a 'cry for help', it is still a highly abnormal piece of social behaviour. We all attempt to maximise our position with other people; indeed, an irate parent may say the teenager was being manipulative, using emotional blackmail to get their own way – equally it may be said by the self-same teenager that that is what the parent is doing to them. But an act of DSH is in another league and highly dysfunctional. The problem is that such an act is seldom or never emotionally neutral, and a parent or a professional faced by a disturbed, impulsive DSH-threatening person is quickly made to feel helpless and not in control. With teenagers, suicide and DSH are associated with the problem of imitation and, occasionally, there are almost mini 'epidemics' in schools, where an especially vulnerable and disturbed young person, mainly a female, acts out DSH in a particular dramatic way. For the next few days or even weeks, there are copycat events, and practitioners are offered guidelines to deal with media reporting in an effort to minimise this phenomenon (Barrickman 2003). Indeed, the impact of the media can be profound, especially when associated with some great public event, for example both suicide and DSH rose significantly in the weeks immediately following the death of Diana, Princess of Wales (Hawton *et al.* 2000). Apparently from a heightened sense of loss in possibly currently vulnerable people, this occurred especially in women aged 24–44, DHS rising 65 per cent and suicide 33 per cent above the average rate. This in part reflects the inevitable high emotionality that will surround either a suicide or DSH.

For the vast majority of parents, their worst nightmare is that their child should predecease them. Therefore, imagine what a parent feels if their child has died or threatened to die by their own hand. The problem for the professional is that we can often see the manipulative behaviour which 'feeds upon itself'. But, such is the parent's panic, they inadvertently reinforce the young person's dysfunctional behaviour, for it is extremely hard, but desirable, to remain calm, concerned but detached in the face of the emotional drama that can surround a DSH incident. Sometimes, tired professionals can fall into the trap of saying 'it's only attention seeking', especially if the 17-year-old girl, rejected by her boyfriend, takes five paracetamol tablets and then alerts everyone to what she has done. If such a situation has happened before, it is easy to dismiss it. With 'personality-disordered' young people, especially vulnerable to DSH (Fombonne *et al.* 2001a,b; Jones *et al.* 2002; Beautrais *et al.* 2003; Conner *et al.* 2003), this is not uncommon, made more dangerous by the presence of drugs or alcohol, but still they survive as the lethal 'dose' was small, perhaps lulling themselves and us into a false sense of security. However, counselling parents who were with their dying daughter who had 'upped the ante' and taken a whole bottle of paracetamol, all shared the parents and her despair that 'she didn't intend it', but the resulting inexorable liver damage proved fatal.

DSH situations are always fraught and, if involved with adolescents under 18, try to reassure the parents and perhaps yourself that the statistics are against the young person dying, but we have to remember that it does happen. It is a cliché but, like all clichés, has a marked element of truth: 'there is no such thing as a safe cry for help', 'there is no such thing as a safe suicidal gesture' and sadly nurses, psychologists, psychiatrists and social workers have found this to their clients' cost.

'John' was a 30-year-old recidivist. Typical of a man with a lifelong history of petty crime, he came from a long line of disturbed and disturbing families. Neglected by his sets of parents, failed by an inadequate alternative child care system, he had been to prison numerous times for nuisance rather than serious or dangerous crimes – though very distressing to his victims. 'Mr Jones', probation officer, had supported John through thick and thin, recognising that John was as much a victim of his circumstances as 'innately bad'. Of course, we are not supposed to differentiate between the deserving and undeserving, but with those very demanding clients, it helps to find some ameliorating exonerating factors. John had got into the habit of making dramatic public suicidal gestures, such as jumping off a low bridge into two feet of water, scaring the public but apparently coming out unscathed and, for a short time, getting a little sympathy in a life that was characterised by an absence of love. John swore by Mr Jones; like many probationers he swore about the probation service, but swore by his probation officer (Ford *et al.* 1997). An objective observer would have noted that John's antisocial behaviour was improving and that he was more able to live independently, albeit needing to rely upon Mr Jones, who was coping well with John's occasional 'low moods', rather than 'depression' because Mr Jones 'didn't believe in psychiatry'. It was late Friday afternoon, Mr Jones was duty officer and John came round, slightly the worse for drink, which made Mr Jones somewhat unsympathetic, not least because he had other crises to deal with. John threatened an overdose unless Mr Jones agreed to see him immediately. Unfortunately, Mr Jones had a bottle of paracetamol tablets in his desk and, in a moment's unthinking exasperation, showed John the tablets and told him to go away and not come back until he was sober. John grabbed the tablets and ran. Mr Jones waited two minutes and then went off in search of the exasperating John. It was too late. In a foolish, perhaps unintended, gesture, John hid himself and took some tablets washed down with cider. He was not sick but collapsed and died in the field in which he was hiding, and died as much from exposure as from the overdose. Mr Jones never forgave himself for his moment's aberration from his usually high standards.

Whenever there is a threat of or an actual DSH incident, we need to review the client-specific situation calmly, focusing upon any new stress points, and with the younger clients, seek to bring some reassurance and to defuse the emotional tension but deal with the 'emotional pressure points'. With the under twenties, especially the under-18s, without the presence of a mental disorder and/or drugs and alcohol, we can be pretty sure that the risk of suicide is extremely low. Therefore, one of our treatment goals is to reduce the likelihood of further DSH becoming a mode of the person responding to stress. Conversely, in a person over the age of 50, DSH is an extremely serious indicator of likely suicide and should be given the highest priority and, in the presence of a mental disorder, urgent treatment will be required and a compulsory admission might need to be considered. The role of the Approved Social Worker under the 1983 Mental Health Act will be examined in a separate chapter, but DSH in the above circumstances must always raise the question of whether the person is a risk to themselves or others and requires the protection that psychiatric legislation provides.

Sexual orientation and DSH

One continuing issue associated with DSH is that of a gay or lesbian sexual orientation; indeed, actual suicide rates of gay and lesbian people still remain higher than those of the general population (Paul *et al.* 1992; McDaniel *et al.* 2001; Noell and Ochs 2001; Botnick *et al.* 2002). This is particularly a problem with younger people who are coming to terms with their sexual orientation. This may surprise some people for, self-evidently, Western attitudes to sexual orientation have changed profoundly in the last 30 years, and although homosexual behaviour was decriminalised in 1967, it was not until the early 1990s in Britain that discrimination against people on account of their sexual orientation was recognised. Nonetheless, research suggests that, for some gay and lesbian young people, it is still an extra life adjustment, with added stress. However, Rutter and Soucar (2002) in a British study found that it was not so much being gay that was associated with suicide risk, as the degree to which the young person felt emotionally and socially supported. Although two large studies, one in the US and another in Canada, found a high degree of suicide ideation in young men, and that over 10 per cent had been involved in a DSH incident, as with the British study, the psychological perturbation was linked to the extent of family support or hostility about their orientation (Paul *et al.* 1992; Botnick *et al.* 2002). In the case of transsexuals, there has long been an association with suicidal behaviour and people wanting to change their gender (Meyerowitz 2001) but, with the greater acceptance and access to treatment, things have improved.

However, comparatively, the transsexual person still faces major readjustment problems, and though rates of suicidal behaviour are not as high as in previous decades, it remains an increased risk until the person is fully established in their new gender (Michel *et al.* 2002; Bosinski 2003).

A key practical problem therefore is how to differentiate between risks of suicide and DSH. Table 10.6 offers guidelines that highlight the differences although there are obvious overlaps. In both types of behaviour, the impact on others – family, friends, neighbours and professional staff – can be very significant with a considerable degree of distress. Wherever there is depression, there is aggression.

Factors associated with prevention

On reflection, one might ask why it is that some people who seem to be faced with major or overwhelming life problems do not commit suicide? Indeed, even though in most Western and Asian countries, it is the over 75-year-olds who die disproportionally more from suicide than any other age group, yet the 353 75+-

Table 10.6 Differentiating suicide from parasuicide/deliberate self-harm

Suicide	Deliberate self-harm
Perpetrator wants to die	No decisions about intent can be deduced
More common in males (2:1)	More common in females (4:1)
Affects all social classes (including professionals) equally	More common in social classs 4 and 5
More common in spring (opposite months in the southern hemisphere)	No variation throughout the year
Divorce++	Divorce
Unemployed++	Unemployed+ and sickness
Living alone	Living alone and crowded
Psychiatric illness (80%+)	Affective symptoms (sadness)
Physical illness	PMT
Stress	Stress
Previous DSH+++	Previous DSH
Alcohol/drugs	Alcohol/drugs
Age group changing but still highest among the elderly	All ages but especially under-35s+
Emotionality and violence	Potential 'gains', hence reactive

Notes
+ indicates strength of factor.
This is a guideline only. There is no such thing as a safe cry for help. When defining DSH avoid post facto 'decisions' about intent.

year-old suicides in England and Wales were equivalent to 0.009 per cent of the elderly population. So what are the factors associated with preventing suicide?

These include being younger, being female, especially women with children, being male and married, not having a mental disorder, not having previous DSH, no easy access to lethal methods, helping people to identify 'alternative' solutions to their stressors and building up a sense of hope (Maris *et al.* 1992) and, crucially, the absence of alcohol or drugs, which always make a fraught situation worse (Testa *et al.* 2004). One theme is not being isolated or living alone, and this reflects a key 'treatment' issue, the importance of 'meaningful relationships' (see below). Linked to this non-isolation, and this crosses cultures, is membership of a faith, especially if they are active attenders (Maris *et al.* 1992). Most important, and this has practical implications, has the person a 'reason for living', which at the moment of crisis has been overwhelmed, but with sensitive counselling can be restored, especially a sense of obligation to the family (Kahn and Faros 2003)? Beck's seminal work on suicide (Beck *et al.* 1979, 1985, 1993a) and Browne *et al.* (2000) highlighted the interaction between depression, hopelessness and suicidal ideation, the key being a persistent sense of hopelessness – shades of Dante's classic 'Abandon hope all ye who enter here' – psychic hell. Therefore, the inculcation of hope to raise the sense of a reason to live is a major preventative/protective factor against suicide. Maris (2002), another major name in suicidology, reminds us that, even with the use of standardised assessment and prediction scales, such as Beck and Hamilton, we still get 30 per cent false positives – conversely, they are accurate 70 per cent of the time, but it appears that it is the change in the sense of hopelessness that may make a major difference. In an ingenious Finnish study on 1,400 adults in the general population excluded for mental disorder, the degree of hopelessness in the general population was measured utilising Beck's rating scale. Its normative element was shown to be clearly associated with major negative life events, which when reduced was associated with a decline in the sense of hopelessness (Haatainen *et al.* 2003). Indeed, the Finnish study showed a fascinating link between money worries, unemployment and hopelessness, which brings together the psychical and social factors – therefore, suicidal behaviour is prevented or reduced when hopelessness is reduced.

Tables 10.7 and 10.8 are a guideline, the emphasis upon guideline, for evaluating safer to unsafe features in DSH and suicide, divided schematically between younger and older people.

Brief points on suicidal behaviour and ethnicity

Most of the research cited has been drawn from the 'Western world' and, while many countries are now multicultural, especially the USA, Australia, France, Germany, the Netherlands and Britain, there is relatively little research specifically upon cultural minorities; nonetheless there are some important differences. Focusing particularly upon research in Britain, three potential variations have to be considered with regard to people from African-Caribbean, Asian and Islamic backgrounds.

Table 10.7 Guidelines for risk of DSH and suicide by age and gender

	Safer		Unsafe	
	Younger (< 40 years)	Older (> 41 years)	Younger (< 40 years)	Older (> 41 years)
	Females (< 18+++)	Females	Males	Male++
	Female with children	Female with children	Women no children	Single women+
	Male married	Female married	Female separated	Male separated+
	No prior psychiatric treatment	No prior psychiatric treatment	Depression++/personality disorder+++/schizophrenia+	Depression+++/schizophrenia++/personality disorder+
	No drugs/drink	No drugs/drink	Drugs/drink++	Drugs/drink++
	Lives with others	Lives with others	Lives alone+	Lives alone++
	In work	In work	Jobless (sacked)+	Jobless (sacked)+
	No prior DSH	No prior DSH	Prior DSH++	Prior DSH+
	No lethal access	No lethal access	Access to lethality+	Lethal access++
	Reason for living	Reason for living	Major role failure++	Major role failure+
	Church-goer	Church-goer	Not social, isolated	Not social, isolated

Note
+ indicates strength of factor.

Table 10.8 Factors increasing suicide risks

Hides behaviour+
Suicide note
Poor problem solver+
HIV positive+
Family history of suicide+
Persistent ideation+
Hopelessness+++
Relationship crisis+

Note
+ indicates strength of factor.

As already noted, African-Caribbean males in Britain are over-represented in 'compulsory admissions', and African-Caribbean people generally receive disproportionate prison sentences compared with white men and women (Brugha *et al.* 1997; Coid *et al.* 2002a,b; Harrison 2002). The issue of suicide, however, is somewhat unexpectedly different.

The history of all immigrants is that initially they are at the bottom of the social pile and experience discrimination, until there is a period of integration. This is classically seen with people from a Jewish background with above average success. Indeed, in parenthesis, Southampton medical school, one of the most oversubscribed in Britain, has almost 30 per cent of its second year students from British ethnic minorities, particularly British-born Asians and Chinese, which is a good example of this historical process. On the other hand, discrimination continues to exist, and this is nowhere more evident than in the USA; when comparing cancer survival rates between white and black Americans, the latter have a 25 per cent worse five-year survival rate than whites, and of course there are proportionately more black Americans in prison than there are in their universities (Evans and Pritchard 2000; US Bureau of Statistics 2004). But, as far as suicidal behaviour goes, it looks as if male black Britons over the age of 35 have a lower rate of suicide than 35+-year-old British whites, whereas in terms of suicide and DSH, there is little difference between blacks and whites in London aged 34 and under (McKenzie *et al.* 2003). Neeleman and colleagues (1997, 1999) explored suicidal behaviour in ethnic minorities in London and found that black and Asian males had lower rates of suicide and/or DSH than whites if they lived in relatively high-density ethnic communities; the converse was the case if they did not. But overall black people had lower suicide rates than white males. A consistent finding has been that young Asian women had relatively higher rates than white women, whereas Irish- or Scottish-born whites living in London had more suicides than the average local rate. One further British variation is with regard to Asian women living in London, who had considerably higher DSH rate than whites or other ethnic minority women (Brugha *et al.* 1997). What this appears to suggest is that there is a socio-evolutionary process taking place as different groups, at different ages and perhaps in different areas and at different stages of 'integration', respond to life stresses and mental disorder in a different way from both indigenous and older compatriots. This may also be due, and it is stressed may be, in part to the psychoses being manifested differently in people of Caribbean origin compared with Caucasians, for certainly there appears to be a different treatment outcome response (McKenzie *et al.* 2001), which may be linked to different underlying premorbid circumstances. For example African-Caribbean people with a psychosis have less premorbid neurological illness than whites (McKenzie *et al.* 2002). This implies that schizophrenia in African-Caribbean people may be more stress reactive than in whites – at present we just do not know.

One fascinating fact from long-term mortality studies in the USA is that rates of suicide in second- and third-generation migrants still reflect their country of origin national rates, although with each succeeding generation, the group rates come closer to the US national average (Holinger 1987). Moreover, despite the long tragic history of oppression of black people in the US, both male and female suicide rates appear to be about a third of white Americans.

With regard to British Islamic people with a mental disorder, suicide remains a serious social taboo.

Yet it is clear from national suicide rates and clinical studies involving Islamic people that they do get depression and have ideas about suicide (Abdel-Khalek and Lester 2002), albeit perhaps less than Europeans, but suicide does occur in Islamic cohorts (Devrimci-Ozguven and Sayil 2003; Pritchard and Amunullah 2006), and we need to be especially culturally sensitive in exploring these matters when working with Islamic people.

Anecdotally, colleagues who have used translators with Islamic clients who have limited English have found that translators might be reluctant to speak of suicidal ideas, especially if there are other family members present, such is the potential response of culturally traditional people about suicide. Where one needs to work through a translator, one needs to discuss with them beforehand the rationale behind questions about low mood and possible suicidal ideation.

Intervention – treatment

Most authorities agree that treatment specific to suicide prevention and suicidal behaviour depends upon dealing with the person's presenting problems (Beck *et al.* 1985; Maris *et al.* 1992; Lester 2001). Consequently, in dealing with the mental disorders, we follow the guidelines outlined in the chapters on depression and schizophrenia, an integrated bio-psychosocial approach, in which the principles of cognitive behaviour therapy will be central (Beck 1988; Warner 2000; Kingdon and Turkington 2002). Thus, after careful assessment, we seek to address the current stressors, paying particular attention to the person's sense of isolation, rejection and sense of hopelessness, as well as any symptoms of the mental disorders.

This should also include a sensitivity to people with a criminal background, being alert to the complicating factor of the person's use of alcohol or illegal drugs, but also being aware of the nature of the person's legal psychopharmacology if they are being so treated. The older antidepressants in particular might still be used, and they carry quite a heavy risk as they can be lethal in numbers (Maris *et al.* 1992; Lester 2001; Baldwin and Mayers 2003). A key practical point is when dealing with the 'homeless' who have extraordinary high rates of DSH, dealing adequately with accommodation needs can yield relatively speedy improvements (Desai *et al.* 2003) (more anon).

At the core of the mental health practitioner's work, as with the mental disorders or other dysfunctional life problems, is the quality of the relationship they can engender with the client. Paradoxically, this can be seen in reverse as King *et al.* (2001) showed that one factor associated with completed suicides by former psychiatric patients was the absence of a key worker at a time of particular stress, e.g. at discharge, be that a psychiatrist, nurse, social worker or psychologist; hence, we are important to our clients.

Of course, the most important persons for the majority of people in trouble are their family members and the quality of relationships there, hence the importance of working with the families as well as the 'suicidal' person (Tarrier and Barraclough 1992; Falloon 2003; Miklowitz *et al.* 2003a,b), which also includes 'psycho-education' of the family, helping them to make sense of what may be occurring within their relative's mind (Warner 2000; Keller and Schuler 2002).

The importance of 'relationship' is seen in many areas of mental health, for example accepting relationship for gay young people by their families considerably reduces suicidal behaviour (Rutter and Soucar 2002), preventative intervention with mentally ill adults to reduce the distress to their children (Ensminger *et al.* 2003) and, crucially, reducing the sense of isolation that people feel (Dekovic *et al.* 2003; Targosz *et al.* 2003). Moreover, it has been shown that the professional relationship can engage the disadvantaged and low-income family to reduce the current stressors (Pritchard and Williams 2001; Pritchard 2001; Brotman *et al.* 2003).

Female suicide has fallen in most Western countries, which may be because of reduced lethality of medicines, but also improvements in community-based services and perhaps an improvement in women's self-esteem generally as the benefits of reducing societal 'sexism' work through the generations (WHO 2001–5; Pritchard and Hansen 2005b). But this means that we have to pay particular attention to the 'reluctant to seek help' male, an argument taken up quite strongly by a Parliamentary committee on suicide (House of Commons 1996).

However, perhaps the most important and difficult form of intervention which aims to relieve the present stressors is that following an actual DSH event.

Post-DSH intervention

There is evidence that appropriate intervention following a crisis can be a key change event or an easy access to client-specific response, e.g. a telephone emergency line (Morgan *et al.* 1993; Aoun and Johnson 2001; Guthrie *et al.* 2001; Cedereke *et al.* 2002; Pritchard *et al.* 2001, 2004b), and this is nowhere more important than in suicide prevention. But we have to take into account the morale of the 'survived' recovered DSH, as the event can be either possibly positively cathartic or further undermining of an already damaged self-esteem 'I can't even kill myself' (Wiklander *et al.* 2003).

These post-DSH interviews are extremely difficult, in part because of the distress of the person and/or their family and because we must not overemphasise and inadvertently reinforce the young person's inappropriate response to stress. There is also the demand upon the therapist not to miss the opportunity that a crisis can become a life-changing event.

The interview has to be concerned with the immediate past, the present and the near and medium future. This means thinking about current risk, current psychosocial resources, intervention plans and any necessary interagency collaboration. One problem for the professional is the time pressure or demands for information from either the family or other agencies, yet when interviewing the person recovering from a DSH needs the most gentle handling, giving them the time and space to review what has happened to them in the most positive light. It is no good congratulating them on their survival if they are still feeling profoundly depressed, under overwhelming pressure, or they really had expected to die. What must take priority is establishing a rapport with them for, without gaining their trust, the necessary risk assessment information may not be forthcoming. Moreover, this may be the time for the beginning of an effective intervention, but we have to respond to the client's emotions. For example, if they are suffering from schizophrenia and under the influence of a command hallucination, it is no good simply saying that the voices are unreal; as mentioned before, we need to address the emotional reality of the delusion and hallucination.

We need the imagination to appreciate what it must feel like to believe that 'I brought AIDS into the world', that the 'Devil is inside me and I am going to destroy the world'. Sadly, there is some evidence that post-DSH interviews are rushed yet, when they are well handled, they can bring relief (Aoun and Johnson 2001; Pirkis *et al.* 2001).

Follow the client, it is a cliché but still very true. Listen to what they think of the situation and build your assessment questions around their experience and, wherever possible, deal with the most pressing practical problem early to show that something is happening, that the situation can be improved, even if you have to give time boundaries. Give no false assurances, but show that the situation can be improved – classically, that their depression will lift – and, after allowing them the expression of their distress, seek the positives to inculcate hope and that alternatives do exist.

Table 10.9 highlights the points that need covering.

Tertiary treatment

Another area fraught with tension is work with the family of a person who died by suicide. In part, this is because of our cultural attitudes to bereavement, compounded by the stigma that still surrounds suicide. It would be fair to say that, until Wertheimer's (1991) work, there was virtually no recognition in Britain of the psychosocial impact upon what the Americans call 'survivors of suicide'.

Table 10.9 Intervention – the post-DSH intervention and risk assessment interview

i	Establish a rapport (note your attitudes and values) Intervention must be client specific
ii	Understand the event – what happened and why now?
iii	Determine current difficulties: social, physical, psychological/psychiatric
iv	Assess coping mechanisms (strengths = process)
v	Prioritise problems
vi	Take a history: ?previous DSH, psychiatric state, usual personality
vii	Assess client's emotional state: self-esteem and hope very important
viii	Note the presence of depression (equates to aggression)
ix	Consider carers' disturbance, disruption, disability, despair and dependency
x	Remember differentiation of suicide and DSH (and where they overlap) and use the guideline to assist judgements

Indeed, it appears from reading Wertheimer that she wrote her book following her own experience and, anecdotally, one still hears of suicide-bereaved families who find themselves isolated and subjectively deserted by neighbours and friends and the professionals who should know better.

We have known since the 1970s that a suicide damages the survivors' health and that, within one or two years of the suicide, there is an association of a relative's subsequent suicide or DSH (Barraclough and Shepherd 1976, 1977), but not until recently has there been any attempt to relieve the distress.

A number of studies have sought to differentiate between bereavement by suicide and other causes. There is some variation in outcome, for example child suicide, sudden infant death and accidental death. All parents seems to have similar patterns of grief reaction, which appears to surround the 'sudden and unexpected' nature of the death (Dyregrov *et al.* 2003), rather than the 'special scar' that suicide survivors experience and is described by Wertheimer (1991).

In the case of children, i.e. under 17 years, being bereaved by suicide, there is still a debate as to whether or not 'all should be revealed' and the child should be told the nature of their loss. The consensus seems to lie with the need to deal child specifically, rather than an absolutist (politically correct) 'one size fits all' approach (Cain 2002). This seems best because, while there is some evidence to suggest that there will be some family psychopathology in families of a suicide (Cerel *et al.* 2000; Pfeffer *et al.* 2000), there will always be a varied family agenda to which different members are likely to respond.

In general, there seems to be agreement that being bereaved by suicide makes particular adjustment demands on the survivors, which will of course vary according to the relationship the survivors had to the deceased. This includes the classic shock, numbness, anger, confusion and then guilt and unresolved anger at this 'ultimate rejection' (Pfeffer *et al.* 2000; Jordan 2001; Wolfersdorf *et al.* 2001).

I remember an elderly lady who was initially told that her husband had died accidentally in the canal, but who in fact had committed suicide. Her words on hearing what had happened three weeks later still echo, reflecting her hurt, loss and anger: 'how could he go and leave me to face old age alone?' From bearing her initial grief with sorrowful dignity, she 'froze' and lapsed into an atypical grief-reactive depression, requiring some months of close counselling before she could cry and be angry at his 'ultimate rejection'.

Recent co-ordinated efforts have been made to reach the families of the bereaved, but there appear to be gaps between what families feel they need and the support they get (Dyregrov *et al.* 2003; De Fauw and Andriessen 2003; Wolfersdorf *et al.* 2001), which in the USA spill over into survivors wanting to 'blame someone' and threats of civil lawsuits are not uncommon (Peterson *et al.* 2002).

Knowing what we know about the impact of 'normal' bereavement upon people, and the extra burden felt by 'survivors', it is clear that we need to reach out, not only in sympathy, but as a preventative measure in restoring their mental health. Any professional who has lost a patient/client from suicide knows the sense of guilt, professional failure, as well as the sadness associated with another's death. Therefore, there is an understandable tendency to avoid them, especially if tensions remain within the family and/or between family and therapist. Yet there seems to be a self-evident case that we should make every effort to provide them with support, not just in the first few weeks, which is the British way of dealing with death, but offer to return in the months ahead to facilitate the normal grief process.

Suicide is final and is one of the persistent anxieties in the field: if we fail to meet the needs of our client and miss the danger signals, then suicide can be the outcome. Yet the mental disorders can be treated, their impact reduced and, in the wider social environment, policies can be developed to improve the mental health of society.

However, the mental health field has one other area of controversy and challenge, in which death may be the inadvertent outcome, the relatively unrecognised problem of the psychiatric–child protection interface.

11 Personality disorders and the psychiatric–child protection interface

A devil, a born devil on whose nature
Nurture can never stick, on whom my pains
Humanely taken, all, all lost, quite lost . . .
So his mind cankers.
(Prospero describing the 'monster' Caliban, *The Tempest*, 4:1)

I am one. . .
Whom the vile blows and buffets of the world
Have so incensed that I am reckless what
I do to spite the world.
                    (Second murderer, *Macbeth*, 3:1)

The controversy surrounding 'personality disorder' (PD) was discussed in Chapter 3 where it was acknowledged that even in psychiatry the imprecision of the concept has been a longstanding cause for concern (Lewis 1955; Clare 1977). Yet there are people whose characteristic behaviour is so self-defeating, so disturbed and disturbing that they are often known to all the agencies, reflecting something of the chaos and pain in their lives. Indeed, Chiesa *et al.* (2002) highlights the cost to health of 'personality-disordered' clients who have had far more different types of mental health treatment than any other group, except for group therapy, apparently because they have such difficulties in relating to other people (Bender *et al.* 2001). The practical issue is, irrespective of definition and assumptions about cause/origin, there are people with 'persistent patterns and characteristic lifestyles who impact adversely upon others and their own lives' (WHO 2000) who are diagnosed/described as 'personality-disordered' (PD). They pose problems that cross the mental health, crime and child protection fields.

There are two broad types of PD. One is the psychologically related: depressed, phobic, anxious or 'schizophrenic-like' as if the mental disorder is not fully expressed and, instead of being episodic, it is persistent and characteristic; these people mainly trouble themselves. The other type spans a range of 'social' related behaviour: being impulsive, aggressive, uncaring, unfeeling, unable to relate to others and troublesome to both themselves and others, sometimes described as 'sociopaths' or psychopaths. As adults, they pose problems for any children in their care. Because of their emotional immaturity and inability to meet the child's developmental needs, children are either 'neglected' or more actively 'abused', emotionally, physically and sexually or a combination of all (Bagley *et al.* 1994; Iwaniec 1995; Read 1998; Newcomb and Lock 2001; Ryan *et al.* 2000; Pritchard 2004). Indeed, Reder and Duncan (1997) speak of 'psychiatry' and PDs as the missing link in child abuse.

There seem to be two distinct forms of PD. Those with the first type demonstrate problematic behaviour from very early childhood, while the second type is exemplified by adults whose difficulties appear to have started in adolescence but have persisted well into adulthood. In both cases, this behaviour becomes characteristic (Rutter *et al.* 1999; Messerschmit 2002). This suggests that PD starting in early childhood may have a greater genetic predisposition of either some dysfunction or an inability to develop personality skills (Van den Bree 1998; Torgersen 2000; Ebstein *et al.* 2000). When becoming problematic as an adolescent, people with PD are predominantly responding to psychosocial environmental adversities (Modestin *et al.* 1998; Parker *et al.* 1999; Ret *et al.* 2002; Siever *et al.* 2002).

This early possibly 'genetic' link is reflected in Prospero's observation about the intractable 'offender' Caliban, as Prospero seeks to justify his harsh treatment of Caliban, whose mother, the witch Sycorax, Prospero killed when he invaded Caliban's island: 'A devil, a born devil, on whose nature Nurture can never stick, on whom my pains Humanely taken, all, all lost, quite lost' (*The Tempest*), the classic stereotypical blaming the victim of discrimination, the justification was that he was 'a born devil' – it was in the blood. Quite ignoring the fact that it was the aristocratic Prospero who was the invader and assailant, not the newly enslaved 'monster', who was considered subhuman because of his appearance. However, Prospero was cleverly appealing to the belief of the times that behaviour was 'in the blood', and that virtue as well as vice was inherited, thus justifying the status quo and the social positions of oppressors and oppressed.

Conversely, the 'environmental' PD might be described by the second murderer in *Macbeth*. He was being quizzed about why he was willing to kill the virtuous Banquo, the ancestor of James I (here Shakespeare was being sycophantic). He justified his desperate plight by the explanation that he was one 'whom the vile blows and buffets of this world have so incensed that I am reckless what I do to spite the world', namely his behaviour was in response to his environment. In other words, he was taking a rational 'alternative market response' to the 'buffets of this vile world'.

Modern research points to the interaction of the two positions, i.e. nurture and nature, as many adults identified as 'personality-disordered' experienced poor parenting, especially with poor parental bonding (Stroud 2003). There are, however, some interesting gender variations: parents of male PDs were high control and low emotional and physical care (Parker *et al.* 1999), whereas female PDs had specifically identified abusive experiences as children and low maternal care (Modestin *et al.* 1998).

In a study of cases in a social services 'At Risk of Abuse' register, it was found that 40 per cent of mothers had some form of depression, ranging from mild to severe necessitating a visit to a psychiatrist (Pritchard 1991), while in a study of a range of behaviour within probation and social services caseloads, practitioners were asked to rate their clients' problems in their last four allocated cases. These problems included 'emotional disturbance', 'mental disorder' and 'depression' (Pritchard *et al.* 1997b). However, 60 per cent of both agencies' clients were considered to be 'emotionally disturbed', 40 per cent were 'depressed' and 25 per cent were 'mentally disordered'. Such patterns of behaviour would be very similar to what psychiatrists diagnose as 'personality-disordered' people, as a range of social disruptive behaviour is allied to recurrent mild depression, anxiety and deliberate self-harm (DSH), very often associated with substance abuse including alcohol (Bender *et al.* 2001; Chiesa *et al.* 2002; Chiesa and Fonagy 2003).

The question then becomes 'is "personality disorder" of the same genre as a 'disease', which implies a medical treatment model?' Clearly, they are not, although there may well be some 'neurological' developmental deficit, which as yet we have no way of assessing. This leaves both psychiatry and social work struggling to deal with disturbed and disturbing people who, because of their longstanding apparently intractable problems, are often regarded as 'nuisances'. However, many psychiatric patients who are described as 'personality-disordered' are also found significantly among both DSH and suicide statistics, reflecting their low self-esteem, loneliness and isolation (Linehan 1993; Marshall 1997; Welch and Linehan 2002). Yet, equally, many PD types of behaviour and personalities are over-represented in prison populations and in the crime statistics (Korbin 1986; Coid *et al.* 2002b; Bird and Hutchinson 2003), which must contribute in part to relatively high rates of suicide and suicidal behaviour in prisons. But the psychiatric–child protection link gets even more complicated with the association of child abuse in people who are later diagnosed as personality-disordered (Bierer *et al.* 2003; Foreman *et al.* 2004). Thus, some child and adolescent 'victims' become 'assailants', damaged and damaging adults, which is the criminological and psychiatric equivalent of the problem of some sexually abused children later becoming abusers (Simon *et al.* 1992; Wyatt *et al.* 1999; Coxe and Holmes 2001).

Violence and personality disorder

There is of course a danger in the circularity of the argument. Because 'personality-disordered' people are found in such 'special samples' of young adults who are clients of probation, social services, police and prisons, such people by definition are statistically different from the 'normal distribution' of the general population. This does not confirm the medical notion of a 'syndrome' as inferred by the PD concept. Rather, these are social constructions, but (and the qualification is important) the patterns of behaviour do exist and are recognisable and, as we shall see, this time patterned behaviour raises practice questions, if or when it comes to questions of their ability to meet the needs of children in their care.

The terms 'sociopath' in the US and 'psychopath' in Europe have been used to describe the extremes of such patterned behaviour, and the overlap with frank mental disorder becomes clear when the extreme statistics of violent behaviour are considered, namely homicide.

Shaw *et al.* (1999), in the British National Inquiry, found that, over an 18-month period, 44 per cent of people who killed another person were found to be suffering from a 'mental disorder', mainly personality disorder and schizophrenia, in that order, a finding confirmed by Woodward *et al.* (2000). Yet Taylor and Gunn (1999) remind us that, over a 38-year period, despite successive media 'moral crusades', proportionally there is no more homicide related to mental disorder than previously, hence the panic over 'risk in the community' is highly exaggerated for, thankfully, such tragedies are extremely rare. Although of course, if you or yours were the victim of such an event, it would be 100 per cent. The fact that road deaths exceeded all forms of 'homicide' by a factor of seven is irrelevant, other than to place in perspective that fatal person-to-person violence is far rarer than road deaths (Pritchard and Butler 2003).

This 'criminal' overlap with PD is seen in the fact that, while proportionally more mentally disordered people are convicted of a crime, the majority of such 'offenders' are personality-disordered (Bourgeois and Benezech 2001). Violence of course creates enormous concern and anxiety, not only in the general public but also among the professionals. It is linked to 'poor anger control' and the 'personality-disordered' person's apparent inability to empathise with others, which overlaps with the abuse of children and domestic violence (Marshall 1997; Myers and Monaco 2000; Pritchard and Bagley 2001; Pritchard 2004; Zink and Sill 2004) and is a pattern that repeats itself often in terms of both victim and assailant.

Woodworth and Porter (2002) highlight an interesting finding. They stress that, while the 'full-blown psychopath' is actually very rare, when comparing types of homicides between the mentally disordered, in their sample of 125 mentally disordered assailants and non-mentally disordered offenders, 93 per cent of the personality-disordered murderers were 'cold-blooded' instrumental assailants compared with 48 per cent of 'normal' murderers. The non-mentally disordered were experiencing emotional relationship crises, crimes of passion if you will, but the PD assailant was simply achieving an end, a robbery, or covering up another crime, or gaining gratuitous sadistic satisfaction. They went on to compare a subgroup of sexual assault homicide assailants, and again found a significantly high scoring on 'psychopathy checklist' (Porter *et al.* 2003). These are the men, predominantly men, that current legislative proposals describe as 'severe dangerous personality disorders'. If one visits homicide assailants in prisons or indeed the 'special hospitals', this cold-blooded aspect, while rare, is noticeable; in one sense, there is a qualitative difference between the person with a psychotic illness and the detached, non-empathetic person who killed almost in an matter-of-fact way. The extremes of such are seen in the even rarer 'serial murderers' as two themes emerge, their sense of omnipotence and dehumanisation – their victims might have been flies (Claus and Lindberg 1999). But the majority of patients of psychiatrists and clients of the community services are a long way from these extremes, and there are civil liberty issues about legislation that is driven by concern over a statistically rare problem, rather than the more frequent run-of-the-mill PD, who essentially is a sad, slightly mad, but not essentially bad person. Psychiatry, however, possibly mistakenly, has a 'half-way house' of PD that includes these mostly self-defeating, disturbed and disturbing people. That is the concept of borderline personality disorder, used to describe the characteristic behaviour of people who do not reach the 'extremes' of the severe dangerous personality disorder paradigm (Linehan 1993; WHO 2000).

In many case conferences where trainee psychiatrists have struggled to understand the form and content of some of their patients, characterised by mild depression, substance abuse, possible DSH and antisocial behaviour, 'borderline PD' is often the designation arrived at. One has stressed that there is more to be gained practically by focusing upon the content of the client's life than its apparent form because psychiatry per se has little effective treatment. In a sense, they are wrestling with people with multiple problems who have 'gone the rounds' and, almost as a last resort and because of the DSH, have been referred to psychiatry (Bender *et al.* 2001). The main, and perhaps only, value in the concept of personality disorder or borderline PD is that it reminds us of the characteristic pattern of the person's life, who may be troublesome but is also troubled; who may be disturbing but who is also disturbed; who is distressing but also distressed. Not surprisingly, such clients in one's caseload can be very difficult and, reflecting Smale's insight of self-fulfilling prophecy, there can be therapist as well as client 'burn-out' as both become demoralised by the series of self-defeating behaviours that undermines everyone's efforts to empower the person (Smale 1984; Linehan *et al.* 2002).

To be fair, however, from the field of clinical psychology and modern psychiatry, predominantly psychosocial approaches are being used to help people with borderline PD, with an adjunct of antidepressants where appropriate, in a treatment approach from the CBT field called dialectic behaviour therapy (DBT) (Linehan 1993; Linehan *et al.* 2002). This approach is very reminiscent of social work at its preventative best, where the first task of the therapist is to establish an effective rapport/relationship with the person, the development of an agreed area of structured work and relief of any stressors. Despite the media image, there is evidence that 'good social work works, with person-enhancing and behaviour-improving outcomes' (Pritchard 1992b, 2001; Capp *et al.* 1997; Ford *et al.* 1997; Rock and Cooper 2000; Pritchard and Butler 2000a,b; Pritchard and Williams 2001). The first objective is to engage the person in a therapeutic relationship, irrespective of what psychosocial approach is being used, with longstanding evidence that creating a 'treatment alliance' is the core of all effective interventions (Lazarus 1976; Ford *et al.* 1997; Pritchard *et al.* 1998; Di Clemente *et al.* 2002). Indeed, on a sample of over 5,000 clients randomly allocated to different psychological treatments, the over-riding theme was the creation of this 'therapeutic alliance' (Di Clemente *et al.* 2002). Thus, people designated 'personality-disordered' can be helped by the use of DBT, especially in reducing the depressive overlay and DSH (Linehan 1993; Linehan *et al.* 2002).

One practical problem with these clients is that, because of the often long-term nature of their difficulties, they are dealt with by many different agencies, as they 'do the rounds' (Chiese *et al.* 2002), which requires that they 'tell their story' again and again, and inadvertently their 'patient/victim' role is reinforced. They may seem to gain insight and knowledge about their particular situation, but insight is not 'curative' unless it is followed by action and efforts to change. There is a rule of thumb that can be of help to the so-called 'borderline personality-disordered' client. The practitioner can spend two or three sessions hearing about the often multiple mishaps and unfortunate parenting they have received, but with adults it must be said that we, unlike the Biblical prophets, cannot '. . . restore the years that the locust hath eaten' (Joel 2: 25) – in other words, we cannot change their past, but help them to manage it better. One must always acknowledge the emotional hurt but then gently, in reviewing their often sad and tragic backgrounds, suggest that, while we have every sympathy and genuinely they have been unfairly treated by life, we cannot take away the pain of yesterday, but we can help to stop them continuing as a victim. Sensitively, without any hint of criticism, we ask them to consider that 'today is your first day of learning to be free from being a victim of your past – your parents hurt you, terribly, unjustifiably, but let's go forward and draw a line under yesterday – the hurt will remain, but you can begin to free yourself from its effects'.

The case of 'Nikki', a 28-year-old woman who was diagnosed by two consultant psychiatrists over a five-year period, highlights how a person could have been a client of the child protection service 20 years ago, and how those child protection issues overlap with borderline personality disorders and require a service today. This is her story, which is fairly typical of the complications of this pattern of behaviour with its invariably complicated antecedents.

When aged nine, 'Nikki' saw her father killed by her mother's lover, who had systematically sexually abused her over the previous two years. Her mother had initially avoided recognising the reality of her cohabitee's abuse, and Nikki's half-disclosure to her natural father led him to return to the family home and become the victim of the cohabitee's violence. Worse, Nikki remained unsure of the degree of her mother's compliance in her father's murder. The cohabitee went to prison and served 12 years, when he returned to Nikki's home.

Nikki had been very disturbed initially by the marital disharmony. 'I can never remember a time they weren't fighting – I was split in two, I wanted to love them both, but they were more concerned with getting at each other than noticing me.' As a five-year-old, she was enuretic (bed wetting) and very difficult at school. 'I have to admit it, I was a bully – it didn't matter what they did to me as long as I could hurt them – I never felt it if they fought back and most didn't.'

At the crisis of her father's death, the school made extra efforts to hold her and postponed her exclusion and transfer to another school. Nikki showed real signs of being depressed and saw child psychiatrists. While there was some improvement at her bereavement, intermittently, Nikki would go on the rampage and, as she told me this, she was smiling.

'I was a little bugger, I suppose I played on it – what had happened to me shouldn't have happened to any kid', and this pattern of emotional distress, followed by huge emotional outbursts, temper tantrums and violence, continued into her adult life.

Nikki saw many different and varied therapists over the years, all concentrating upon her past and, in my view, inadvertently colluding and reinforcing her position as 'victim'. Of course, anyone would have to be saddened and sympathetic at what had happened to Nikki, but they failed to appreciate that she was developing a characteristic patterned way of dealing with any normal life stressor: 'I admit, I go over the top' but, when she tells you this, it is reminiscent of a naughty child or adolescent, with a twinkle in her eye. By the time I met her she was enjoying her notoriety and the mayhem that surrounded her, which included crimes related to her illegal drug misuse, very heavy drinking of an almost compulsive nature, sex working, and promiscuous sexual relations. On two occasions, only 'manly pride' prevented her victims from pressing charges after she seriously assaulted them by hitting them over the head with a bottle. Clearly, Nikki's behaviour was self-defeating and, though in a sense 'explicable', she was unsure of her worth, etc., she virtually offered sex to every man who came into her orbit, including therapists, as she played manipulative games and, despite the distress she created, was obviously a very unhappy distressed person. Crises were building up in her life, as she oscillated between minor criminality, socially inappropriate behaviour, including extreme threats of violence, with bouts of self-loathing and despair and suicidal ideation. At our fourth session, after I had tried in the previous session to help her to repossess her life by enabling her to move out of the 'victim' mood, she attended late, half-drunk and under the influence of illegal drugs. She was alternatively sexually and physically threatening, shouting that 'you don't care about me' that 'you're a lousy therapist . . . and not a real man' or otherwise 'you would have enjoyed your opportunity' because she was a good, etc., etc., etc. I was able to keep calm, avoid any response to her deliberate provocation and crucially avoided arguing with her or, by my response, adding to her anger. I spoke in a quite deliberate measured voice, recognising her underlying distress, but pointed out that no-one was forcing her to see me and, while I wanted to try to help, I could only do so if she really wanted to change. This was the key as, at the end of our previous session, she had not welcomed my approach that this is the time to end being a victim, because otherwise I truly feared for her. The fourth session was drawing to a close reasonably quietly but with real tears and expressions of remorse and apology. This was the time to reinforce the positives in her life: she was an attractive person, was clearly intelligent and with great potential, and life really could be worth living. Over the next months, we explored her self-deprecatory behaviour but focused always upon the future and what she could do to change things. We identified together what she wanted from life and confronted the reality of the horror of suicide – namely, we had to have a whole session of disabusing her of the romantic ideas of death from an overdose. Later, she told a colleague that I was a 'rubbish therapist', despite continuing to see me over a six-month period, and slowly some aspects of her life became less chaotic. Our relationship was always fraught, and one felt on a knife edge that she would explode or damage herself in a dramatic gesture, but patiently she came to realise that she did have goals to achieve and that she could achieve them.

She established independent living, with the help of her mother 'who I manipulate, but why not after what she did to me?' There was no more talk or behaviour of deliberate self-harm, she stopped her coquettishness, at least with me, she held down a job and, what proved to be an enormous boost, gained a promotion. She stopped using any hard drugs, only occasionally used cannabis and handled alcohol much better (there had been times when she was endangering herself with binge drinking plus drug misuse).

The second great step forward was when she found an older man with whom she began a reasonably mature relationship. She used me as an agony aunt, although her new partner, 'John', did seem to want to settle down and with help was able to tolerate her extremes of mood, which she was able to manage better; she was much less inclined to be demanding because she was a victim. The relationship, with storms, lasted another six months, when she triumphantly came to our last session, stating that they were moving in together and were to be married.

Nikki's life history may be familiar to colleagues who work in child protection – certainly, as a child, Nikki would be a familiar case for child protection workers. So let us turn to another dimension in the mental health–child protection interface, something of the nature of the abuser, rather than the abused victim, for unless we better comprehend the abuser, we will be less equipped to break the cycle and/or reduce reoffending behaviour that can lead to a damaged and distressed adult.

Psychiatric–child protection interface

In 1962, Professor Richard Kempe and colleagues shocked the Western world when he alerted us to the extreme consequence of child neglect and abuse. Until his time, there was a tacit assumption that neglect and abuse were predominantly associated with poverty, and the extreme, the death of a child, was predominantly associated with post-partum depression and the assailant was almost by behavioural definition 'mentally disordered'. Kempe's work highlighted the fact that child neglect and abuse occurred across all social classes and ethnicities and, to emphasise the ubiquity of the problem, he played down the mental disorder link (Kempe and Kempe 1978). It is now appreciated that that the 'causes' of child neglect and abuse are multiple and complex, and while it can occur within any social grouping in society, including the educated middle class, the main factors are essentially psychosocial; while 'poverty' is an important contextual issue, it is poverty of mind and spirit, a 'psychological' poverty, that is the key. That is, a failure of parental bonding for 'within family' neglect and abuse, or inappropriate, exploitive and abusive behaviour by 'extrafamily' abusers (Utting 1997; Corby 2000; Pritchard 2004). Britain still has 'infanticide laws', which recognise that severely depressed women, who unrecognised and/or undiagnosed develop a puerperal psychosis, and at the extreme of the so-called 'baby blues', might harm their child. Because of the mother's depression, she fails to bond and may either neglect the child or develop a psychotic delusion. She misinterprets what is occurring, and she might kill the child because it is 'possessed of the devil' or it's 'not my child' or because of the dreadful depressing world around her, the mother kills her child in love to 'protect' it from a worse fate (d'Orban 1990; Bourget and Labelle 1992; Stroud 2003). This 'psychiatric' link with child protection is self-evident, and modern treatment is to develop mother and baby units via a partnership with paediatrics. A study from Manchester describes the successful treatment of the mother's underlying mental disorder and assistance in bonding with the child (Armstrong *et al.* 2000). More than 60 per cent of mothers had a formal mental disorder, mainly depression (43 per cent) and schizophrenia (21 per cent). Interestingly, while staff perceived the mother with schizophrenia to be more physically dangerous, in fact, she harmed her child no more than did the mothers who did not have schizophrenia. Crucially, there was a good outcome in 78 per cent of cases; the less good results occurred where there was a combination of negative factors such as lower social class, poor relationship with the partner or the partner also had a mental disorder, findings similar to a later British study (Abel *et al.* 2005).

It is also known that children of mothers who have depression in the child's early years may have more psychosocial problems than those of non-depressed mothers (Mowbray *et al.* 2001; Hammen *et al.* 2003; Maki *et al.* 2003; Targosz *et al.* 2003). And of course poverty and mental disorder often go together, with negative outcomes for the child (Famularo *et al.* 1992; Lipman *et al.* 2001).

Hence, wherever there is a mental disorder in a parent, the psychiatrist and/or the mental health practitioner should ask, 'what of the child?' How is the child/ren's needs being met? Equally, the child protection team should ask themselves the question, 'is there a mental health problem here?' and think actively of involving the psychiatric team.

Is this overprotective? No, for when we look at those rare cases where a child has died, from numerous enquiries, two themes emerge, first the well-known one of a lack of effective interprofessional communication (Noyes 1991; Lamming Report 2003), and the less well recognised, the presence of a mainly male abuser, whom we would now recognise as having a personality disorder (Noyes 1991), 'mad, bad and dangerous to know'.

Here is the good news. In the early 1970s, when Britain woke up to the problem of extreme child abuse, as highlighted in the Maria Colwell enquiry, England and Wales had the fourth highest rate of 'child murder' in the Western world; by the end of the century, over the 30 years, we gradually declined to become fifth lowest (Pritchard 1992c, 1996c, 2002; Pritchard and Butler 2003). In parenthesis, it should be noted that, while our adult homicide rate has remained fairly constant, we had a major reduction in children's homicide, whereas the USA, with a declining adult murder rate, increased their child homicide rate by more than 40 per cent (Pritchard and Butler 2003). Unlike Britain, where relatively child protection services have had a degree of resource protection, this was not the case in the USA. We explore the extremes of child abuse and neglect and any mental health dimension in an analysis of who are the people who go on and kill children.

At the extremes: who kills children?

Police, social service and suicide register records regarding child homicide over a ten-year period have been analysed in two English counties with a population of 2.6 million people, equivalent to 5 per cent of the total population of England. The results enabled some reasonably firm conclusions to be drawn (Pritchard and Bagley 2001; Pritchard 2004).

First, between 80 and 90 per cent of all assailants were 'within-family' offenders, all parent 'figures', a common finding throughout the Western world (d'Orban 1990; Bourget and Labelle 1992; Stroud 1997). All assailants from outside the family were male child sex abusers with histories of multiple criminality, including at least one conviction for violence.

Examining the 'within-family' assailants first, over the ten years, 64 per cent of the assailants were blood mothers, 18 per cent blood fathers and 18 per cent stepfathers or cohabitees (note that child homicide is very different from adult homicide). The assailants could be categorised into those with a 'mental disorder' (55 per cent), mothers on the 'At Risk of Abuse' register (27 per cent) and men with a previous conviction for violence (18 per cent), all of whom were stepfathers or cohabitees (Pritchard and Bagley 2001).

Thinking of the high media profile of child abuse deaths and the decade these figures came from, a population of 2.6 million people, off the top of your head, guess how many child murders there were? Was it 100 over the ten years, 200 or 50 or fewer?

In fact, over the ten-year period, there were 22 'within-family' child homicides and five murders by assailants outside the family, who together killed 33 children over the period. It might be thought, as suggested by McDonald (1993), little valid information can be drawn from such small numbers of cases, especially from such a large general population, but this is not the case. Murder is so rare that it also occurs only among people who belong to a 'special' category, like the four designations we identified.

A simple 'common-sense approach' to statistics highlights how we can draw reasonable conclusions about differential risk between 'within and outside' family assailants and between the different categories of offender.

Using an epidemiological approach, we ask the simple question 'How many people belong to our various categories or to the potential sample of child homicide assailants and how many deaths per million of population did this produce?'

Based upon the ages of mothers who actually killed (19–34 years), to find one random child killer, we would need approximately 144,000 women, a rate of seven per million p.a., whereas, as shown in Table 11.1, in fact the 14 female assailants, eight of whom were mentally disordered, based upon a potential population of 8,022 women in the general population with a severe mental disorder (Jenkins *et al.* 1998), killed at the rate of 100 p.m. p.a.

Although these mentally ill mothers (MIM) were the most frequent assailants of our four categories, based upon the potential size of population, they killed at a lower rate than the men with previous violent offences, who killed at a rate of 440 p.m. because, based upon police records, there were only 901 such men in the general population. In terms of numbers of assailants, there were four such men living with a child under 5 who was not his blood child.

Table 11.1 Rates per million of child homicide assailants by category

Assailant category	Estimated population	Homicide rate (p.m.)	Ratio to mentally ill mother
Within family			
Mentally ill mother			
Fathers aged 24–69	13,419	40	0.4:1
Mothers aged 19–34	8,022	100	1.0:1.0
Violent males aged 20–33	901	440	4.4:1
SSD mothers			
Alone 18–34	723	280	2.8:1
With cohabitee	723	830	8.3:1
Outside family			
Types of sex abuser			
Sex only aged 19–69	93	None	
Multiple sex abuser	49	2,040	20:1
Violent multiple child sex abuser	46	8,690	86:1

Source: Drawn from Pritchard (2004) based upon police and SSD records.

Among the 723 mothers on the 'At Risk of Abuse' register (SSD mothers), the child homicide rate was 830 p.m., but only if the mother was living with the violent offender, as in four cases both mother and cohabitee were jointly convicted because the jury could not determine who was the main assailant. A review of the sentences subsequently imposed shows that the cohabitees typically received much more severe custodial sentences, indicating that the judge thought them the most likely offender. Without her 'violent' partner, the SSD mothers' homicide rate fell to 280 p.m. Thus, in terms of 'frequency', the most frequent assailant actually had a lower rate than the others.

With regard to men who killed a child in the two countries aged 19–64, to find one random assailant would require more than 370,000 men.

This highlights the fact that the 'extrafamily' assailants killed least frequently, five compared with the 28 children for 'within-family' assailants, based upon the types of child sex abusers within the general population (Pritchard and Cox 1990; Pritchard and Bagley 2000). There were 46 p.a. male multicriminal abusers with previous conviction for violence, who killed at a rate of 8,690 p.m., 80 times the rate of the mentally ill mother!

These rates help to put into context the level of risks of the different categories. Even among these categories, the extremes of child abuse are quite rare; for mentally ill mothers, it was 0.01 per cent, for the violent males 0.44 per cent, the SSD mother with a cohabitee was 0.08 per cent and even the most dangerous of all, the violent male child sex abuser, was 0.87 per cent; thus 99 per cent of these most dangerous men had not killed. But self-evidently, they are a far greater physical risk to children than the mentally disordered parent. Thus, comparatively, the identified categories of child homicide assailants are highly dangerous, especially the 'extrafamily' violent multiple criminal child sex abuser. However, it has been strongly suggested from the most authoritative source, UNICEF (1999), that the violent death of a child is but the 'tip of the iceberg' representing the minimal extreme of abuse.

Of course, not all child neglecters or abusers are mentally disordered. Yet, reading the records, it is reiterated that, if the psychiatrists had asked themselves the question about whether their patients were involved with children, or the social worker had asked themselves is there a mental health problem, then it would be reasonable to assert that probably half the children who died might have been saved by an integrated interdisciplinary approach. Social workers in child protection teams should consider the risk that the presence of a non-blood father male, with a history of violence, poses to child and mother with a chaotic lifestyle.

It cannot be overstated that, in view of modern treatment for the mental disorders, these conditions are eminently treatable, the personality disorders less so.

This might be considered controversial and a threat to an individual's civil rights, but personality-disordered people are unlikely to change their behaviour significantly within the time in which the child's developmental needs are to be met; these two facts have major practice implications.

Parents or child carers who have a mood disorder or schizophrenia can be helped by a bio-psychosocial form of intervention, and the presence of their mental disorder should not automatically be a case for removal of the children.

However, with the personality-disordered, can they adequately meet the needs of any children in their care? It is appreciated that many such people were themselves victims of disadvantaged and deprived and abusing families, but what of the needs of any children? It is unpalatable and against classic social work values (Pritchard and Taylor 1978), but we should give serious thought to considering whether any children could be better looked after, and we should do it earlier in an effort to maximise the child's life chances and break the potential cycle of child neglect and future personality-disordered adults. When examining Noyes' (1991) catalogue of child protection disaster reports, any objective reader would begin to appreciate that the most abusive of the parent figures reviewed would fit the PD label by virtue of their life-long characteristic chaotic lives. Self-evidently, each situation would require the most detailed and in-depth consideration to avoid any further compounding of that person's situation. Reviewing our decade of child homicide cases, if there had been a greater awareness of the child protection–psychiatric interface, then children could have been better protected and an integrated approach to those with a severe mental disorder could have halved the fatalities.

Social science and social work might not like the PD category, with its admitted imprecision, but its value lies in reminding us that there are people whose life patterns are such that, apart from their own distress, in positions of power over a child they cannot reasonably be expected to meet the child's developmental needs. Furthermore, if there is the antisocial dimension present, they may be an active abuser, rather than the feckless neglecter.

As regards potential extrafamily assailants, the male child sex abusers, we need to differentiate the type of sex abuser, as they carry very different physical risks to children.

Out of a two-year cohort of 374 men convicted of a sexual offence against a child, 50 per cent were 'sex only' offenders, i.e. they had no other criminal convictions, whereas 26 per cent of the sample were multicriminal and in every case had more non-sex criminal convictions than sex offences; the remaining 24 per cent were multicriminal and also had a least one conviction for violence. Grossman *et al.* (1999) ask the question: are child sex abusers 'treatable'? In brief, there is evidence that probably the 'sex only' men might be helped to reduce the number of offences against children (Beckett *et al.* 1994; Paradise 2001). Members of the middle group, 'multiple criminal child sex abusers' require control and management; as yet no good evidence of effective intervention with these chaotic men has been found. However, in the case of multicriminal violent sex abusers, reviewable sentences should be considered until they can demonstrate that they are safe to live among us. And of course these men, while having the highest child homicide rate of our four categories, 80 times the rate of the 'mentally ill mother' (MIM), killed far fewer children than do we motorists! For every extrafamily child homicide in England and Wales, 22 children die on our roads (Pritchard 2002) but, of course, few in the media or the political establishment would contrast such risks as, although statistically extremely rare, sexual homicide assailants are especially violent, sadistic and dangerous and more than 80 per cent of them scored on a personality disorder checklist (Porter *et al.* 2003).

What can be said about convicted child sex abusers is that the majority appear to have life-long patterns of characteristic behaviour and whether they should be included in the personality disorder paradigm is a debate for the future, when research helps us to understand better and, therefore, prevent perpetuating the cycle of abuse.

As if this chapter was not controversial enough, we now turn to the final two areas relevant to the psychiatric–child protection interface, about which the individual worker will have to make their own judgements.

Suicide and child abuse

The link between being a victim of child abuse and later mental disorder, including suicidal behaviour, is increasingly being understood (Fromouth 1988; Bagley and Ramsay 1997; Hawton *et al.* 2001, 2003). In a study of a two-year cohort of all men convicted of child sexual abuse (Pritchard and Bagley 2000), it was noticed that a number these men had committed suicide. This paradoxically seemed to have some treatment implications in that a key deficit in child molesters is that they appear to have little empathy for their victims and treatment aims to restore or inculcate a proper appreciation of their victims' distress (Simon *et al.* 1992; Beckett *et al.* 1994). Hence, if some of these men are suicidal, it may be indicative of a degree of remorse, albeit mixed after being detected, but such remorse may be worked with.

Bringing together coroner's, police, SDD records and a Regional Suicide Register, suicide rates in the general population were explored, and those with a mental disorder, victims and/or perpetrators of child sex abuse, were identified (Pritchard and King 2004). It was then possible to identify 'mental disorder-related' (MDR) suicides and 'child sex abuse-related' (CSAR) suicides and compare them with the general population suicide rate (GPSR). It is readily admitted that identifying 'victims' in the CSAR suicides was problematic, and there may have been more suicides of 'victims' of abuse, which was not shown in official records, whereas the 'perpetrators' in the CSAR suicides were very easy to confirm via police records, although of course there may have been other perpetrators who were unknown to the police. Nonetheless, this is, as yet, the hardest data available from de facto court-decided suicides.

The results were surprising and have important practice implications.

The male GPSR was a little higher than the national average, at 153 per million. With both male and female victims of abuse, CSAR suicides were more than twice the rate of the GPSR, but not as high as the MDR suicide rate, which for males was 12 times and for females 15 times the GPSR. The big surprise was that the perpetrator CSAR suicide were significantly higher than the MDR and more than 40 times the GPSR as shown in Table 11.2 (Pritchard and King 2004).

These results confirmed our earlier impression that male child sex abusers committed suicide significantly more often than the general population (Pritchard and Bagley 2001). However, the practical implication was that all the perpetrator CSAR came from one type of child molester, namely the 'sex only' offender, indicating some remorse. This, Paradise (2001) argues, can be a starting point to reach out to these men, a number of whom regret their orientation, and in this sense are 'treatable'. Grossman *et al.* (1999) explores the hard reality of whether these men are treatable; they argue that, in view of the antecedents of many child abusers, i.e. they themselves were victims, we should reach out in compassion and understanding to those who would end their depredations on children. However, they also conclude that some offenders are not treatable, but offer no recommendation about what to do with them.

Conversely, in the suicide study, not one of the multicriminal violent child molesters was engaged in suicidal behaviour (Pritchard and King 2004), and whether they wish or are able to want to change is questionable, and therefore requires a different approach until they are ready to take up their humanity again.

Nonetheless, we should not forget the victim CSAR suicides as a reminder of the extreme consequences that can be associated with prolonged abuse and that, possibly, because the abuse in childhood may not have been disclosed by a depressed adult, the victim CSAR suicide rates are probably an underestimate.

Munchausen syndrome by proxy

Munchausen syndrome by proxy (MSBP) is currently at the centre of a major controversy, and the question is being asked, does the syndrome exist and, of pressing import, has the use of the syndrome led to cases of miscarriage of justice where parents have been falsely accused of the death of their child and/or children have been taken away on the advice of 'experts' (Pritchard 2004)? If nothing else, the controversy shows the power of the media, ever wishing to simplify and dumb down for a population that allows itself to be fed pap, for 'there is nothing either good or bad but [the media] makes it so'. From the start, the main protagonist of

Table 11.2 CSAR and MDR suicide rates compared with the general population suicide rate (GPSR) (per million)

Group	Number	Rate (p.m.)	Times GPSR
Male general population	757	153	1.0
Female general population	260	48	1.0
MDR			
Males	167	1,820	12
Females	101	78	15
CSAR victims			
Males	5	340	2.2
Females	4	120	2.4
Male perpetrators	16	6,130	40

the concept, Professor Roy Meadows, acknowledged its imprecision, but argued that there were a rare number of parents who, seemingly to attract attention to themselves, fabricated illness in their children (Meadows 1977). Indeed, the current term is 'fabricated illness syndrome' but, for common usage, we shall use MSBP.

In brief, Munchausen syndrome is a rare adult syndrome in which the person presents themself as sick and, as the WHO states, is 'a condition best interpreted as a disorder of illness behaviour and the sick role' (WHO 1992). It falls into the PD category but a few people end up later presenting psychotic-like behaviour.

Meadows was confronted by a series of parents who behaved a little like Munchausen patients in attention seeking, but the focus was upon their child being presented as ill. The consequence of this illness-inducing behaviour for the child could be quite serious, leading to disability and even death (Bools *et al.* 1993; Tenny *et al.* 1994; Meadows 2002; Tessa *et al.* 2002). An ethically questionable study of 'suspected' parents having MSBP by Professor Southall *et al.* (1997) nevertheless demonstrated that using covert TV to observe parent's behaviour when alone with the child showed in many, but not all, cases actual physical damage by the MSBP suspected parent, a finding that was repeated elsewhere (Tenny *et al.* 1994; Hall *et al.* 2000).

The pattern of fabricated illness has been found in 25 countries (Feldman and Brown 2002) and in non-Western cultures (Al-Lamki 2000). But, all in the field would admit that the syndrome is very imprecise and, indeed, perhaps Meadows' core problem was to try to use a label from adult psychiatry to describe what he seemed to be observing. Discussing informally with a number of consultant psychiatrists, they point out two key features. First, it is very rare, as is adult Munchausen's; second, they accept a child-damaging pattern exists but they question whether there is a syndrome per se, but rather it is a ragbag of severe personality disorders, atypical mood disorders and/or atypical schizophrenia, and that Meadows' mistake was to try to define a syndrome with such questionable parameters.

Social workers from the child protection field might have some sympathy with paediatricians, as they know only too well that the media condemns them for being either too intrusive or not intrusive enough. What certainly must not happen is that 'sudden infant death syndrome', i.e. the so-called cot deaths, must not be automatically assumed to be covert neglect or abuse, which has happened in the past (Pritchard 1995) and, thankfully, the pendulum has swung away from the earlier kneejerk reaction, but a rare minority of parents do damage their children and present it as a cot death. What can the practitioner do with such conflicting and complex messages? Do we throw out the idea of a pattern of behaviour described as 'fabricated illness' and assume that all those professionals in the different countries were jumping on a bandwagon, or that experts were not looking carefully enough at specific cases and were making generalised assumptions leading to miscarriages of justice? Or rather the syndrome is an artefact and should be abandoned? Indeed, recently, Professor Meadows, although retired, has been struck off by the General Medical Council for 'unprofessional practice'. Yet it is conjectured that Professor Meadows' real 'failure' was that, after years of exposure of the extremes of child neglect, he began to think less like a detached academic and practitioner and perhaps more like a policeman, and started thinking the unthinkable? Certainly, this researcher and practitioner never dreamed that the research evidence would lead them to reject, for a very small minority of men, deeply cherished social work values of being 'non-judgemental'. Yet, after being exposed to police records of child sex offenders and child homicide assailants whose behaviour showed that they had laid aside their humanity, I was 'damaged' by this research. The evidence seen meant that I would not want to risk these men living among us until they could prove they were safe to do so. Consequently, although cautioning against accusations of child abuse in cases of 'cot deaths' as early as 1995, objectively it seems that Professor Meadows has been harshly treated, although recognising that there could be few worse things in life than being falsely accused of killing your own child.

But how real and dangerous is MSBP?

In an effort to estimate the incidence of MSBP, McClure and his team (1996), including Professor Meadows, reviewed all cases in Ireland referred to a paediatric surveillance unit. Over a two-year period, there were 128 cases, of whom 85 per cent were mothers and 58 appeared to be possible MSBP. Sixty-eight of the children suffered severe illness and eight died over the period. So what does this mean?

Extrapolating from McClure's results, two figures emerge. First is that, if we assume that all the Irish cases did have elements of MSBP, then this is equivalent to an incidence of 0.008 per cent MSBP in the general population, far lower than our extreme male child molesters. However, the eight deaths represent a mortality rate of 62,250 per million or 6.3 per cent. The immediate fact is that 92.7 per cent of these parents were not associated with the death of a child but, based on an epidemiological approach in estimating extreme physical risk, the Irish sample of MSBP parents had a mortality rate seven times the violent multicriminal child molester, who was 80 times more fatal than the most frequent assailant, the mentally ill mother!

It is not an easy area, and certainly not one for simplistic, scapegoating media, and we might await the next tragedy, where the professional will be castigated because they did not suspect the unthinkable.

As with all statistics, the above figures can only be a guide, being based upon 'groups' rather than individuals. So that, for example, X condition might have a 90 per cent outcome, but invariably your client might well belong to the odd 10 per cent. What this controversy should do is to take us back to basics, that the professional seeks to offer this person a personalised service based upon current evidence-based knowledge, applied to their circumstances, and provide person-appropriate 'techniques'. Life becomes complicated when our clients cross different expertise/agency boundaries, as they do in the psychiatric–child protection interface.

Our task therefore is to be aware of the different knowledge bases that might be relevant to our client's needs; self-evidently, we can seldom if ever be categorical, absolute in our practice, because our clients, like ourselves, are never like the textbooks, which should inform, guide but can never offer the definitive answer for this person at this time. It has been said that 'happy families resemble each other, each unhappy family is unhappy in its own way' (Tolstoy, *Anna Karenina*); perhaps this is a good approach in seeking to serve in the mental health social work field.

We now turn to those control issues within mental health and, in particular, the role of the Approved Social Worker, where social workers daily face some of these recurrent dilemmas.

12 Statutory mental health social work

Care and control dilemmas and role of the Approved Social Worker

> Sometimes I stand and think – this is a sick plan to control a special person who's been fighting stuff a long time. 'Notice the difference, when you treat me right!' I shout. Does no harm. It is better here, than years ago. Same label – but they ask about the colour of the bricks in your wall.
>
> (Southgate 2000)

Objectives: by the end of this chapter you should:

1 know the most often used sections of the Mental Health Act 1983;
2 be familiar with the controversial proposals for a community treatment order;
3 have some idea of the needs and limits of 'compulsory' care;
4 understand the potential therapeutic role of the Approved Social Worker in the statutory process.

As discussed previously, mental health is an area in which care and control go side by side. This chapter aims to outline the core tasks of the Approved Social Worker (ASW) and the tensions involved in this statutory role, where care and control issues interface. It has been written in conjunction with a senior ASW colleague who prefers to remain anonymous – in part so that they can 'tell it as it is'. It aims to show how the new legislative proposals may influence the nature of the work in the future. It will draw upon examples from practice to illustrate the often complex nature of the ASW's decision-making task.

Introduction

The role of the ASW was introduced by the Mental Health Act (MHA) 1983. This Act replaced the existing 1959 Act and emphasised the desirability of community-based care over hospital-based services. If hospital admission was indicated, if necessary by compulsion, the 1983 Act was clear that this should only be under specific circumstances, and that there should be no better alternatives.

The primary gateway to compulsory admission would necessitate two registered medical practitioners both independently concluding that a patient required hospital admission. But this alone would not suffice. It would be the role of the ASW to 'satisfy himself that detention in a hospital is in all the circumstances of the case the most appropriate way of providing the care and medical treatment of which the patient stands in need' (Section 13(2) MHA 1983). It concluded that, if this was the case, the ASW was invested with the responsibility of making a legal application for the compulsory admission of the patient and that this was the 'safest' and least restrictive option. If the ASW could not concur with the two medical recommendations for compulsory admission, then he/she was under no obligation to make such an application. Herein lies part of the dilemma and tension in the role of ASW – the need for the careful weighing of medical evidence vis-à-vis the individual's own personal choices, social circumstances and human rights, reaching the 'safest' decision. This safety element is central to the ASW's decision-making role, within the context of risk assessment and risk management – the decision needs to take full account of the potential risks of the patient to themselves and to other people. This consideration is vital in informing the final decision whether to make an application or not. Fundamentally, it is these 'tensions' that provide the challenge to the ASW – the challenge of making a balanced and reasoned decision in the midst of often chaotic circumstances, often without having all the information one would wish, while always ensuring that there are medical, ethical and legal bases for the decision reached.

But the role of the ASW is not specific to situations requiring assessment for possible admission to hospital. ASWs also have the responsibility for making applications under Section 7 for individuals to be received into guardianship, and are also involved in making recommendations as to whether a patient should be subject to aftercare under supervision (Section 25A). More will be said about these later.

The most commonly used sections of the Mental Health Act

Section 1 – Defining mental disorder

No individual can be detained under any section of the MHA unless they fall (or are believed to fall at the time of detention) into one of four categories of 'mental disorder' as defined in Section 1 of the Mental Health Act 1983. These four categories are 'mental illness' (not actually defined in the MHA), 'mental impairment', 'severe mental impairment' and 'psychopathic disorder'. People may not be categorised as mentally disordered 'by reason only of promiscuity or other immoral conduct, sexual deviancy or dependence on alcohol or drugs' (Section 1(3)), which was to guard against the pre-1959 MHA situation of people being incarcerated for decades primarily because of sexual behaviour (Jones 1959). Furthermore, chaotic or criminal behaviours alone are not grounds for detention under the MHA, yet sometimes it will be these behaviours that bring an individual to the attention of their GP, the police or mental health services in the first place. And it is known that many people in prison have a 'co-morbidity' of a mental disorder (Korbin 1986; Bhui *et al.* 1998; Hoyer *et al.* 2000; Ramsbotham

2001). While 'mental disorder' per se is not defined in the Act, each of the four categories of mental disorder is defined. Under new proposals likely to replace the existing Act by 2005 or 2006, these four categories are to be replaced by one single definition. Some are concerned that this will bring more people within a widening net of compulsory powers.

Section 2

Admission under Section 2 is a compulsory admission for assessment. It is one of the major 'civil admissions' so does not involve the court system in any way. The order can last up to a maximum of 28 days and cannot be renewed thereafter. During the period of assessment, an individual may receive medical treatment for their psychiatric illness against their will, subject to the 'consent to treatment' laws. Part IV of the MHA outlines the 'consent to treatment' laws. In order to be admitted to hospital for assessment, the individual has to be 'suffering from mental disorder of a nature or degree which warrants the detention of the patient in a hospital for assessment (or for assessment followed by medical treatment) for at least a limited period' (Section 2(2)(a)) and 'ought to be so detained in the interests of his own health or safety or with a view to the protection of other persons' (Section 2(2)(b)). In order to make an application for a Section 2 order, the ASW must have two medical recommendations in the prescribed form. The nearest relative (NR) may not object to the use of Section 2 and has no recourse to the Mental Health Review Tribunal (MHRT). However, the patient can apply to the MHRT, and their nearest relative may use their powers to request discharge of the patient. This power can only be blocked by the Responsible Medical Officer (RMO) if the person's discharge from detention, 'would be likely to act in a manner dangerous to other persons or to himself' (Section 25(1)). This applies also where a person is detained under Section 3, which is reviewed below.

Section 3

Section 3 allows a patient to be compulsorily detained in hospital for treatment for up to six months. Thereafter, the Section can be renewed for a further six months and then on an annual basis. In practice, a Section 3 is used where an individual is already known to services and a treatment plan is already established in the community. The ASW again requires two medical recommendations in order to make an application for a person's admission to a specific hospital. The ASW must, if 'reasonably practicable' or if it would not 'involve unreasonable delay', consult with an individual's NR about a potential admission under Section 3. As we shall see in the example of Mr X (below), a NR can object to the use of compulsory powers under Section 3, but can also have their function as NR removed by the County Court, thus having their views as NR over-ridden. Under present legislation, no-one can choose their nearest relative – the NR is defined by Section 26. If a person's NR is an abusive parent, this places the ASW in a difficult position ethically. Under the 1983 Act, the ASW must still consult with an abusive NR but, with the advent of human rights legislation, this is being challenged. It remains a grey area. Under Section 3, both the patient and their NR are entitled to apply to the MHRT for the detention to be considered by this independent tribunal. This can result in the making of recommendations for a person's treatment or a patient being discharged from their Section. In the case of Section 3, an ASW should only make an application if they conclude that a person's mental disorder 'is of a nature or degree which makes it appropriate for him to receive medical treatment in a hospital' and if 'it is necessary for the health or safety of the patient or for the protection of other persons that he should receive such treatment and it cannot be provided unless he is detained under this Section'. The ASW must seek the 'least restrictive alternative' to ensure the health or safety of the 'patient' and the 'protection' of other persons. Hospital admission need not always be the result of a Mental Health Act assessment. In fact, we shall see that legislative proposals afoot suggest that compulsory treatment 'in the community' (the 'community treatment order') is planned for the future. Table 12.1 shows the more common sections of the MHA 1983.

'Mr X' is the carer for his wife 'Mrs X'. Mrs X has been a user of mental health services for approximately seven years and has been admitted to psychiatric hospital on numerous occasions, often under a Section of the Mental Health Act. The perceived treatment of his wife while an inpatient at a specific inpatient unit has led Mr X to become very disillusioned with this health service provision. Some months later, Mr X's eldest son (aged 22) is also admitted to hospital with a very similar presentation to his mother (Mrs X). Behaviours include aggressive outbursts, overdosing on over-the-counter medications, superficial ligatures around the neck and attempts to abscond from the hospital ward. At this point, the son X is under Section 2 (28-day assessment order). The RMO later makes a recommendation for a Section 3 to be applied for by the ASW. Unlike when being assessed for an admission under Section 2, the patient's NR (see Section 26) can make an objection to the application for a Section 3 treatment order. If they exercise this right, an application cannot normally be made by the ASW without recourse to the County Court to have the NR displaced. A Section 3 can only be applied for where the ASW has first taken the case to the County Court to have the NR removed and another person or the local authority appointed. However, this can only occur where there are specific reasons under law for the NR's removal. Mr X did object to the use of a Section 3 order but not because he objected to his son's need for compulsory detention in an inpatient setting. His objection was due to his anger that the NHS Trust would not agree to placing his son in an inpatient unit other than the one which he perceived as having provided a very poor service both to Mrs X and to the son X. The local authority subsequently took the case to the County Court and requested that Mr X be displaced as NR and the local authority appointed to exercise this function. This application was accepted by the court and the son was subsequently detained under Section 3 at the hospital that Mr X objected to. This ensured that the son received the treatment deemed necessary but did not endear the NHS Trust to Mr X who essentially desired the same outcome for his son as the ASW and recommending doctors.

Table 12.1 The more common sections of the Mental Health Act 1983

Section	Criteria	Action	Power
Section 2: Admission for assessment	Need for detention in hospital for risk assessment to health or safety of self or others	Either ASW, nearest relative plus medical recommendations from two doctors, one approved under Section 12	Patient can be detained for a maximum of 28 days for assessment and treatment to be started
Section 3: Admission for treatment	Severity of disorder requires medical treatment in hospital	ASW, not nearest relative, plus two doctors, one approved	Can be held for six months and is renewable
Section 4: Emergency admission	Urgent admission for assessment	ASW or nearest relative plus one doctor, ideally GP who knows patient	Can only be held for 72 hours but can be transferred as per above to another section
Sections 5 (2): Change of status	An informal patient who requires detention because of risk to self or others	RMO or designated deputy	This can last 72 hours but treatment cannot be started unless transferred to another section
Sections 5 (4): Power of hospital nurse	Informal patient considered to be at risk to self or others requires detention	Qualified mental health nurse	Lasts up to six hours – in effect, emergency holding for a patient who has suddenly deteriorated
Section 58: Treatment (needs second opinion)	Section 3 patients who may require ECT or other treatment after three months of care	RMO or independent doctor who certifies that the patient has agreed to the ECT treatment to prevent deterioration	Course of ECT or drugs given for longer than three months

One wonders whether such an outcome would have occurred if this situation had concerned a person with a physical illness?

Special sections

Section 13 – Duty of ASWs to make applications for admission or guardianship

The MHA outlines the duties of the ASW in Section 13. Where concerns are expressed for an individual's mental health, there are occasions when an ASW is required to co-ordinate a Mental Health Act assessment. This can result in an application being made for a person's compulsory admission to hospital or reception into guardianship. But the ASW must first be satisfied 'that such an application ought to be made' and only after the patient has been interviewed in a 'suitable manner'. This can be particularly challenging to the ASW where the person being assessed is a child or if the person is deaf or communicates in a different language or belongs to a different culture – remembering that it is the professional's responsibility to communicate adequately with the patient, not vice versa. A Mental Health Act assessment is a specific legal process involving specific individuals. The intention of this process is to assess fully an individual's mental state in order to form an opinion as to whether they require hospital admission, if necessary, under compulsion of the Mental Health Act. If an application for hospital admission is being considered, the ASW must be satisfied 'that detention in a hospital is, in all the circumstances of the case, the most appropriate way of providing the care and medical treatment of which the patient stands in need'. Where hospital admission is not felt to be necessary or appropriate, an assessment can also serve the purpose of clarifying what services, if any, will assist an individual. In this situation, the ASW can provide the necessary information regarding access to potentially helpful mental health services.

When an ASW is asked to co-ordinate an assessment, it is often to assess a person previously unknown to the ASW. It is a specific time-limited piece of crisis intervention work. After a decision is reached, the ASW may have no further personal involvement with the patient's care, which is not very satisfactory or good practice, bearing in mind the importance of the client–therapist relationship (Lazarus 1976; Pritchard *et al.* 1998; King *et al.* 2001; Pritchard and Williams 2001). If an ASW applies for a person's detention under the Mental Health Act, they then facilitate the admission on the receiving hospital ward and then leave the care to the nursing staff. Often ASWs are not afforded knowledge of 'what happened next'. This can be a frustration of the role and perhaps against the spirit of the original 1983 Act.

'Mr A' is a 20-year-old man living with his parents. He has become increasingly reclusive over several months and is no longer attending to his personal care. He has become obsessed with alien life forms and is expressing many paranoid ideas. He is depressed and at times has expressed the desire to die. He has no specific plans to end his life. There is a history of depression in the family. His mother and maternal uncle have both been treated for depression. The consultant psychiatrist has seen Mr A in his outpatient clinic for some time and both he and Mr A's GP are keen for the use of Section 3. The ASW is minded to agree. However, the father (nearest relative), while supporting the urgent need for hospitalisation, has some key questions regarding the proposed treatment plan. The concerns centre on the parents' belief that Mr A's uncle died as a direct result of undergoing electroconvulsive therapy (ECT). This cannot be verified, but the ASW is concerned to offer the family some reassurance about Mr A's treatment before making application for the Section 3. The father is wishing to exercise his right to object to the use of Section 3 unless he is given reassurance that ECT will not be used. However, clinical decisions are outside the remit of the ASW. The ASW attempts to discuss the treatment plan with the consultant psychiatrist but the consultant will offer no guarantees about possible treatment options for Mr A. The consultant says that he does not at this time consider ECT to be a likely treatment option. Both the NR and ASW are now in a quandary. Both feel that Mr A should be compulsorily detained in hospital to ensure he receives the appropriate care. But how can the situation be resolved to each party's satisfaction? And, amidst this dilemma, how can the ASW ensure that the rights and dignity of Mr A are upheld? This dilemma is not untypical of the situations that can face the ASW.

In the above example, the ASW had no further dealings with Mr A or his family. After negotiation with the NR, a Section 3 application was made. The NR agreed to an application for Section 3 primarily because he did not feel that he and his family could cope with Mr A returning home that day. The ASW later found out in a hospital ward round that ECT had subsequently been considered for Mr A.

Sections 135 and 136 – The place of safety

There are occasions when a person will deny the assessing doctors and ASW access to their home. In this scenario, the ASW must consider going to court to seek a warrant under Section 135(1) – only then can the ASW legally enter the premises with a police constable executing the warrant and, if necessary, remove the individual to a 'place of safety' for assessment.

Under Sections 135 and 136, the Act allows for individuals to be removed to a 'place of safety' under certain conditions and in the interests of their own or others' safety. Section 136 gives police constables the powers to detain an individual (who is found in a public place) 'who appears to him to be suffering from mental disorder and to be in immediate need of care or control' if he or she feels this is 'in the interests of that person or for the protection of other persons'. Removing a person to a 'place of safety' can serve several functions. It provides a 'safe' environment where an individual can be closely monitored and provides a contained environment within which a Mental Health Act assessment can be undertaken within a period of up to 72 hours. However, the local authority or NHS Trust for whom the ASW works will determine where the agreed 'place of safety' is. Herein lies a dilemma. Best practice dictates that a 'place of safety' should be a hospital or medical suite. However, the 'place of safety' is often an agreed police station. The person may not have committed any crime and yet could be forgiven for thinking that they are being punished. For an individual suffering from psychosis, the added stress of being placed in a police cell may prove intolerable.

This concerns the assessment of a man in his early thirties – 'Mr G'. He had been picked up on a S136 and was being held at a local police station in a holding cell. He had lacerated his upper torso prior to his coming to the attention of the police. He had become aggressive with police officers and been physically restrained. Having attempted to make ligatures out of his clothing, he had been stripped naked and was huddled in the corner of the cell. The interview soon established that here was an extremely vulnerable man who would benefit from a time of assessment under Section 2. An assessed risk of violence determined that he should not be admitted to an open ward. However, the local psychiatric intensive care unit (PICU) was full to capacity, so a bed was sought elsewhere under an extracontractual arrangement. This would mean Mr G being hospitalised against his will in another town or city. The problem was that a bed could not be found elsewhere either because there were no vacancies or because units would not accept Mr G given the description of his current presentation. With no bed, it was not possible to complete an application and Mr G remained in the custody of the police for at least another 24 hours before arrangements were in hand for his transfer to an inpatient unit. Naturally, this delay was far from ideal for his care and treatment and safety.

Future challenges for the ASW: the proposed community treatment order

Compulsory treatment in the community was not a provision of the Mental Health Act 1959 and is not a part of current legislation (Mental Health Act 1983). This is set to change, with the proposed introduction of community treatment orders (CTOs), which in part is a 'political' response to a rare but tragic case, where a Mr Clunis killed a total stranger, Mr Zito – hence the Zito Trust who have argued for more restrictive legislation – shades of the child protection situation and the dangers of overdefensive practice as touched upon in Chapter 8. Frank Dobson (a former Secretary of State for Health) stated in 1998 that 'failure (in community care) has been caused by . . . an outdated legal framework, which failed to support effective treatment outside hospital' (Department of Health 1998: 3). As we shall see, Dobson was keen to promote policies that would be seen to address perceived gaps in the service – gaps that were widely felt to have contributed to the occurrence of well-publicised tragedies involving mental health clients.

In 1991, the Conservative government had published their consultative Green Paper *The Health of the Nation*. It claimed that the arrival, in the 1950s, of more advanced psychiatric drug treatments meant that mentally ill patients who would previously have faced long-term institutional care could now be 'treated in the community' (HMSO 1991: 86). For those patients who accepted or responded to community-based treatments, this was perhaps the case. Otherwise, the law afforded little alternative other than to compulsorily admit people into hospital if their mental health deteriorated such that they met grounds for hospital detention under the existing legislation.

The new Labour government of 1997 promised a 'root and branch' review of the 1983 Act and appointed an 'Expert Committee', chaired by Genevra Richardson, to make recommendations for change in key areas – including how to manage those patients who cannot, or refuse, to comply with community treatments once they've left hospital. A Green Paper was published on 16 November 1999. What was promised is 'The biggest shake-up in mental health services for 40 years' (Democratic Health Network 1999); as we shall see later, this was 'media needs led' rather than based on the evidence. Although the final framework still remains unknown at present, Department of Health officials have made it clear to the House of Commons Select Committee on Health that 'the principle of compulsion in the community is regarded as non-negotiable', that is not 'whether' CTOs will be implemented, but 'how' they should be implemented (House of Commons 2000: para. 140). In July 2000, Professor Louis Appleby (the government's mental health tsar) confirmed that plans to introduce CTOs were 'in the pipeline' (BBC 2000). But what is this proposed legislative development based upon and is it universally welcomed? To reflect on this question, we will first briefly review the current policy context and some of the key legislative developments in mental health policy over the past decade or more.

Current legal framework

At present, the statutory framework for managing mental disorder is enshrined primarily within the Mental Health Act 1983 and its accompanying Code of Practice (most recently revised March 1999). The 1983 Act allows for compulsory treatment – but as we have previously outlined – only under certain grounds and ultimately in the hospital setting under Section. Sectioned patients on leave from hospital (under Section 17) are still 'liable to be detained' and can be recalled from leave if it is felt they need their treatment programme to be more closely monitored and enforced. However, once discharged from Section, it is practically impossible to ensure ongoing compliance with a treatment programme. In view of this, and arguably in response to the recommendations of the 'Ritchie Report' (HMSO 1994), Supervision Registers were introduced in 1994 as a means of attempting to ensure that the best possible aftercare arrangements were in place for the higher risk category of discharged patients. This was in addition to the relatively new Care Programme Approach, introduced in 1991, which again had a focus upon ensuring that thorough aftercare arrangements were in place post discharge. Schneider (1993) argues that the Care Programme Approach was a government reaction to the 1988 'Spokes Inquiry' that investigated the circumstances leading to the killing of hospital social worker Isabel Schwartz. In passing, there was virtually no discussion about how relatively the effective resource budget was cut to mental health between the early 1980s and the mid-1990s (Pritchard *et al.* 1997a) – any tragedies are all the fault of 'inadequate' professionals or systems, not lack of resources – we are being ironic.

In 1996, the provisions of the Mental Health (Patients in the Community) Act 1995 came into force as an addendum to the 1983 Act. This allowed for the responsible medical officer (RMO) to make an application for certain catego-ries of detained patients to be discharged with their aftercare under supervision. However, this legislation stopped short of legalising enforced compliance with treatment in the community, despite allowing the supervisor legally to convey the patient to 'any place where the patient is required to reside or to attend for the purpose of medical treatment, occupation, education or training' (HMSO 1983: s25D (4)). While the boundaries of Supervised Discharge and Guardianship (S7/S37(2) (a)(ii)) helped to encourage compliance and to promote effective aftercare provisions for some, others continued to experience mental stability only when compulsorily detained and rapidly deteriorated once 'lost' back into the commu-nity. Section 25A had been specifically targeted at 'the small group of so-called "revolving door patients"' (Jones 1999: paras 1–265), but the current proposed policy developments imply that the government wants to provide further legal measures to provide for this higher risk category of discharged patients. But what is the motivation for this current policy of compulsion?

Frank Dobson, speaking at a fringe meeting at the 1999 Labour conference, gives us a big clue: 'I want to be able to look Jayne Zito in the eye and say that our mental health strategy might have stopped her husband being randomly stabbed' (Dobson 1999). Jonathon Zito had been killed by a discharged patient – Christopher Clunis – and in the above-mentioned 'Ritchie Inquiry Report', mental health services had been criticised for their lack of provision of effec-tive aftercare. In the keynote document, *Modernising Mental Health Services* (Department of Health 1998), published the previous year, Mr Dobson made it clear that the government intends to bring the laws on mental health 'up to date' – to ensure that patients who might otherwise be a danger to themselves or to the general public 'are no longer allowed to refuse to comply with the treatment they need' (Department of Health 1998: 6). It is clear that Mr Dobson had no concept of what 'random' means or the relative risk of looking citizens in the eye after a road death, for his motivation has arguably been driven by government reaction to the media portrayal of the alleged dangers of mentally ill patients 'left to flounder in the community'. In passing, a simple statistical comparison of the numbers of Clunis–Zito tragedies and the number of road deaths is revealing. Four hundred children die annually on our roads, more than 2,000 adults (Pritchard 2002), but dare politicians deal with this 'internal civil violence' on a comparable basis? Certainly, they do not appear to look at the evidence, nor does the media, who are afraid to offend readers who might be motorists.

The National Service Framework (NSF), introduced in September 1999, is an attempt to monitor standards in mental health policy and practice. According to one commentator, the NSF was motivated 'as expected' by the mental health 'mantra' – 'risk, risk, risk' (Davidson 2000: 5). Genevra Richardson from the 'Expert Committee' feels that the links between mental disorder and violence have been emphasised disproportionally in the media and 'really fear[s] that the Green Paper has almost accepted that without question' (House of Commons 2000: para. 127). The government have said that the mental health services should be 'safe, sound and supportive' in order to 'protect the public' and to provide 'effective care for those with mental illness at the time they need it' (Department of Health 1998) – not just at the time they 'want' it. Admirable objectives if they were backed by adequate resources at the point of crisis. The evidence and practice tend towards making one cynical.

George Bernard Shaw is reported as having commented that scandal has a much more immediate effect on policy than research (Spicker 1995). So, is the government's insistence on CTOs a crude reaction to media scandal or is it founded on clinical research? It is also important to establish whether service users and professionals welcome the proposal or we are getting the issue out of perspective. For example, what about the annual toll of suicides in most Western countries and its link to mental disorder? There are more suicides annually in Britain than died in the Twin Towers tragedy on 11 September 2001. While nothing justified the taking of innocent life, the tragic toll of 3,074 of 9/11 is exceeded every fortnight in the USA by homicide, suicide and road deaths; it is far too easy for governments to over-react to a media-led panic and get the problem out of perspective (Pritchard and Wallace 2006).

Surveying the evidence

We should first note that 'treatment' as defined by Section 145 (1)(c) of the 1983 Act 'includes nursing, and also includes care, habilation and rehabilitation under medical supervision' – it is not confined solely to 'medication'. However, despite this broad definition, the House of Commons Select Committee on Health, in their review of the Green Paper and Expert Committee Report, felt that the 'discussion of compulsory treatment tended to focus primarily, if not exclusively, on pharmaceutical treatments' (House of Commons 2000: para. 139). This is highly significant as 'non-compliance' has also tended to focus primarily on 'medication' compliance, rather than a broader 'treatment compliance'.

Most are agreed that there are potential problems with non-engagement from treatment (in the broadest sense) for individuals with more severe mental health problems. However, while the government has arguably focused primarily on 'risk to others', others have highlighted the 'risks to self' and the tragedy of mental health difficulties being prolonged or exacerbated through people's avoidance of statutory services. Mental health interest groups are concerned that the threat of compulsion will increase the likelihood of people avoiding services that could potentially help them cope with their illness. Without these supports, most agree that the risks to the public and the individual are increased, and the resulting crises are likely, through media coverage, to further increase the stigma still surrounding mental illness.

In the case of *R v. Hallstrom* (1986), it was ruled that a person liable to be detained, but who had been on s17 leave for a majority of their Section, could not have their Section renewed. Prior to *Hallstrom*, the so-called 'long leash' procedure had been commonplace among psychiatrists and had allowed a de facto CTO to operate for a number of years (Bean and Mounser 1994: 72). This is once again the case, as the *Hallstrom* case law was over-ruled by the Court of Appeal in 1999 (*B v. Barking Havering and Brentwood Community NHS Trust* 1999). Many psychiatrists would prefer to see a CTO with accepted 'sanctions' introduced rather than adopting the so-called 'long leash' policy which, in any case, cannot adequately provide for compulsion in the community, or enforce compliance. Research from the Zito Trust has also claimed that officials in health authorities overwhelmingly support the drawing up of protocols for 'forcing patients to take their medication' (BBC 2000). Research supporting CTOs has also come from Professor Louis Appleby, director of the National Confidential Inquiry into Suicide and Homicide by People with Mental Illness (Department of Health 1999a). Recommendation 25 of the inquiry report states that the new Mental Health Act 'must allow treatment in the community at the earliest point in case of high risk' (Department of Health 1999a). They argue that high-risk patients with mental illness who become non-compliant with treatment or show increasing signs of risk must be treated compulsorily 'even in the absence of clear signs of relapse' (Department of Health 1999a).

Mind (National Association for Mental Health) is concerned about this proposal because it does not see 'non-compliance' as automatically synonymous with relapse – yet the proposals could attract a significant sanction. It also fears that it may risk breaching the European Convention on Human Rights (Article 5) because, if someone was forcibly conveyed for the compulsory administration of medication, the likelihood is they would then require at least a brief admission for observation, and it would have to be shown that hospital detention was warranted – which it may not always be at the time of non-compliance (Pedler

1999a: para. 10.1). Mind have headed a significant lobby against the introduction of CTOs. Primarily they fear that CTOs will drive service users away from mental health services for fear of being forced to accept medication even if not sectioned into hospital. They suggest that the ideal of a therapeutic relationship between service user and professional will be undermined through fear of compulsion to accept treatments that can still have 'serious and irreversible side-effects' (Pedler 1999a).

Crucially, compulsion under current legislation is already proven to be used disproportionally against black and ethnic minority service users in the case of Sections 2, 3, 4 and 136, and such groups are more likely to be diagnosed with schizophrenia and detained in locked wards (HMSO 1996; Coid *et al.* 2002a,b). In fact, the total number of patients compulsorily admitted to hospital, standardised for age, gender and ethnicity, rose by over 30 per cent between 1997 and 1999 (Soliman and Reza 2001), and some have suggested that the political climate has led clinicians to lower the threshold at which patients are judged to require 'sectioning', as 'defensive practice kicks in' (Lelliott and Audini 2003). Some argue that the threshold for 'compulsion in the community' will be even lower and that more black service users will be compelled to receive treatment (Democratic Health Network 1999). A prediction of net widening has been mooted by the civil libertarian lobby, i.e. first a few 'chronic schizophrenic' patients will be placed on CTOs but then soon another 'group of patients' will be identified and 'they too', it would be argued, 'would also benefit' from a CTO – 'Do not all control systems have inbuilt tendencies to enlarge themselves?' (Bean and Mounser 1994). Others have argued that people subject to CTOs are more likely to be kept on medication longer term on the basis that 'they are doing so well in the community while subject to compulsory medication' so a CTO might as well continue (Parkin 2000).

Compliance with medication is often implied to be the ultimate goal of treatment and non-compliance as a clear sign of mental ill health. In the Rooney Inquiry (Department of Health 1992: para. 33), it stated that, 'There is no power to force a person to take medication even though the failure is caused by the illness which the medication is designed to treat'. This assumption, argue Mind, lacks an appreciation that an individual may rationally choose to refuse medication on the ground of distressing side-effects (Pedler 1999a). On this point, the Expert Committee are appreciative of Mind's approach, but made it clear that 'in certain circumstances, such as the existence of substantial risk to the safety of others, an individual's competent refusal of treatment could be over-ridden' (Department of Health 1999b: para 5.95). Pat Guinan of the British Psychological Society has given examples of patients who have stopped taking medication against medical advice 'and were able to maintain their recovery' (House of Commons 2000: para 140). Evidence for the positive outcomes of non-compliance is scant, however, and most agree that seriously mentally unwell patients benefit from being engaged in services, and that positive engagement, in turn, serves the welfare of the community. The question being asked is whether CTOs are the appropriate response to this group of individuals.

Practical implications

The opinions are clearly divided and the agenda varying. Nevertheless, the government has assured the mental health services community that CTOs will form part of a future and forthcoming Mental Health Act. So, what will be the implications for ASWs and other mental health workers?

First, the issue of who would make an application for the CTO has not been fully addressed in the proposals. If, like a guardianship order, it is to be an ASW, service users' confidence in social workers may be further challenged. Secondly, at what point does one intervene to enforce the conditions of a CTO? If a patient is refusing medication but not visibly deteriorating, is it ethical to convey them against their will to treat them forcibly, and would this be at a hospital, GP surgery or an alternative community medical facility? The government does not envisage a situation in which individuals are forcibly treated in their own homes (Department of Health 1998: 40), so how could compulsory treatment be facilitated? Would the assistance of the ambulance or police services for the purposes of conveyance become necessary as with many current compulsory admissions to hospital? And what effect would this have upon the 'therapeutic alliance' so valued by users and professionals alike? At best, it is likely to strain the therapeutic process. At worst, the person requiring treatment and care becomes more difficult to engage in the future – increasing risks to self and others if 'lost' in the community. This might further necessitate an increased role for the new assertive outreach or crisis resolution approach as persons with mental health problems increasingly avoid contact with workers perceived as coercive and overly powerful.

Here, the resource implications are huge if assertive efforts are required to monitor this potentially increasing population. One regional ASW interest group is also concerned at the increased risks to professionals involved in enforcing CTOs (ASWIG 2000). Many are already avoiding social work as a career option because it is seen as increasingly coercive and inconsistent with the therapeutic ideal, and as attracting risk of aggression towards the worker as a result.

On the other hand, all are concerned with reducing risk and perhaps the CTO, for some service users, might provide a viable alternative to a hospital admission. Many would sooner accept compulsory treatment at home than be away from family and friends in the confines of a hospital ward. For some, much like guardianship or supervised discharge, a CTO may provide the legal and psychological boundaries required to persuade them to comply with a care programme – and may help to ensure that the community team remains actively involved in providing services. But, for this to occur, adequate resources would have to be forthcoming. This view is largely consistent with the Expert Committee's principle of 'reciprocity', i.e. if subjected to compulsion, quality services should be available as a paramount entitlement (Parkin 2000: 5).

If this 'reciprocity' principle were to underpin the proposed CTO, there is a continued danger of resources being targeted principally at high-risk groups. But might this not be at the expense of other users of mental health services? Resources, as workers are frequently reminded, are not limitless. Might not the targeting of resources at preventative practice with crisis response, assertive out-reach and creative alternatives to hospital admission and patient care avoid the need for CTOs?

A principal concern has been that the Green Paper ducks the key issue about CTOs, namely what to do if people don't comply with an order (Pedler 1999b). Yet there is some evidence that, although patients who have experienced 'restrictions' under the Mental Health Act 1983 are ambivalent about their treatment, there was nonetheless a degree of understanding that their disturbed behaviour at the time had to be dealt with (Canvin *et al.* 2002). However, attempts to 'enforce' compli-ance when 'non-compliance' is interpreted so widely by service users, mental health interest groups and professionals might risk breaching Human Rights Act legislation in terms of an individual's right to liberty and security. In practice, it is likely that persistent non-compliance with a CTO would lead to a hospital admission. Essentially, this is no different from the situation facing professionals when patients subject to supervised discharge fail to comply with the conditions of their discharge. If it is felt that an individual is not complying with the condi-tions of their supervised aftercare, and that the person should be readmitted to hospital for treatment, there are no powers of recall under s25A – the person must again be assessed under the Mental Health Act and a new application for hospital admission made by an ASW.

Some believe that the motivation for CTOs is primarily driven by the desire of psychiatry to re-establish its power base in the community now that the power of the large institutions has been eroded through the policy of downsizing hospitals and hospital closure. Bean and Mounser (1994) argue that CTOs are about help-ing to provide psychiatry with a new platform. They comment, 'Emptying the mental hospitals seemed wonderfully progressive but it left the psychiatrists with no forum on which to exercise their authority'. CTOs would arguably provide a powerful legal platform for psychiatry, at least in principle. Yet a recent survey of South London psychiatrists did suggest that their main criteria for compulsory admissions was still risk to the patient or others (Dazzan and Bhugra 2001).

It remains to be seen exactly what form CTOs will take and whether or not they will be workable in practice but, I would suggest, divided opinion is likely to continue to surround this controversial legislative proposal. For some, the CTO is welcomed as a means of enforcing treatment for those patients who would otherwise be untreatable without recourse to a hospital admission. Others believe that the introduction of the CTO would add little to powers already available because, they feel, the resource implications of enforcing compliance are so great and the practicalities of supervising CTOs unrealistic and damaging to the patient/professional relationship. For others, the CTO is perceived as a misjudged piece of media-driven policy, which stands to discriminate against a group in society with mental health difficulties, who nevertheless choose to lead their lives independently of mental health services. The potential introduction of CTOs is set to increase the scope of legal powers currently available to mental health professionals. If CTOs are set to become enshrined in the future Mental Health

Act, effective rights of appeal will be crucial in ensuring that individuals are not indiscriminately targeted for CTOs.

The problem appears to be understanding and responding realistically and proportionally to the risk of violence. Yet a quite recent study confirmed what has long been known, that depressed people and people with schizophrenia in the main are not violent against others; indeed, violence among psychiatric male inpatients was almost exclusively related to personality-disordered patients who had previous violent episodes (Soliman and Reza 2001; Craig and Hodson 2000; McNeil and Binder 2005; Monahan *et al.* 2005). While the inadequate resource issue for mental health service persists, paradoxically, for those patients with a history of antisocial behaviour, there has been an identified shortfall in long-term medium secure facilities and allied services, and efforts are being made to reduce the shortages (Riordan *et al.* 2002); perhaps yet another example of governmental priorities following the overhyped media concerns?

Concluding thoughts

The role of the ASW is complex. It requires a firm grasp of legislation, organisational acumen and a sensitivity to the particular circumstances of an individual and their family/carers/community, etc. The role also requires the worker to be knowledgeable about modern psychiatry and evidence-based practice of 'what works' in this field.

Ultimately, the ASW must decide whether it is appropriate to make an application for a compulsory admission. If it is decided to detain an individual, the ASW must make all the arrangements for that person's admission. This can often necessitate the presence of the ambulance and/or police services. Often work priorities of the emergency services differ from those of the ASW. This can increase the stress upon an ASW when managing a risk situation. The strong emotional feelings shown by a person being detained can range from extreme distress to almost complete passivity to raging anger. Often the ASW will be walking into the unknown. The completion of a Mental Health Act assessment is often emotionally and physically draining, taking several hours from start to finish. Having the opportunity to 'debrief' should be central to any post-assessment supervision. However, some ASWs find this supervision inadequate or, at worst, absent. As one of our previous examples showed, once an assessment is completed, the ASW may never get to find out 'what happened next' – was the admission fruitful? – did the individual benefit from time in hospital? – how long was the person detained for? There can be a feeling of 'incompleteness' about the process for the ASW.

There can also be a sense of being 'caught in the middle'. If a recommending doctor is adamant that an individual should be detained and the ASW does not feel that the making of an application is appropriate, it can lead to unrest between health and social services colleagues. On the other hand, if the ASW concurs with the two recommending doctors, then the 'patient' can assume that the ASW is simply colluding with the medics. Either outcome can be disconcerting. That 'tension' is ever present in the role of the ASW. If, in the future, the CTO is introduced, there are going to be new challenges for the ASW in terms of how, practically, they monitor a person's treatment compliance and decide at what point such a person should have their liberty eroded further by being compulsorily treated within a hospital setting.

At present, the Mental Health Act allows only social workers to assume the role of the ASW. This at least ensures that an application is made by someone employed independently from those making the medical recommendations. The specific training of ASWs generally promotes a strongly social model perspective of care, which can, at times, provide the necessary balance against a sometimes strongly medically biased perspective. Under the newly proposed legislation, it is likely that the current ASW role will be revised and a new role – approved mental health practitioner – introduced, also available to non-social work professionals. Many interest groups are concerned that this will potentially dilute the current value of having a non-medical professional as a key member of the assessing team. This proposal introduces some uncertainty to the future of the ASW role. Yet, despite all these pressures, there can be tremendous satisfaction in working in this field, not only when effective social work avoids an unnecessary compulsory admission, but the frequent occasions when we really make a difference to the lives of our clients and their families when, even if we control, we do so because we care.

13　The accommodation dimension

Housing and mental disorder

Rebecca Pritchard

> Poor naked wretches, wheresoe'er you are
> That bide the pelting of this pitiless storm,
> How shall your houseless heads and unfed sides,
> Your looped and windowed raggedness, defend you
> From seasons such as these? Oh I have ta'en
> Too little care of this! Take physic, pomp;
> Expose thyself to feel what wretches feel . . .
> And show the heavens more just.
>
> (*King Lear*, 3:4)

Objectives: by the end of this chapter you should:

1　recognise the interface between homelessness and mental health;
2　understand the accommodation problems for people with a mental health problem;
3　understand the different range of accommodation provisions;
4　have some grasp of the role and contribution of the voluntary sector.

This chapter seeks to identify some of the main accommodation-based environments likely to be encountered by social workers today.

It highlights some of the key legislation that governs the rights that people have in different accommodation settings, and identifies some of the different funding sources for such services. Social workers need to have a broad understanding of these legislative and funding regimes in order to make informed choices about services for their clients. It presents models of good practice, emphasising the benefits to clients and providers alike of effective joint working, and draws on case studies of good practice.

The importance of such an approach is underlined by reference to recent Inquiries where joint working broke down or was not adequately established.

Historical perspectives: cycles and circles

As demonstrated in earlier chapters, the accommodation of people with mental health problems in the 1800s and first half of the 1900s was focused essentially upon control, being concerned to protect the wider community (Jones 1959).

The Mental Health Act 1983 introduced the concept and model of community care, promoted integration and support in a community setting and began a programme of reprovision of the old mental health and learning disability institutions to a range of different accommodation-based settings in the community.

Community care has been said to be very expensive. Providing quality support and supervision for individuals or small groups of service users in the community lost the economies of scale achieved through the mental health institutions. However, this excuse is hugely questionable. At a microlevel, those requiring hostel accommodation cost, at 2000 prices, £104 per week (p.w.), a 'special' hostel placement costs between £442 and £508 p.w., which is expensive, until these costs are contrasted against the cost of an ordinary place on a general psychiatric ward at £1,925 p.w. and an 'intensive psychiatric care' bed at £2,310 p.w. (Pritchard 2000).

A comparison of expenditure on mental health within the NHS budget between the early 1980s and mid-1990s found a massive saving, as it moved from 19 per cent to 11.5 per cent, in an ostensible attempt to utilise the benefits from switching from care in hospital to the community. The government of the day allocated £500 million to social services departments (SSD) to facilitate this, apparently substantial input into 'care in the community'. However, the 'savings', at 1994 prices, were equivalent to £3,500 million. A fair interpretation would be that there had been an effective reduction in funding for mental health care (Department of Health 1995; Pritchard *et al.* 1997a).

One possible unlooked for consequence has been that, in study after study, former psychiatric patients have been found to be over-represented in cohorts of homeless people, with multiple pathologies, substance misuse, suicidal ideation, etc. (Scott 1993; Pritchard and Clooney 1994; Odell and Commander 1999; Eynan *et al.* 2002; Park *et al.* 2002). Indeed, the multiplicity of risk to women who have been mentally disordered is considerable, including homelessness, which is associated with a fivefold lifetime risk of being a victim of domestic violence (Zachary *et al.* 2002). Furthermore, inadequately resourced support accommodation is, in part, why mentally disordered people within the community are more often victims of crime, including violent crime, than the general population (Marley and Buila 2001).

Hence, accommodation is a central practical issue for effective mental health social work, a fact that cannot be overemphasised.

Reprovision initially focused on those with lowest needs, leaving an increasingly residual and marginalised population behind. Although there remains a commitment to care in the community, with some of the most recent hospital closure programmes delivering the resettlement of some very institutionalised individuals into the community, the pace of reprovision has slowed over the years.

Through the 1990s, reprovision became ever harder for the remaining very damaged and high-needs individuals. User and advocacy organisations such as Mencap are now having to campaign against hospitals being redesignated as 'community villages' – as the process of reprovision and moving people into the community slows down.

In the mental health sector, the lack of resources and poor communication between organisations involved in the care and support of individuals have resulted in a series of high-profile disasters (e.g. Magdi E, Jonathan Newby, Christopher Clunis).

The forthcoming mental health legislation is widely predicted to include more stringent treatment in the community orders, and may seek to establish places of safety for those without a treatable condition, but whose personality disorder means that they pose a potential (but as yet unrealised) threat to the community, the so-called 'dangerous severe personality disorders' (Bindman *et al.* 2003).

These latest developments may well have an impact upon the role of the social worker in the community – and could shift clients' perceptions from one where the worker is seen as a positive source of support to one where they have a more controlling supervisory role in their lives. Are we reaching a point where, once again, accommodation-based services for those with mental health difficulties are focused on control and the protection of others, and less upon the needs of service users themselves?

Introduction: accommodation-based environments

Social workers' relationships with their service users do not develop or exist in a vacuum, but will be influenced by the context and settings in which contact takes place. The accommodation occupied by a client will form a key part of their environment, and will potentially have a strong influence on the dynamics of the relationship, and the role and resources that the social worker will be expected to bring.

For example, a social worker with a client on a section in hospital will expect the client to be 'in' when called upon, and accessible – whether on an open ward or in a private room. The worker will have considerable power if they are part of the team assessing whether the individual service user is 'ready' to leave the ward, and the requirement to comply with the risk assessment and treatment programme may be a significant aspect of the relationship for both worker and client.

Conversely, a social worker visiting a client in their own home (whether a tenant or an owner occupier) in the community will be seeking to establish a relationship, which recognises their greater autonomy. Different approaches are required when assessing and encouraging clients to comply with medication regimes and regular appointments with psychiatrists if these take place in the client's own home. The role may be different again if the social worker is the client's main source of support and contact in an otherwise isolated environment.

A 'middle way', which is extremely important for social workers seeking to support clients with mental health needs, is the role that supported housing (often provided by the voluntary sector) plays. This sort of accommodation includes a diverse range of models of provision. High levels of support (usually 24 hours with waking staff cover) are provided in registered care homes (for which a social services funding package agreed through care planning is required). Lower levels of support (which can still include 24-hour cover in some cases) exist in shared houses, cluster flats and 'outreach' or 'floating' support provided in the community by peripatetic workers. In these contexts, the social worker is part of a team, and must work with others to deliver a package of support and services that meets users' needs.

Legislation and rights: an accommodation perspective

Most social work training does not include any consideration of the different rights and levels of security that different types of accommodation and legislation confer on individual people. This is a serious practical gap, as even among the high-profile cases of child protection, one in five mothers had chronic and recurring accommodation difficulties (Pritchard 1992c) and, with one or two notable exceptions (Scott 1993; Bughra 1996), psychiatry does not give homelessness the practical priority it deserves.

This has led to misunderstandings between different professionals involved in an individual's care and support – and potentially puts the ill-informed social worker at some risk, as well as their client.

Generally, in accommodation settings where housing-related support and care are offered as part of a 'package', the amount of control an individual exercises over their accommodation is influenced by the level of their needs and/or the length of time they are expected to stay in the accommodation.

Table 13.1 sets out the likely relationships between needs, duration of stay, type of accommodation and the housing rights the individual is likely to enjoy. This table does not seek to provide a comprehensive guide to housing legislation, but offers an indication of some of the accommodation-based issues that a social worker might need to consider when planning care and support for their clients.

For example, knowledge of the rights that a client's tenure gives them enables the social worker to advocate more effectively on their behalf and offer a more responsive service. Knowing that the serving of a 28-day Notice of Seeking Possession order does not end the tenancy and mean that the tenant is homeless, but that it gives notice that the breach (whether non-payment of rent or behaviour) must be resolved in the time period or the landlord will proceed to court to seek to end the tenancy, empowers the social worker and their client to take informed decisions and appropriate action.

Table 13.1 sets out the type of accommodation that clients with mental health problems may be living in, sets out the likely occupancy agreements/tenure that may be used for that type of accommodation and describes the accommodation rights and arrangements that accord with the tenure.

As noted above, it is important for social workers to be aware of the type of tenure or occupancy agreement that their clients enjoy, as this does affect the practical delivery of services.

For example, a social worker visiting a client in hospital or in a hostel where they have a licence agreement could gain access to the client's room – even without their permission. This might be important if an assessment of their ability to manage independently was being undertaken. The condition of an individual's room in a hostel might be a good indication of their current mental health – there could be considerable hoarding activity and very poor sanitary conditions suggesting that someone was not coping or functioning well. Good practice would expect the worker to be able to operate co-operatively with the client, even though possibly disturbed. However, if the individual had a tenancy agreement, their permission would be needed before a social worker (or other professionals) could gain access – and this could be withheld.

The rights of individuals in terms of the tenure they enjoy is set out in a number of pieces of legislation: the Protection from Eviction Act (1977), which sets limits on the level of 'force' that can legitimately be used in evicting someone without a tenancy agreement; the Landlord and Tenant Act (1985), which sets out the mutual responsibilities and duties of the landlord and the tenant – key in terms of ensuring that a property is well maintained and repaired; and the Housing Act 1990, which introduced assured and assured shorthold tenancies.

The social worker does not need a comprehensive knowledge of this legislation for their day-to-day work, but some awareness of the different rights of people in different forms of accommodation is useful to inform their chosen practice and approaches.

Two other key pieces of legislation that have a bearing upon accommodation are the Care Standards Act 2000 and the Homelessness Act 2002.

The Care Standards Act 2000 governs the level and quality of service that should be provided in registered care homes. This sets out minimum room sizes and facilities and minimum staffing levels, as well as governing the inspection regime, which falls to the newly independent Care Standards Commission, established in 2002. Social workers arranging care packages and placements in residential care should have a working knowledge of this Act, and should ensure that they develop appropriate relationships with the inspection teams. Although recent research with respect to carers of people with learning disability showed that they had little understanding of the Carer's Act (1995), ostensibly designed to help such people in long-term situations (Robinson and Williams 2002), it is to be hoped that this will not be the fate of the Care Standards Commission.

The Homelessness Act 2002 sets out the categories of people to whom local authorities have a duty to provide accommodation, and requires local authorities to develop Homelessness Strategies that focus upon both prevention of and responses to homelessness in their areas. These should be developed in conjunction with social services and other stakeholders – such as voluntary sector organisations – and should provide for both physical accommodation and advice and support required by people with mental health needs to prevent homelessness and to secure for them appropriate accommodation.

Social workers whose clients may be vulnerable and at risk of losing their accommodation because of their poor mental health should ensure that they are familiar with their local authority's strategy – and the resources they may be able to provide to assist service users.

Table 13.1 Relationships between needs, duration of stay, type of accommodation and housing rights

Type of accommodation	Likely tenure	Rights/level of security
Hospital	None – a patient may be on compulsory section	Limited rights – cannot deny access to own room
Registered care home	Licence agreement	Licence agreement gives basic 'permission to stay'. May be asked for permission to enter own room as a courtesy, but staff have the right to enter even without permission – usually because of the need to provide care or cleaning services or to check on someone's welfare. Can be asked to leave without requiring a court order, usually if needs change and where the individual no longer requires the level of care offered, or where their needs cannot continue to be adequately met. The social worker should be involved in these decisions and may be required to secure funding and arrange an alternative placement
Permanent or long-term supported shared accommodation (own room; shares bath/kitchen/living room)	Licence agreement	Licence agreement – if support needs are such that access to the individual's room is required to provide support and personal cleaning, then a licence agreement is the most likely form of tenure. As described above, this gives service users only limited rights to stay. Once they are given notice to quit by the accommodation providers (landlords), they will be required to leave. Notice to quit must be for a reasonable period. Generally, this will be 28 days' notice. However, what is a 'reasonable' notice period may depend upon the cause of the decision to ask the client to leave. If there is a serious and potentially dangerous breach of behaviour agreements included in the licence agreement, immediate notice to quit may be issued

Accommodation	Tenancy	Description
Temporary supported shared accommodation	Licence agreement	As above
	Assured shorthold tenancy	Assured shorthold tenancy gives a tenant full rights in the first fixed period (usually 6 months) when only a court order can end the tenancy on prescribed grounds. Thereafter, a court order is still required after a two months' notice requiring possession is served, but the court has no powers to withhold this order
Hostel	Licence agreement (may be an assured shorthold tenancy)	Likely to be a licence agreement, excluded from the need to gain a court order. This enables hostel managers to take people about whom little is known, as they are able to manage the risk by requiring someone to leave immediately if their behaviour cannot be managed safely in the hostel
Cluster flat (self-contained flat in a block/designated group for people with support needs)	Assured shorthold	An assured shorthold may be used if the accommodation is not intended to be permanent once someone's health is stabilised and they are expected to be found permanent accommodation in the community
	Assured tenancy	As above
Self-contained flat	Assured tenancy (if the provider is a housing association)	As above
	Secure tenancy (if the provider is a council)	Secure tenants have similar rights (slightly enhanced – e.g. the right to buy) to assured tenants
	Assured shorthold (if in the private rented sector)	Assured shorthold – as above
Owner-occupied house	Owner-occupier	Relationship is with mortgagor – may lose accommodation if default on mortgage repayments, but otherwise have full control over who has access to their accommodation

Funding accommodation-based services

In practical terms, securing funding for appropriate accommodation-based services for people with mental health needs may be one of the greatest practical challenges facing social workers in an environment of constrained resources.

For periods of hospitalisation, the local health authority or primary care trust (PCT) will fund the costs. Once someone faces discharge into the community, however, the situation can be very complex.

If someone is returning to the community via a stay in residential care, this will need to be funded from social services' community care funding resources – always under pressure. A social worker will need to make a good case to secure this funding in a 'competitive' environment, so he/she should research the care home in question, compare with other alternatives and match this to the individual service user's needs.

If residential care is not required, the client may be returning to his/her own home (owner-occupied or rented) or to a supported accommodation project provided by either the council or a voluntary sector provider, although the social worker should be thinking ahead if, through their disturbed behaviour, this accommodation becomes at risk (Craig 1995; Diaz 2000). In the first case, returning to their own home, there will be no requirement to fund the accommodation from social services resources. However, if mortgage payments have lapsed because of a prolonged stay in hospital, the social worker will need to assist the client to renegotiate payments, and potentially make a claim for financial support with the interest payments via the Benefits Agency. Local authority housing advice centres or Citizens' Advice Bureaux should have the expertise to assist with this process if the social worker is unfamiliar with debt counselling and the benefits system.

If the client is a private or social housing tenant, they may require assistance to restart a claim for Housing Benefit to pay for the rent of their property. These forms are held by the Housing Benefit Department of a local authority (usually accessible via the town hall, and located in either the Housing or the Finance department). A Housing Benefit claim needs to be accompanied by proof of tenure and liability for the rent (i.e. a copy of the tenancy agreement) and proof of income (whether in employment or on benefits). If the tenant is already claiming, then the Housing Benefit department needs to be notified of a change in circumstances, e.g. a return from hospital. Wherever possible, social workers should inform the landlord that these claims are being made – as Housing Benefit administration is often poor and may take some time before a claim is assessed and in payment. Many landlords prefer that tenants request that payments are made directly to the landlord – so their bank details will need to be obtained. If tenants prefer to receive the Housing Benefit directly, they should be encouraged to set up standing orders (where they have bank accounts) in order that regular payments to the landlord are made, and rent arrears – that could put their home at risk – avoided.

Where clients are returning to the community and moving into new flats, they may have little in the way of personal possessions. Applications to the Social Fund – administered by the Benefits Agency – can be made for people leaving institutional care (either hospital or registered residential homes). Payments are awarded as Community Care Grants or Social Fund Loans for basic furniture, white goods and other household goods.

Social workers may find this level of detailed involvement in the benefits system daunting or beyond their resources in terms of time. If this level of practical assistance is not feasible, social workers should consider referring a client to a voluntary organisation for such assistance. These may provide support through user-led day centres or through a range of 'floating' visiting support services. These latter services will be primarily funded through the Supporting People grant regime that came into effect from 1 April 2003.

The paradoxical issue of funding accommodation is that, in the south-east, a standard place in a hostel costs £130 per week (2002 costs), a 'special' mental health hostel, £480 p.w. (£550 p.w. in an equivalent London hostel) but a standard inpatient psychiatric bed costs £2,200 and £2,500 p.w. for an 'intensive psychiatric care' bed – five times the cost of a specialist hostel place. If the general public lose confidence in maintaining people who have had a mental disorder in the community, and some of the public hostility is related to homelessness as much as mental disorder (Wolfe and Stuber 2002), then the scrimping underfunded accommodation policy may well be very expensive in the medium term.

Social workers should be aware that Supporting People teams in every local authority (or possibly at county level in two-tier authorities) have been required to map and compile databases of every service offering housing-related support in their area as part of the process of preparing for the introduction of the Supporting People funding regime from 1 April 2003 (for further information, visit the Office of the Deputy Prime Minister's dedicated website: spkweb.org.uk).

These databases are extremely useful sources of information about the range of resources that might be available to support clients with mental health needs in the community – and social workers should ensure that they have access to the information held by the Supporting People teams.

Each authority will have compiled a Supporting People strategy, which is required to reference and support other strategic provision in the social care, health, probation and community safety fields. Social services, health and probation are all represented on the commissioning bodies that oversee and agree the development of these strategies, and mental health social workers should strive to develop mechanisms to influence the commissioning decisions set out in these strategies, as they are a key resource for those with mental health needs seeking to sustain independence in the community.

Supported housing projects, which may include shared accommodation, cluster flats or visiting support to people in their own homes, are likely to be funded by Supporting People grants from April 2003.

Supporting People funds the housing-related support, which includes practical advice and assistance with benefits, helping people understand their obligations and maintain their accommodation, support and guidance to develop the skills required to live independently in the community and assistance with using community-based services. Supporting People will not fund personal care or 'clinical' interventions (such as drug detoxification and intensive or specialist counselling) but will cover emotional support to help people cope with mental health needs.

In addition to Supporting People grants, supported housing providers will also require occupants to claim housing benefit, and they may have to contribute towards some of the costs (such as their personal use of heat, light and water) from personal income. In addition, 'top-up' funding from social services may be required for domiciliary support.

'Kevin', 56 years of age, has a history of alcohol abuse as well as of mental health problems and has poor physical health and low motivation. He has spent time sleeping rough and was recently discharged from hospital into a supported flat. Table 13.2 shows the different funding streams to help him.

The above example shows the range of different funding streams involved in a typical supported housing setting – and the need for community care funding packages even where the main services are funded from elsewhere. There is evidence that people such as Kevin, despite some of the limits and pressures of living in the community, have a much more positive perspective on their lives compared with when they were in hospital (Okin and Pearsall 1993; Pritchard and Clooney 1994; Kingdon 1996). Consequently, Kevin's support worker not only enhances his client's life by maintaining him in the community, but there are also considerable 'savings' to the public purse, £325 p.w. compared with £2,200 p.w. for a

Table 13.2 Different funding streams involved in a typical supported housing setting

Services	Funding source
Accommodation – rent for his flat, with communal cleaning of the shared lounge and corridors and windows	Housing benefit paid by local authority (*c.* £60 per week)
Support – a worker is on site and helps Kevin attend appointments, complete benefits, reminds him to take medication, helps him budget and supports him to cook a meal twice a week, liaises with his social worker and GP	Supporting People grant paid by local authority Supporting People team to the provider (*c.* £230 per week)
Personal heating and lighting and water rates – paid for by the accommodation provider, but collected from Kevin as a weekly personal service charge	Kevin's personal income likely to be income support, disabled living allowance (DLA) or incapacity benefit (*c.* £6.50 per week is a fairly typical average cost for heating, lighting and water rates in a shared property)
Domiciliary care – two hours weekly to help Kevin keep the flat clean	Social services pays from community care budget (*c.* £30 per week)

Total: £326.50 per week.

standard psychiatric bed; these are arguments that managers should be making to both central and local government treasurers.

Accommodation settings: choices and practice approaches

As indicated above, social workers' advice and choices about accommodation options for their clients, and the approaches they take to their clients, may be influenced by the rights that service users have over their accommodation.

If a client requires a high degree of monitoring and supervision, then a placement in a self-contained flat with only visiting support might not be ideal. Such individuals may benefit from a supported accommodation setting with on-site staffing, who can be the 'eyes and ears' of the statutory services, able to alert psychiatrists, community psychiatric nurses (CPNs) and, in view of the psychiatric–child protection interface, child protection to changes in behaviour and functioning.

Someone who poses no risk to others and very little to themselves may be seen as 'ideally suited' to a self-contained property that maximises their independence. This will only be appropriate, however, if they have access to formal or informal support networks and are confident in using community-based facilities – if they are not in this position, they may become very isolated and withdrawn with adverse impacts for their good mental health. Placing such individuals in shared accommodation where they can benefit from contact with others or, alternatively, linking them into 'befriending services' may be necessary to ensure that appropriate accommodation and support is offered for the individual's needs, for there is considerable evidence that a factor in secondary mental health breakdowns is a sense or actual lack of key relationships, being unsupported and being isolated (Craig 1996).

Other choices may involve placing clients in 'permanent' supported accommodation, or services, which are intended to be transitional and temporary.

In temporary placements, service users need to be enabled to feel secure and stable, but not put down 'roots' that would impede their moving on. This involves action planning that focuses upon the longer term objectives of achieving independence, being clear that moving on will take place – and is desirable (even where it may be to accommodation of a lower physical standard).

Even in permanent placements, it is important for social workers to seek services that have an ethos that encourages and supports people to develop independence, albeit in small and incremental steps. Services that work with, rather than for, users and which provide a sense of purposefulness, constantly checking users' motivations and aspirations, are essential if people are to recognise their potential and avoid being 'warehoused'.

Care managers should regularly review the continued suitability of such placements – and not assume that permanent placements will continue to meet needs of users – even if funding packages can be maintained.

Accommodation services: good practice

Voluntary sector providers can offer a way in and enable effective engagement with clients who may distrust traditional social workers, whom they may perceive as having undesirable power and control over their lives. Voluntary sector providers do not have the same 'enforcement' role as statutory staff, and can be more flexible and creative – offering needs-led services such as meaningful occupation, informal learning activities and befriending.

The case studies highlight models of good practice where accommodation-based services have been designed to be flexible and responsive to a range of needs, and the roles of the statutory and voluntary sectors complement each other.

Indeed, the example from the Richmond Fellowship reflects the longstanding quality contribution that the Fellowship has made to people with mental health problems.

Joint Working: Richmond Fellowship–West Sussex Joint Rehabilitation Service

The service comprises a nine-bed registered care home, three small shared houses (each with three occupants) and a floating support scheme (which offers visiting support to people in their own self-contained flats in the community).

The target client group is people who have spent (often long periods of) time on acute psychiatric wards and who require a period of rehabilitation before living independently in the community.

Support is delivered by a multidisciplinary team, managed by the Richmond Fellowship on behalf of the local Mental Health Trust. The team includes a psychiatrist, a CPN, social workers and housing support workers.

The Richmond Fellowship, a voluntary organisation with many years' experience of providing accommodation and support for people with mental health needs, is accountable for the management of the team, including its budget. It provides assets in the form of accommodation and has expertise in housing management, tenancy law and benefits. Its housing support workers understand the perspectives of the local housing providers who offer longer term accommodation, and can liaise effectively with them to ensure that clients meet their obligations as tenants and manage their tenancies well.

The mental health professionals bring expertise in mental health legislation, the workings of the health system, access to medication and clinical interventions. Being part of the multidisciplinary team enables them to respond swiftly to the needs of clients supported by generic housing staff, who can alert the CPN or psychiatrist to changes in functioning and ensure early interventions which prevent service users' mental health deteriorating to crisis point.

One of the key requirements for effective joint working is clarity about individuals' roles. Misunderstandings about what different professionals can/should do are often the cause of ineffective joint working.

In a typical supported housing project (such as that described for 'Kevin' above), the 'roles' shown in Table 13.3 might be expected.

Accommodation staff in the voluntary sector are unlikely to be mental health experts, even though many of their services users have experienced severe mental health problems (Scott 1993; Pritchard and Clooney 1994; Davidson 2000; Craig and Hodson 2000), so social workers will have an important role in enabling them to understand how the mental health system works.

Social workers can also offer support and advice to staff who are dealing with particularly challenging behaviour (such as self-harm) and can increase the capacity of the voluntary sector to respond to these needs (Bird and Faulkener 2000).

Social workers are also likely to have specific training in the assessment of clients – something that is often lacking (or not provided in depth) for voluntary

Table 13.3 Roles in a typical supported housing project

Statutory sector: social worker (and/or CPN)	*Voluntary sector: supported housing worker*
Assessment of needs	Input into assessment of needs
Access to resources (community care funding packages)	Advice and assistance with benefits and resources such as household goods
Monitoring of care package/placement	Practical advice and assistance on managing accommodation/using community facilities
Advice for generic support workers about managing difficult behaviours/risks	'Eyes and ears' for other professionals – day-to-day contact with the service user enables close monitoring of their behaviour and functioning
Advice on the mental health 'system' – and access to psychiatrists for further assessments/interventions	Input into care planning – attending CPAs – to advise on the individual's functioning and the limitations of the support offered directly by the support service
Advice on and access to medication	Information about compliance with medication; reminders to attend appointments and take depots, etc.
Sectioning and referral on to more specialist care	Alert to changes in risk-related behaviours
Training and support for generic staff in the voluntary sector	Training for statutory services on housing law, voluntary sector resources

sector staff (Park 2002). Trained social workers can therefore support and guide voluntary sector partners in the assessment process, ensuring that assessment is an effective and ongoing, dynamic process of intelligent enquiry that is led by the needs of individual service users and results in effective planning and responses (Renshaw 1987; Middleton 1999).

Thames Reach Bondway and 'START'

Thames Reach Bondway (TRB) is a voluntary sector organisation that works in central London with rough sleepers and has specialist accommodation for those with mental health and dual diagnoses. They have worked closely with the dedicated mental health team for single homeless people (START) in south-east London.

TRB established a number of accommodation-based services for people with mental health needs. One of these, 'A&G', comprised two sites where self-contained bedsits/flats were built around a communal courtyard, with central 'lounge area' and offices. Staff were on site from 8.00 a.m. to 8.00 p.m., with an out of hours on-call service and the flexibility to provide waking or sleeping in cover if individual tenants went into crisis.

Access to the service was through community care assessments carried out by START. This engendered a high level of commitment to the service from mental health professionals, and TRB staff were routinely involved in community psychiatric assessment (CPA) reviews.

On one occasion, a member of START spent several days in the project informally observing a tenant about whom the project staff had considerable concerns, but who refused to meet with the START professionals. This joint working enabled effective risk arrangement strategies to be put in place.

On another occasion, a service user was discharged from hospital after being diagnosed with an untreatable 'personality disorder'. TRB was supported by START in raising their concerns about this decision with the Trust concerned – START's psychiatrist had direct links with the relevant clinical staff in the Trust.

START was also involved with TRB in agreeing referrals to a newly developed block of supported flats in another part of the borough. They played a key role with TRB staff in liaising with local GPs, who had expressed concern about the demands that were likely to arise from eight new patients with long-term mental health needs moving into their area.

Social workers can benefit greatly from the input of voluntary sector workers, whether on site in staffed accommodation-based services or in the form of 'floating support' to clients in the community.

Voluntary sector workers may be able to respond more flexibly to users' needs and requests – and support their personal and social development through a range of activities and accessing meaningful occupation (from training to leisure activities) in the community.

Voluntary sector support workers are more likely to have informal time with service users, assisting them with the day-to-day 'human' aspects of life, such as shopping, budgeting and developing relationships. This places them in a good position to be able to feed back to social workers on the level of functioning of service users and provide valuable insights into the needs of users.

Many voluntary sector services, when adequately funded, can offer relatively high staff–client ratios, which enables providers to get to know service users well, establish trust and be able to respond flexibly and with varying support levels as needs change through time.

Flexible support: Richmond Fellowship, Liverpool, grouped flats

A housing support team provides services to 90+ tenants in cluster flats (three to ten flats in stand-alone blocks in the community). The team offers a ratio of 1:6 and is large enough to vary support if tenants' health deteriorates.

Thames Reach Bondway – Managed Accommodation Team

A team of housing support workers provides support to tenants in cluster flats (blocks of six to nine flats). Most blocks have an office with staff toilet and shower which can be used as a sleep-in room in an emergency. Although usual support is offered in office hours, the budget is set to allow additional cover in times of crisis. This has enabled the team to provide sleep-in cover for a week following a user's discharge from hospital, and to employ a locum to provide 24-hour cover at a new scheme whose first tenants moved in just before Christmas 1999.

Centrepoint – Support and Development Model and Multiple Health Needs Team

Centrepoint is a charity working with homeless young people. Its direct services in London work with over 1,500 young people each year. A significant proportion of young people using Centrepoint's services in this period identified factors that put them at risk of longer term poor mental health. These included:

- disrupted family support networks (running away from home before they were 16 years old);
- poor educational attainment (no qualifications; problems reading, writing and with numeracy);
- experience of the care or youth justice systems.

Many young people fear the stigma associated with a 'label' of mental health problems, and this is increasingly recognised by professionals. Mental health difficulties in young people using Centrepoint services range from anxiety and depression to severe bipolar disorder. Co-morbidity with drug and alcohol use is also a distinctive feature of many young people presenting with poor mental health. Many statutory mental health services are not able to respond effectively to such complex needs, and there are still situations in which young people are passed between different services, failing to receive the holistic support they require.

In 2001, Centrepoint commissioned a King's Fund-supported research project to review and improve the way in which it worked with young people with mental health problems (O'Connell and Grimbly 2002). Based upon this and further evaluative work during 2002, Centrepoint has developed two key responses to the needs of the young people it works with:

- establishing a specialist Multiple Health Needs Team to work with young people with drug, alcohol and mental health needs;
- developing a service model/approach to working with young people, which built on theories of risk and resilience (Furnam 1998; O'Connell and Grimbly 2002) and also incorporated best youth work practice and the techniques of motivational interviewing – rooted in the dependency sector.

Centrepoint's Multiple Health Needs Team

Centrepoint's specialist Multiple Health Needs Team provides three key services:

- direct work with young people with drug, alcohol and/or mental health needs;
- advice, training and 'consultancy' to generic support and development staff in the accommodation-based services;
- referrals to, and links with, community-based specialist statutory and voluntary sector services (such as the community mental health teams).

This approach enables Centrepoint to offer specialist interventions to young people. The team works to an integrated model, which recognises the incidence of dual diagnosis (the presence of both mental health and drug or alcohol needs) (Drake *et al.* 1996; O'Leary 1997).

The model is based around cognitive behavioural therapy. This uses motivational interviewing techniques and focuses upon presenting issues, supports young people to understand the (distorted) thoughts that lead to (undesirable/damaging) behaviours and works in a structured way to help young people develop skills and strategies to alleviate the 'symptoms/behaviours' (Beck *et al.* 1979, 1993b; Miller and Rollnick 1991).

Centrepoint's support and development model

Centrepoint believes that dealing with the social exclusion of homeless young people requires an integrated approach, starting with the provision of a safe home and building on these firm foundations. Socially excluded young people need security, stability and support, but also need to be challenged and empowered to fulfil their potential.

Many of the young people working with Centrepoint have no stable and meaningful relationships in their lives, and the quality of the relationships they develop with Centrepoint staff is critical to their ability to benefit from the services and opportunities offered. Interventions should enable young people to improve their lives by developing sustainable skills, which they draw upon throughout their lives – long after they have left Centrepoint services. Young people need to see themselves as 'learners' if they are to develop and become independent.

Centrepoint's 'curriculum' – or service offer – focuses upon young people's personal, social, educational and vocational development. Good mental health and emotional well-being are key to personal development and have a significant impact upon social functioning and development, as well as learning and work opportunities.

Centrepoint's support and development 'curriculum' includes the key building blocks for independence and also supports young people's long-term development and learning. The curriculum approach moves beyond the traditional supported housing service. The support and development model enables young people to have their basic needs met, to work with Centrepoint to address specific needs, issues and challenges in their lives and to benefit from wider opportunities to improve their lives (Table 13.4).

While the generic social worker, or even the mental health specialist, will not be able to be fully conversant with the details of every voluntary sector organisation in their area, it is evident how effective partnership working can extend the resources available to social work professionals. It also indicates the level of expertise available within the voluntary sector that effective partnerships can harness to the benefit of all service users.

Table 13.4 Centrepoint support and development model

Centrepoint curriculum: firm foundations

Housing – understanding and enjoying the rights and responsibilities of living independently

Income – welfare rights advice; support to improve earning potential

Health and well-being – looking after yourself, diet and lifestyle, physical fitness, good mental health including being able to cope with stress appropriately, managing the use (or reducing/stopping) of alcohol and drugs

Basic skills and life skills – literacy and numeracy for everyday situations, developing the ability to listen and communicate effectively, self-advocacy

Education, training, employment – guidance, advice and support with education, training and employment opportunities

Centrepoint curriculum: sustainable futures

Emotional intelligence – self-awareness, self-esteem, motivation and sensitivity to others, handling a range of relationships

Creativity and enterprise – feeding and expressing imagination, recognising and solving problems, calculating and taking risks, thinking laterally, applying knowledge and experiences

Citizenship – social responsibility, getting involved, making a contribution and being influential, finding a voice and a place

---

Contingency planning

Planning for contingencies and crises is vital if accommodation services are to respond effectively to changes in users' needs. This is something that can be done most successfully through joint working – involving service users as well as professionals from the statutory and voluntary sectors.

This is especially important for service users with dual diagnoses and complex needs, and often challenging behaviour, often compounded by substance abuse problems (Wasylenki *et al.* 1993; Zachary *et al.* 2002). Trust between all the parties (statutory, voluntary and user) is central to this – and many voluntary sector providers are skilled at providing a bridge between different parties, identifying shared agendas and crossing boundaries to enable 'shared care'. Social workers are encouraged to foster and welcome such approaches.

Effective planning will involve workers close to the service user being trusted to describe symptoms and behaviours, and getting immediate responses from skilled social workers and psychiatrists (Smith and Leon 2001).

Successful contingency planning will enable rapid responses and interventions that effectively manage risk, prevent accommodation arrangements breaking down and avoid clients being evicted and hospitalised or faced with homelessness.

At their best, voluntary sector staff should be able to offer service users a level of 'therapeutic' support as well as practical day-to-day assistance. This 'therapeutic' work is basically managed, 'boundaried' emotional support. This will draw upon effective, active listening skills, the ability to assess users' needs through skilful and sensitive questioning. Techniques such as motivational interviewing enable workers to assist users to recognise the difficulties in their lives, identify some underlying causes, aspire to change and work towards changing behaviours. This involves reflection and learning, and good training is required to underpin such approaches. This may well be an area in which both the voluntary sector and social workers should develop further.

Practical support and advice is also critical and should not be underestimated. People with mental health difficulties can find themselves involved in the criminal justice system. At best, a custodial sentence does not mean that someone will lose their home. For example, Housing Benefit can continue to pay for someone's rent – even if they are in custody – as long as they are expected to return to their home within 13 weeks. Social workers and support providers need to be aware of these aspects of the benefits system. Those with short custodial sentences of less than a year are at greatest risk of losing their homes, as they are unlikely to be able to maintain Housing Benefit payments and will not be assigned a probation worker on release. Wherever possible in these situations, mental health social workers should maintain some contact, or establish links with HM Prison Service to minimise the disruption that will face clients on release. Increasingly, a number of voluntary sector organisations are offering outreach and resettlement services into prisons to address these needs.

Challenges of accommodation-based services

Working in someone's home, regardless of whether they are licensees in a hostel or tenants in their own flat, can engender a range of tensions and sources of potential conflict. Tensions may involve the following areas.

Users' rights versus risk management

Housing providers are encouraged, for best practice reasons, to offer the highest level of security of tenure wherever possible, which maximises users' rights. However, where little is known about someone's history, or there is significant risk of relapse and mental health is associated with risk behaviour, providing accommodation on a licence basis may actually empower providers to accept people with a higher level of risk. Insisting upon tenancy agreements may deter providers from accepting people whose health and behaviour could deteriorate.

Support versus compliance

Housing support providers often have dual roles – they are there to offer practical and emotional support and assistance to service users, but also to ensure house rules and tenancy conditions (such as the payment of rent, non-harassment of neighbours) are complied with.

A skilful worker will be able to establish clear boundaries with users from the outset, and explain why they need to assist the user in keeping their obligations – as failure to do so will put their ongoing accommodation at risk.

The combination of support and housing management will also reduce the number of people that a service user needs to deal with – and enables 'key working' and co-ordination of services to be dealt with more effectively.

However, there will be tensions in a relationship where support and compliance are involved in the same worker – something that social workers themselves may recognise!

Sharing and peer support versus stress and lack of privacy

Shared housing may offer some service users the opportunity to establish positive relationships with others who have shared experiences and can offer informal peer support. Conversely, having to share accommodation and facilities can create additional stresses and result in loss of privacy for some individuals. Where a user's behaviour is likely to impact upon others, shared accommodation may not be suitable, and accommodation options that offer both self-contained units and close supervision/support are needed.

Good design examples

Thames Reach Bondway – Lambeth High Street

Lambeth High Street provided a complex comprising a small shared hostel for rough sleepers with mental health needs and a group of self-contained bedsits, with their own entrances. The bedsits enabled users whose behaviour made it too difficult for them to share accommodation and facilities to live as independently as possible, with 24-hour staff on site. One client who was often very aggressive and threatening was excluded from the office in the hostel by the use of an injunction, but still enabled to live in his bedsit, continued to receive support from his CPN and prevented from returning to the streets again – because of the design of the property.

Richmond Fellowship – Mixed Provision Service

This service comprises a courtyard development of a registered five-bed shared project and five self-contained bungalows, with an office on site. The clients in the shared accommodation are catered for in a large communal dining and kitchen area. Those in the bungalows are expected to self-cater. However, at times of poor health, people in the bungalows are able to be included in the arrangements for the shared house, which enables people with quite frail mental health and low levels of practical skills to live as independently as possible.

Some group homes – especially those developed in the mid-1980s as part of the first tranche of hospital reprovision, often staffed and managed (initially) by social services or health authority personnel – can be quite large and appear relatively institutional. Poor design means they can be easily identified and may be stigmatised within the local community. Social workers need to be sensitive to these issues when seeking to place people with mental health needs, who may prefer the relative anonymity of smaller group homes provided by the voluntary sector, for it is reiterated that the stigma of homelessness compounds the stigma of mental disorder (Marley and Buila 2001; Ryan 2003; Schulze and Angermeyer 2003).

Conversely, some clients who have long histories of institutions may find comfort in the relative anonymity of larger homes and hostels.

Independence versus isolation

Service users may wish to have their own accommodation in the community to maximise their independence and autonomy. However, this can lead to isolation – so social workers should be aware of voluntary sector providers who can offer visiting staff and informal peer support and befriending services, as 'isolation' is a very important fact associated with the extreme consequence of mental disorder, namely suicide (e.g. Scott 1993; Duckworth and McBride 1996; Appleby 1997; Pritchard 1999); hence, the special focus on the accommodation dimension.

Confidentiality versus joint working

Sensible sharing of information policies is required for joint working to be effective. The service user should be informed with whom information will be shared from the earliest possible moment – ideally when a placement/referral to an accommodation-based service is being arranged.

Staff in residential settings are not always valued by statutory colleagues and may be perceived to have low skills. This should not be an excuse to keep relevant information on risk, support needs, etc. confidential to the statutory services, but would indicate the need for very clear protocols on what information needed to be shared and arrangements for passing that information on to third parties (Park 2002).

Definitions: high/medium/low support

One area of tension between professionals is misunderstandings about high, medium and low support definitions – these often surface when voluntary sector providers refuse referrals from social workers.

These definitions are moveable feasts – and social workers should enquire further rather than taking definitions and descriptions at face value.

Key questions to ask when assessing whether an accommodation service is suitable include:

- What hours are support services provided (office hours from on-site staff/ weekly or daily visits . . .)?
- Is there waking or sleeping night cover?
- What training does the staff team have (general mental health awareness or skills in assessment, motivational interviewing, risk management, etc.)?
- What level of observation/supervision can be offered (does this match the needs identified in the client risk assessment)?

If a project appears suitable, but staff are reluctant to accept a referral, it may be worth social workers investing the time in developing relationships with staff – explaining the risk assessment process in detail and advising on the support that social services will provide (many voluntary sector agencies may have been 'let down' in the past). An offer of additional training and support may well open doors to new and highly beneficial resources for social services and clients alike.

Social workers should also be aware of the anxiety that individual clients and their carers may be living with, where the client lives in the family home with ageing parents, and it is acknowledged that these arrangements may not be sustainable into the longer term as the carers age and become more frail. It is essential for social workers to plan ahead with clients and their carers for such inevitabilities, and it is incumbent on all social workers to ensure that these 'future needs' and demands for services are fed into the departmental planning systems of health, housing and social services through the community plans (now replacing the community care plans) and Supporting People strategies.

Wherever possible, information should be given to carers and clients about the range of options available to them. It is possible to arrange for the family home to be put into a legal trust for the service user to enable them to remain living there after their parents have gone – and to arrange for a package of visiting support/care to maintain their independence. Alternatively, supported accommodation services can be identified and even visited in advance, so that a client may be settled before their current living arrangements become untenable.

When it goes wrong

There have been a number of high-profile inquiries into instances of suicide and homicide by people with mental health problems in the last ten years, and these have all highlighted the need for effective joint working and noted the central role that stable and appropriately supported accommodation plays in caring for people with mental health needs (Baker 1997; Burrows 1997; Department of Health 1999a, 2001). In Department of Health (1999b), particular concerns were noted about the risks posed (to themselves and others) by people who were disengaged from services, and the Inquiry found that homeless people were disproportionately represented among those not in touch with services.

The Newby Inquiry (Davies 1995)

Jonathan Newby was a voluntary organisation worker and was alone in the accommodation project's basement office when he was stabbed to death by John Raus, a resident at the scheme. In the weeks leading up to the incident, John Raus had started drinking and using drugs again, and had made threats to his social worker. None of this information was adequately discussed with the project, which had put in place no adequate risk management procedures.

Christopher Clunis

Christopher Clunis was mentally ill when he carried out an unprovoked attack on Jonathan Zito in a tube station in north London. The subsequent inquiry found that communication between the professionals involved in Christopher Clunis' care had broken down. This was exacerbated by the fact that Mr Clunis had a long history of homelessness and unsettled accommodation – only a few months before the stabbing, he had been in a large (192 bedspaces) hostel in south-east London, which was wholly unsuited to his needs at the time.

The Dixon Inquiry

Magdi E had a history of unsettled accommodation, hospitalisation, failure to comply with medication regimes, and had a forensic history, which was showing a pattern of increasing aggression. Again, communication between services broke down as he moved from Croydon to London to Brighton and back to central London again. Despite the interventions of a voluntary organisation, which referred him to mental health services in a new area, after a central London local authority housing department discharged their duty to provide accommodation by placing him in bed and breakfast in east London, he lost touch with mental health services. He was unwell and in a friend's flat when police broke into the property to try to arrest him after another incident involving a knife. During the 'storming' of the flat, Magdi E once stabbed the policewoman who led the entry into his flat. Magdi E is in a secure unit.

It is unlikely that the inquiries referred to above would have been avoided simply and easily by the provision of suitable supported accommodation and effective joint working between voluntary and statutory sector providers. However, in all three cases, the perpetrators (who are also victims themselves) were in touch with voluntary sector accommodation services, but the appropriate joint working with statutory social and health services did not occur.

These case studies show the importance of effective communication between sectors – and the fact that the voluntary sector does not work with only 'low needs' mental health users. However, for balance against these tragedies, we need to remember that the mentally disordered citizen, especially when isolated and/or homeless, is far more likely to die by their own hand than damage others (Appleby 1997; Shaw *et al.* 1999). Nonetheless, when we get it wrong, it can be fatal for someone, perhaps even ourselves?

Conclusion

There are a range of different models of residential provision for people with mental health needs – and social workers are likely to work across the spectrum, from hospital and registered care through shared housing and hostels to self-contained supported accommodation in the community.

The voluntary sector is increasingly the provider of accommodation and basic support, and their contribution and roles must be appreciated by social workers, as they are key partners in providing effective care and support to vulnerable people.

The statutory sector – social workers – are key players in carrying out community care assessments, undertaking care management and enabling access to clinical resources and therapeutic interventions.

Social services and voluntary sector providers need to work together. The voluntary sector provides benefits and can complement the role of social services, but also requires support in the form of training, advice and information sharing.

14 The vortex of mental disorder

The client speaks

Objectives: by the end of the chapter you should:

1 Understand the client's perceptions of the mental health crisis.
2 Explore strengths and weaknesses of mental health social work intervention.

It is a truism, but nonetheless true, that every case is different. Indeed, experienced practitioners know that they are more likely to make mistakes with a client they think they know particularly well, as we fail to notice possible significant changes that alter the situation, moving it from a potential crisis to emergency.

But what of the experience of the people involved? With the greatest care to maintain confidentiality and disguising their identities, clients describe their perceptions of a mental health crisis. Throughout this chapter, we hear the voice of the person in the crisis themselves, with minimal editing.

Dilemmas in depression

It can sound cynical and exploitative to say that we learn from our clients, but in a true sense that is what practice is about. No matter how long we have worked in the field, we still have much to learn, not only about the specific person with whom one is working, nor even about oneself, but about the unfolding field of mental health practice if we can keep an open mind.

A simple example, but one that has stayed with me over the years, was when I was a young lecturer in the Department of Psychiatry at the University of Leeds. There, all the disciplines had at least one and a half days a week of practice, but this case was an 'accident'.

My car had broken down, and I had missed and tried to thumb a lift, which at 8.15 a.m. was unlikely. My luck was in as a large Daimler pulled up and an immaculate BBC voice asked me was I in trouble? I explained I wanted to go to the university, four miles away, and fortunately it was on his way.

He was an obviously intelligent man in his late 40s, very well turned out and seemingly a man of authority.

'I don't usually give lifts, but you're obviously a professional chap (best suit for a big meeting), so I thought I'd enquire.'

The traffic was heavy and slow moving and we chatted about Yorkshire cricket, which we both mourned. He then asked me to which part of the university I belonged. By this stage of my career, I had grown out of the desire to gain new clients, and my usual answer was fairly non-committal, 'teacher' – however, it seemed churlish not to be open so I mentioned the Department of Psychiatry. He expressed pleasant interest and said that he knew my professor. I assumed that he would know him from some finance committee or other as 'Mr Z' had told me he was in 'finance' so I made the mistake of asking him how he knew Professor Hamilton.

'Oh professionally, he was extremely helpful with my wife.' It transpired that she had had a depression. 'Hamilton was quite excellent and Dr X has taken her on for psychotherapy in addition to antidepressants and things are really going well now.' I expressed satisfaction and then, almost without thinking, said that it must have been a difficult time for him as the family also had to bear the pressure, how had he coped?

Suddenly, the car began to swerve across the road alarmingly, I could see that he was distressed; for a moment, I thought he was having a heart attack. He pulled over to the side of the road, switched on his emergency lights as he sought to regain his self-control. I could see he was crying.

'You know, you're the first person to ask me how I was. We have a good marriage and, when my wife first began to be depressed, I thought that something was wrong with us. I felt hurt, rejected, shut out and, when she began to speak about leaving me or even dying because she was not worthy of us, at first I didn't realise that she was ill. She then collected some tablets and nearly died. Of course, we then appreciated that she was ill, that all her negative talk was not because she no longer loved her family but because she was ill. But no-one, not one person, asked how I was coping.' Everyone assumed that a man of his social stature could carry on: 'They simply ignored the sight of one's wife collapsing before one's eyes, you know the effects of depression are contagious. We were all affected, our children, not only my wife, and I had to carry on as if nothing was happening, that our lives were not being torn to shreds by this hideous psychological cancer . . . That's what it's like you know for the family – the depression drained all her emotion but, until you appreciate what's happening, it eats into your mind, making you doubt everything.'

He gathered himself, apologised for burdening me and was reluctant to agree to a further meeting.

'No, that's kind of you. I think I'm all right now I know my wife is OK. Only do tell your colleagues to think beyond the patient. I'm glad I picked you up, you've actually been very helpful and I promise, if I feel I need help for myself, I'll get in touch.'

He apparently did not need any further help and discreet enquiries about his wife proved positive. Two months later, I received a Xmas card from them both.

Here was a dramatic example of the 'contagion' of depression and the paradox, which is often missed, that we men suffer from sexism. We are not good at expressing ourselves, at seeking help or support, which is often missed by busy professionals. Yet, after care and treatment for the primary client, nothing is more important than maintaining the client's family networks, for that is where they still gain the greatest prolonged level of support.

The vortex of suicidal behaviour

Dilemmas in schizophrenia

The following detailed example was written in close conjunction with 'Alan' who, for reasons of privacy and confidentiality, decided not to have his authorship acknowledged.

'Alan', aged 34 at the time of the crisis, was an arts graduate who had worked part-time on a research project in the university. He had a turbulent adolescence, massively underachieving academically and receiving a mixture of diagnoses of early schizophrenia and unipolar affective disorder, characterised by being withdrawn and agitated; his earlier persistent school 'phobia' had led to his admission to an adolescent unit. Alan perceived part of his problem as the complexity surrounding his relationships with his parents for, although his mother tacitly accepted his gay orientation, his father found this unacceptable, and they were diametrically opposed. Alan being slightly built, non-sporty and an ardent socialist was opposed to his right-wing, six-foot-six, former rugby-playing, scientist-trained father. However, Alan appeared to absorb his family and cultural attitudes to homosexuality, and he was never 'out' and bitterly regretted something 'I can't help – I have never been able to see what other men see in girls, they've never interested me'.

Alan made major progress in the unit, being symptom free for four years, and finally 'caught up' and entered university as a 22-year-old student.

At the end of his student days, Alan had a possible 'psychotic' episode following the break-up of his only long-term lover relationship. His symptoms were possible auditory hallucinations, with marked persecutory ideas, but no overt delusions. He was successfully treated with respiridone and was supported by his social worker on a minimal dosage of respiridone for prophylactic purposes very successfully for the next six years. At times of particular pressure, Alan saw me for formal counselling, with increased respiridone; otherwise, a monthly to six-week maintenance contact, back on the lowest possible dosage was sufficient; thus he had virtually no side-effects.

The second big crisis was when Alan took a post-graduate programme out of the region. He achieved very creditable results, but again at the end of the university period, an unresolved love relationship led to his first frank and overt episode of schizophrenia, leading to an informal hospital admission. He experienced auditory hallucinations and for a short period was intensely paranoid deluded. After discharge, he returned home and made contact again, and 'long-term' support was resumed along the lines outlined above. He took up work but not at the level he was capable of, but nonetheless he was well regarded by his colleagues and, in effect, he decided not to attempt to achieve his potential because he recognised that, for him, stress was a precipitant. All was well for three years to the extent that Alan decided he should have a 'clean start', got himself a flat and a job in London away from the restrictions of rural England, and also hoped to find a close long-term relationship.

I lost touch with him for the next two years and this is his story of what led to our next meeting.

'I'll try to make sense of what happened, but of course I'm talking with the benefits of hindsight. My GP had increased my dose and, like the passive idiot I am, no problems with non-compliance with me – so I took it and started to put on weight and got some twitchy side-effects, which made me very unhappy. I started to get anxious, I really ought to have known the signs but you weren't about and I didn't trust my GP. Then I realised that he fancied me but I didn't fancy him and, as he had suggested I increase my medication, I knew he was up to no good. I heard the whispers; there were a number of incidents when I saw people talking about me – they'd look away, snigger but I knew – once I nearly got into a fight as I asked him did he think I was gay. I couldn't sleep, couldn't think straight, the whispers became worse and then I heard them. I knew they were trying to kill me, they wanted me to kill myself, I was terrified. I stayed in all day, only went out late at night to get food from the 24-hour shop. I realised suddenly and knew that it was true that the police and my GP were talking together, that they were signalling on TV but not just against me but all gays, only I was the worst, because though I've never practised unsafe sex they accused me of bringing AIDS into the world. Wherever I went they were watching, talking about the coming pogrom to rid the world of gays and the voice kept telling me that I'd be the first to be killed.

'I fled from London, got home but they didn't believe me, we had a row and I ended up in hospital. This was a trap, because the voices were still there, and I knew that it was part of the plot and the fights and shouting on the ward were all part of the plan to take me off guard, and I knew I was even more at risk there despite their smiling faces. They talked down to me as if I was a little boy. I asked for seclusion and they gave it to me and, when they closed the door I was able to break out, it was a horrible journey but I'd nowhere else to turn so I came to you.'

Alan arrived one winter Sunday evening about 5 p.m., ringing the doorbell in an agitated way. I was totally surprised to see him. He looked distressed, agitated, clearly frightened; his first words were 'They're killing all the gays, I'm the only one left, I don't know what to do.'

I asked him in, took him to a quiet room and calmed him down but first excused myself to tell him I was going to call my wife. I went to her explaining he was not well and, dependent on how things went, could he share our meal; the professional she is took everything in her stride and told me to return to Alan.

I asked him what he thought was happening. He poured out his beliefs and fears and how he feared 'they're trying to kill me, it's true, they've followed me home, I wish I was dead, they keep telling me I'll only be safe when I'm dead and keep asking why don't I kill myself and do everybody a favour'.

I did not try to challenge his delusions, but acknowledged the reality of the experience of his voices and, of course, avoid the temptation to explore who 'they' were and responded to his real fears, giving full recognition to his emotional reality – he was terrified for his life, as would we all be if we experienced what Alan was experiencing. Slowly he calmed, and I decided that the most appropriate action would be to 'normalise' the situation and, as he knew my wife socially, invited him to stay to supper. We agreed not to 'alarm' my wife, so we would not discuss the reasons for his unexpected arrival.

Of course, here was the professional dilemma, how to get him the treatment he needed and, in his present state, anti-psychotic medication, which it emerged he had stopped months ago, and the legal 'responsibility' of returning him to hospital, especially as he had been admitted under Section 3.

While I was trying to work this out, I called in my wife to reinforce the 'normality' of the situation and of course Alan behaved like the perfect gentleman he is. I had ascertained that his parents did not know his whereabouts and suggested that I ring them to let them know he was safe. This made him extremely suspicious but I said that he should let them know he was here, while my wife reinforced my approach by stressing how she, as a mother, still worried about our grown-up children, and his mother would be equally worried.

Alan accompanied me to the phone, standing by the door as I rang the parents from the hall phone. I was very brief, said who I was, gave them Alan's greeting and told them that he was with us. The father asked did I know Alan had absconded from hospital. I said yes and asked could Alan come home. His answer was very panicky, 'We can't cope, he's frightening us – he'll have to go back – I'll get the hospital to get in touch with you'. Here was a real dilemma, I could not explore that any further without alarming Alan; I quickly ended the conversation as I could see it was disturbing Alan, so I compromised. While self-evidently Alan needed help, did he need compulsory admission – someone had thought he did? Should I offer to take him back to his parents? On balance I thought this too problematic in case he panicked while I was driving. So I sought to 'normalise' and reinforce Alan's positive social behaviour and asked did my wife need me for anything in the kitchen and, as she did not, I poured us all a sherry.

I gave Alan further time to express any worries, trusted him to use the bathroom and sought to transform the 'crisis' into as normal a social interchange as possible.

Albeit that Alan had clear paranoid delusions, I was confident that, provided he did not feel threatened, he would not be a risk to anyone; indeed, as he had no history of violence or aggression, I felt that the only person who was vulnerable was Alan.

Furthermore, I decided that alcohol was appropriate, that it would not clash with any medication, for it seemed he was not on any, so my wife and I sought to transform the situation into a pleasant social occasion, with an intelligent, courteous, socially aware young man who happened to be experiencing a psychotic episode. The one potential expression of his underlying bizarre feelings and fears was when my wife asked him 'how old are you now Alan'; his reply was 'If I'd lived to my next birthday I'd be 35'. I decided not to pursue this, but it reminded me that along with his delusions were suicidal ideas.

At 9.30 p.m., the evening was disrupted by less than tactful hospital staff, whose patronising and condescending language was an eye-opener. Alans' reaction was one of both fear and anger, 'You've let me down, you've betrayed me, and you're like them'. He then refused to say another word and looked desperately fearful.

I escorted him out to the hospital car, held his hand, reassured him of my regard and best intentions and promised to see him the following day. He had become totally withdrawn, refused to look or answer me. But I reiterated my regard and promise, acknowledging that he was angry with me and that I felt very sad about this because I really did want to help and would want to help next week, next month and, if he wanted, in the months ahead. I did not expect a reply, nor did I get one but realised that I would need to began to repair the inevitable break in the therapeutic relationship.

My wife summed the situation up: 'I don't think I've ever seen anyone so afraid. I can hardly believe he was the same person', and she worried whether we had done the right thing, especially in view of the response of the hospital staff.

Visiting the following evening, I was saddened but not surprised to see the poor quality of the atmosphere of the ward. Initially, Alan wanted nothing to do with me but, relying on Alan's core character, reminding him I had come a distance, we spent half an hour in a quiet room and had only a few monosyllabic replies, in part because of the heavy dose of medication he had received and in part because he was still angry at my 'betrayal'. When I left him, we were at best at a stage of benign neutrality.

After a week, it was possible to discharge Alan home and, while he was very cautious in his response to me, we re-established a working relationship. He was assigned an excellent community psychiatric nurse (CPN) and I resumed my secondary support role.

Alan re-established his links with his family. He was reconciled with his father and was an excellent support to his mother during a long illness. We maintained a distant quarterly support contact, in part to supplement the CPN's role.

Phyllida Parsloe wrote many years ago that long-term support of mentally disordered people means the creation of a long-term support relationship, which might be described as 'professional friendship' (Plant 1968) because of its boundaries. I do not feel that is inconsistent, for relationship means a degree of interaction and reciprocity, which over time can appropriately erase the unnecessary hierarchy.

Mania

Another example of the dilemmas that often surround mental health practice was when a lady referred by Mind came to explore the possibility of 'compensation' for 'wrongful compulsory' admission. In order to prepare for our first meeting, she forwarded a memorandum of what she described as 'the outrage'. Indeed, she pressed me to accept the history as a case example: 'For your students to appreciate just how terrible compulsory admission can be'. With her permission, I have repeated her story, without comment, but will ask you to consider the 'rights and wrongs' of the case at the end of her narrative.

She was a widowed lady aged around 60 and the chairperson of a major family business, which she had run with her husband for many years until his death and then alone. She was a professional person in her own right and, as this situation was some years ago, she was one of the relatively few female graduates of her generation. She was competent, capable, highly intelligent and a sophisticated person and, in her own words, 'always had the energy to do three jobs [family – profession – an executive director in her firm], which would probably overwhelm most average men'. She lived in a large house, in three-quarters of an acre of grounds in a very affluent commuter village, which was the scene for much of her story.

The outrage

On a hot and peaceful afternoon last June, I was gardening in solitude when there suddenly appeared the two partners in the local GP practice, together with a stranger, who it later emerged was an 'Approved Social Worker' (ASW).

After initial polite greetings and a good deal of hedging, they announced that I was obviously ill and in need of 'treatment'. To my profound amazement, no amount of reasoned argument would deflect them from their polite insistence that the purpose of their visit was to commit me to the local mental hospital.

On returning to the house, I realised the seriousness of my position and their intent. When I saw lined up in the village street a large ambulance, complete with two uniformed attendants, a police car and two private cars. I found it difficult to believe in the reality of my situation [shades of Kafka and *The Trial*].

The doctors filled in a form, and they both signed it without disclosing its contents, except that I understood I was to be in hospital for two days for observation.

After further delaying tactics on my part and equally determined countermeasures on the part of the escorting team, I was finally led down the path by the two large ambulance attendants. I was wearing my gardening clothes, but was allowed to take a cardigan and my handbag. I insisted that I travel in the police car and, to my surprise, the two men dropped their grip, but the ASW felt thwarted for he immediately attempted to jump into the back of their car, but the policeman firmly shut the door as I was anchored by the safety belt. We then drove ten miles in procession to the hospital. Police cars were placed at every strategic position on the route. I remained silent during the journey and my driver equally so. I was delivered to the hospital followed by the ASW and the empty ambulance.

The Chief Officer received me courteously in his office and filled in a detailed form. He asked what had led up to the present position. I maintained that I was angry and bewildered, that I lived alone and moreover had a dinner party that night for which I had had my hair done.

I was then taken to the observation ward and asked to undress for a physical examination. This was efficiently carried out by a polite Indian doctor and nurse, and I then returned to the office where the doctor took a detailed account of my past history, which included two stays in mental institutions after the death of my husband. The first had been in similar circumstance when I apparently acted in a highly elated way for a short time when staying in Essex, and the local doctor committed me to a state mental hospital where I was forcibly made to take drugs and given shock treatment thrice weekly. I was freed after six weeks and in another six weeks had so lost confidence and identity that I asked my own doctor to send me to a private hospital. I was again given shock treatment and drugged so much that I remember very little about it. Due to the strenuous efforts of my family and friends, I soon recovered and was able to take on and hold a responsible post in a hospital.

The Indian doctor put me through the usual psychological tests, and I was then taken to the dining room and given a cup of tea. No further explanations were tendered. I joined the rest of the 'patients' seated around the walls of the television room and remained there for the rest of the evening; no-one spoke to me other than a brief visit from kind friends who brought me my night things. At 9.30 p.m., I was shown to my cubicle in the observation ward. Sleep was impossible as the two nurses on duty kept up an incessant conversation. About 2 a.m. I asked for food and I was given a cup of tea and a biscuit at 6 a.m. I dressed and from then onwards sat once more in the television lounge. The boredom and misery were infectious and my sense of frustration was acute. Having seen the food that was offered, I refused it up to 5 p.m. I was at length persuaded to co-operate by the Indian nurse and joined the others in the dining room. I asked the Chief Officer if there was a single room and he was kind enough to allocate one to me.

On the Monday morning, I was seen by the consultant psychiatrist, whose attitude was interrogating and punitive. He presumably filled in another dossier and I was then committed to the statutory 28 days laid down by the 1983 Mental Health Act.

During my stay, I resisted all pressures to take drugs. I was prescribed three different varieties by three different doctors. Shock treatment was not proffered this time owing to the resistance put up by my son (a solicitor) and myself. Those who did accept this 'treatment' gradually became dulled and institutionalised in spite of the fact that, for the most part, they appeared to be quite well on admission.

I involved myself in the life of the community in which I found myself but the boredom at this time was quite excruciating. We were expected to attend 'occupational therapy' on weekdays but, at the weekends, no form of recreation was available. Two tennis courts stood idle, but it was impossible to break through the system to make use of them.

On two occasions, I was quite involuntarily involved in trying to help patients who were being persecuted and, after each incident, was summoned to a doctor's presence, interrogated and warned not to get 'involved'.

The tensions at times were acute – the rational result of a group of intelligent people being herded together in such an unnatural situation. Visiting was allowed but no place to receive visitors was provided.

During my stay, the weather was good and I was able to walk every inch of the spacious but too tidy grounds.

The staff were mostly kind but dutiful. Their position must have been extremely invidious. The Chief Officer was highly efficient and I liked him, even though he had to take several blood tests and, on several occasions, inject me with Largactil when I refused to take the drug orally. His face was a mask until the last day when I went to thank him. I would have flung my arms around him and hugged him had he given me the slightest encouragement.

In conclusion, the experience was valuable. I made some new friends and there were a great many amusing incidents, which lightened the burden. I am saddened when I think of the many who have been and must necessarily be there for many years. My own fate could have been the same had not my son and daughter been behind me. I am still seething with anger at the misuse of power on behalf of the doctors and psychiatrists and the state. The loopholes in the Mental Health Act are glaring and obvious and need attention.

Postscript

The culminating incident, which led to my apprehension, was the fact that, while trying to gain entrance to a neighbour's house in order to protest at his gross rudeness, I somewhat injudiciously and accidentally broke a pane of glass in a French window. This could have been dealt with under civil law had he really wished to take the matter further and would have been dealt with by the police.

Had I not resisted every attempt to make me take the drugs so forcibly offered to me in hospital, I have not the slightest doubt that I would not have escaped at the end of the statutory 28 days.

Her account is graphic and perhaps all too familiar. Whatever the 'rights and wrongs' of the situation, her recall of the boredom, the apparently inexplicable behaviour surrounding her, the apparent dichotomy between staff and patients has an authenticity that cannot be ignored. One could not fail but to be charmed by her many talents but was she so 'ill' that she really did require admission? Was she suffering from a bipolar affective (manic) episode? In remonstrating with her neighbour because of his 'rudeness', according to the son, our lady was shouting the odds about the incompatibility of her friend with her husband, as well as making derogatory remarks about his sexual prowess. This was a case in which I found myself 'on the wrong side', but also on the side of the solicitor son. To my relief and surprise, he appreciated that his mother had to 'exorcise' the 'outrage', not least because he thought that, while the admission was necessary at the time, her experience highlighted many shortcomings and, though he had advised her that legally he did not think she could win her case, he was willing to support her through the exploration. Mrs 'W' reluctantly accepted that 'I can't win, and you've been very helpful and sympathetic but I still aver that we really should not treat people in such an unsympathetic and high-handed manner. We really should do better.' Who could disagree with her?

Family burden and complexities of schizophrenia

While there is overwhelming evidence that families bear a considerable burden in their support of their mentally disordered relative, it must be remembered that young teenagers can sometimes pose particular problems for the 'family', by virtue of age and situation. To highlight the psychiatric–child protection interface, the following case illustrates the complexities that can follow. My role was initially supervising the social worker involved and latterly utilising my position to be an advocate for the family. The story of 'Jag' also illustrates a core theme within this book, that people do not always fit 'the textbooks' but rather spill over the boundaries of problem categories and agencies. Thus, from one perspective, we are looking at a school problem, from another, a possible case of child sexual abuse and, from another, the ramifications of a person with chronic schizophrenia.

At point of referral, 'Jag' was 15 years 1 month and was the 'delight and bane' of his secondary school teacher, who found herself exasperated by the obvious 'almost deliberate' educational underachievement of an obviously bright young man. 'When he wants he can be an absolute delight and, on occasions, reminds you why teaching is a great job and, on others, why one thinks of early retirement.'

Jag came from a single-parent family. His mother was aged 45, a quiet, shy woman, known to have 'mental problems'; it later transpired she had had three serious episodes of schizophrenia and two short admissions to psychiatric hospital in the past six years. The father had left after the first hospital admission and, apart from the paternal grandmother looking after Jag and his older brother, 'William', when mother was away, he had severed all contact with the family. The mother had no family herself in the region and, when she worked, often had jobs not commensurate with her ability. Her strengths, however, were that she was a graduate and an intelligent woman, who was undoubtedly committed to her boys and, when well, keen to re-establish independent living.

'William' was 18 and was learning-disabled. He attended an adult training centre and was very much dependent upon Jag, treating him as an older, rather than a younger, brother. He was very close to his mother and dependent upon her and Jag.

First crisis

Jag was obviously unwell and refused to see a GP; however, at his teacher's insistence, he saw the school nurse. She found he had a urethral infection and a sore bottom, and began to suspect sexual abuse. Jag told her that he and William 'were just messing about'; this indeed seemed to be the source of the irritation. In addition, Jag admitted that he was worried about his mother, who was again unwell, and that he was anxious what might happen to William and himself, as he did not want to return to his grandmother should his mother be readmitted. Jag's priorities were 'to get some cream to stop the itch' but, more importantly, some help 'for me mam so she doesn't have to go away again . . . she's fine when she's well, we're all right if people will leave us alone. When she's working, we can manage.' He negotiated that he would talk to a school social worker (SSW) in confidence as he admitted, 'that when her muttering gets bad, it worries me'.

Resolving the crisis

The social worker successfully engaged with Jag and his mother and liaised with the community mental health team (CMHT), the GP and the consultant psychiatrist, and it was agreed that the SSW would be the key worker for the family and take advantage of mental health supervision.

The SSW was also in touch with the child protection team, whose team leader was initially dubious about Jag staying at home as he might be 'at risk' of abuse from William, not least because, if anything went wrong, 'it would look bad if we were thought not to have handled the problem appropriately'. Based upon a number of interviews with the two brothers, the team leader was persuaded by the SSW that, despite the age difference between the boys, Jag did not appear to be a 'victim' in any way. Furthermore, 'fears' about Jag's sexual identity were allayed by the fact that Jag had girlfriends and had promised to avoid any further sex play with William.

The SSW helped the mother to recommence her medication and agree to depot treatment, at a minimal dose and with help to tolerate the mild side-effects. She especially valued the support of the SSW, as he could visit more frequently than the community psychiatric nurse or the CMHT, and she was able to contact him at the school if necessary: 'it's such a comfort to know I can call him . . . he's very good, I can always get a message to him'. In fact, she hardly used the facility.

It became clear that, over the past two years, the exacerbation of Jag's misbehaviour had coincided with his mother's mental state, as he struggled to hold the family together.

Second crisis

All went well for the next six months; the mother's symptoms reduced with minimal side-effects, and she was able to take up a job in a supermarket and valued the supportive contact with the SSW, and the SSW's support of Jag, whose school work was improving; he was looking set to entering for GCSEs, which was in keeping with his undoubted intelligence and mother's active support.

Jag had been encouraged to be involved in a couple of school projects that brought him into contact with more stable youngsters and he left behind his previous 'truant' group (truancy is often an activity of alienated pupils; Pritchard 2001) and developed appropriate and socially confirming friendships. Crucially, he had a 'steady' (3 months+) girlfriend, 'Mary', a classmate who shared with Jag her ambitions to go to university.

The crisis blew up when Jag and his girlfriend were found in flagrante by Mary's military father, who was 'outraged' and said that he would 'demand the law'. The incident was surrounded with claims and counterclaims; Jag sustained bruising to the face and there was broken furniture in the girl's bedroom. Mary's father went to Jag's mother and was very threatening, and she buckled under his threats that Jag would be sent to prison 'for rape'; the situation completely destabilised her and, within a week, she was expressing frank paranoid ideas and was failing to cope.

The situation worsened as Mary's father 'interviewed' William in a highly questionable illegal manner. He learned about the earlier sex play with Jag and that William had an adult friend at the Training Centre and, according to the father, their mutual sexual activity was 'tolerated' by the staff, which was again 'outrageous'.

Jag was greatly distressed and concerned for Mary, who he loved – 'I wouldn't do anything to hurt her . . . he's got a dirty mind . . . there was nothing wrong, we love each other' – and played down the beating that Mary's father gave him because 'I don't want to make it worse for her'. Jag's anxieties increased as his mother's mental state deteriorated, but matters became more confused when Mary came to stay at Jag's home, with the approval of Mary's mother, to save her from the father's wrath, which now included corporal punishment, which Mary's mother thought was unacceptable. It later transpired that Mary was on 'the pill', with her mother's approval, but unbeknown to her father.

All the agencies involved were now faced with a complex legal and practice problem. Undoubtedly, Jag was guilty of having underage sex, although Mary was 15 years 4 months and Jag 15 years 7 months but, along with the knowledge of William's behaviour, the professionals were afraid of being seen to condone this behaviour. Jag's mother's mental state was very parlous and, unfortunately, Mary's father was using this against Jag's family and the agencies, threatening to 'expose you all' to the media. Worse, the father, quite illegally, had gone in uniform to the Jag household threatening both William and the mother with the police, and it appeared that he deliberately provoked her into a panic response so that, for the first time in her history, she was 'violent' and threw something at him. But as he was six feet tall and built like a second-row forward and she five feet nothing and slight, there was little damage. Mary's father, however, was threatening to charge her with assault and, when Jag came home from school, he found both mother and William in a state of mute, frozen shock. Fortunately, he caught the SSW before he had left and he was asked to come and deal with the crisis.

The SSW was faced with two severely shocked and withdrawn 'adults' and an angry confused adolescent who feared for his family. Jag was also close to panic, fearing the loss of Mary, his mother and therefore William and what he perceived was the threat of a custodial outcome for himself. In the background was the 'loose cannon' of an irate father and at least two agencies that were ambivalent about the whole situation.

Some practice questions
- The first dilemma was who is/are the social worker's client/clients?
- What do you think of how the situation has been dealt with so far?
- Do you think we have underplayed the 'at risk' of sexual abuse issue?
- Have we colluded with an offence?
- Can there be a multidisciplinary consensus?
- What is the most pressing problem?
- Can there be an optimal solution?
- What would you recommend?
- Prefer to deal only with unidimensional single category/diagnostic cases?

Outcome

It was decided that the family should be seen as 'the client' with the interests of Jag being pre-eminent. However, it was recognised that the mother's mental state was central to everything and that the core longstanding problem was how the mother could be helped to deal with her schizophrenia. And, despite the 'child protection/educational welfare/delinquency/learning disability' aspects of the case, in essence, it was a 'mental health social work 'case. Hence, every effort should be made to maintain the mother at home and avoid any custodial outcome for the boys. Jag's and William's interests would also be best served by maintaining the family unit. To this end, it was agreed that William would attend the Training Centre daily instead of only three and a half days per week as previously the case. However, the most pressing factor was to reduce the stress precipitants on Jag's mother, which meant trying to deal with Mary's father.

It was appreciated that the underlying emotions of Mary's father and his response would have to be dealt with to avoid antagonising him further, concomitant with helping to restore relations between him and his wife and daughter, in order to get him to withdraw his pressure on Jag's mother.

Working through Mary's mother and police contacts, the father was helped to see that, despite 'being hurt' by what had happened and 'like any father, I would want to protect my daughter', his contact with Jag's family and his threat to go to the media would be counterproductive to him and to his relationship with his wife and daughter. Equally, it was decided that there would be little to gain from confronting the father with the possible illegal and questionable behaviour against Jag and the mother. Working with him was an example of the importance of being able to see the perspective of someone with a markedly different orientation to oneself and to acknowledge his cry 'just because they all do it at their age doesn't mean my daughter has to do it'.

He was placated and Mary returned home but continued to see Jag. A mini-crisis arose when we needed to treat Jag's mother more intensively at home, rather than admit her to hospital. The judgement was made that, with close support, all could be safely maintained and the need for the boys going into some form of residential care could be avoided if their mother was readmitted. So a new equilibrium was re-established.

Jag's mother strongly encouraged his schoolwork and he eventually went to university, with his mother's active blessing, as Jag was apprehensive about leaving her. Jag and Mary continued as 'an item' up to 'A' levels, which was a real boost to Jag's commitment to his studies, but later they moved on into different relationships. Jag's mother continued her prophylactic medication and was able to maintain herself and William.

I am quite certain that, without the excellent social work support the mother received, which included the interests of all, but centred upon the mother's mental health needs, this family would have splintered, and Jag would have been heading for a career of educational underachievement and delinquency. This is an excellent example of how, in the living world of practice, individuals and families seldom fit just one textbook, and how mental health social work is paradoxically very often 'generic'.

ASW conundrums and dilemmas

While 'forensic' cases are always a minority in mental health practice, they do emerge, and create disproportionately enormous demands and anxiety for all involved, often complicated by the conundrums of unclear 'diagnosis' and the dilemma of a clash of rights. While they may not always work out totally satisfactorily, there is much to learn from these situations if we can keep calm, focused and an open mind.

Some years ago, a 22-year-old man, 'Stan', walked into a police station and told the desk sergeant that he had raped and then strangled a four-year-old girl and thrown her body into the canal. It later transpired that he was physically very roughly handled when thrown into a cell. The horrified police immediately went to search the canal and made frantic calls to discover whether such a child had been reported missing. Within 24 hours, Stan, a singularly nondescript young man, apologised and told them it was all a mistake and that he had made up the incident. Apparently, he was again 'roughed up', threatened with wasting police time, which did not seem to alarm him, and then thrown out of the police station.

Two months later, Stan, a former long-term resident in one of the largest children's homes still left in the country, returned to another police station and repeated his story, with more or less the same results. A frantic anxious search by the police and then, with another negative result, Stan was unceremoniously thrown out of the police station; a third similar incident occurred a few weeks later.

At this stage, all that was known about Stan was that he had been taken into care as a four-year-old and had stayed there until 16. Apart from the most minor 'delinquencies', when he sought to avoid bullying and gain favour by being 'cheeky' to the staff, Stan's stay was singularly uneventful. Indeed, he was described by the Head of Home, who had known him for almost a decade, as 'the most unmemorable lad one could imagine. He was just below average at everything. He was easy to miss in an empty room. He seldom spoke to anyone unless they spoke to him. He was the classic hanger-on, because hardly anyone noticed he was there.' If this sounds 'judgemental', 'I'm sorry, but he was so passive, docile, unobtrusive, and he virtually never laughed or cried.' This was reflected in his school record, where he hardly seemed to leave a trace. Stan left the children's home and his social worker had found him the 'perfect' digs and landlady. She was large, homely, demanded total obedience and compliance and ruled the other four long-term lodgers with an affable authoritarianism. Stan was an ideal lodger, and she ensured he was punctual at work in a factory, organised him and changed his clothes, and Stan seemed happily dependent upon her. Four months before the first incident, the landlady had died unexpectedly and Stan had to find new accommodation, which was a single bedsit, but without any type of external support.

The third visit by Stan to a police station with the rape and murder story led to an emergency psychiatric referral and admission to a psychiatric unit. Stan was examined and was passively co-operative in that he answered any questions calmly and fully but would say nothing about his story other than 'it were silly, I don't want to talk about it'. The police had found nothing incriminating in his bedsit, no pornography, indeed no books or magazines of any kind. Initially, the duty consultant psychiatrist, who in the circumstances had responded immediately to the police request at superintendent level, initially said that he could find no evidence of a 'mental disorder' under the Mental Health Act and therefore could offer no further treatment but perhaps refer Stan to a forensic psychiatrist, if Stan would be willing to go. The superintendent, who had consulted with his senior officers, had their backing to 'demand he be admitted'. As Stan was perfectly willing to be admitted informally, the immediate agency clash was avoided.

The police position was perfectly clear. They dare not risk Stan continuing in the community while he appeared to have these dangerous ideas for, irrespective of what the Mental Health Act said, they felt that, if Stan should commit such a violent sexual attack on a child, then the community would rightly be highly critical of them. They rejected the counterarguments that the only 'offence' Stan had committed was wasting police time and that the courts could deal with it accordingly. The police argued that, even if a court decided upon a custodial sentence, it (a) would not be long and (b) would not deal with Stan's presenting problem, which alarmed everyone. Furthermore, if such bizarre behaviour was not considered 'mad' by the professionals, it certainly would be by the public, and there was a hint that they might go to the media, implying that the psychiatric services were not concerned enough to put public safety first.

Stan was duly admitted and was the most compliant and accepting patient. He joined in all occupational therapy activities and otherwise listened to the radio or watched TV. While he had little to do with other male patients, he did respond in a quiet way to female patients.

Needless to say, Stan's case caused enormous controversy within the psychiatric department, and theories flew thick and fast, but Stan could not confirm any, as he was not depressed, miserable, resentful or anxious, and the clinical psychologist who was delegated to be his key worker by virtue of being closer to Stan's age resolutely 'defended' Stan as, in a whole range of tests, nothing had been found to suggested anything amiss. His IQ was of course 100; it was determined that he was heterosexual; on the Eysenck scale, he scored more on the introvert scale but not clinically so; there was no suicidal ideation, his Hamilton Depression rating scores were not significant nor were his scores on the Maudsley obsessive–compulsive or the Worry Anxiety Questionnaire, although it should be borne in mind that such tests are not as conclusive as some of their scoring suggests (Freeman and Graham 1999). The psychologist said, 'I'm sorry to say, I can find nothing wrong with him except that he's boring, which is hardly a scientific diagnosis. He simply clams up when you ask him about the events, and other than that he is totally unremarkable. He shouldn't be here, there should be some form of ongoing care for him. I know I should not say it, but "he's a pudding". And except for scaring the police, and us, he seem totally harmless.'

Who could disagree with such a conclusion except that the police felt some longer term solution was needed that was 'psychiatric' in view of the repeated bizarre stories. The department was so concerned that they invited Stan to undergo abreaction, under sodium pentathol, an anaesthetic. In this procedure, the subject is taken to a presleep stage and, theoretically, is at their least conscious resistance. Stan complied but, once the question of his 'stories' was raised, no matter how close he was to unconsciousness, he resisted all efforts to gain any further understanding. The social services department (SSD) and we suggested that a place be found for him in a mental health hostel, which had a degree of supervision, and that he continue for another six months with support counselling with the clinical psychologist. It quickly became clear that this was not acceptable to the authorities so a multiagency case conference was called, chaired by an adult psychiatrist. Stan, who declined the invitation to attend, was 'represented' by the psychologist, I 'represented' the department, and the charge nurse, a senior manager from the hospital and assistant chief officers from police, probation and the SSD also participated.

The case was put that, from what we knew of Stan, we could not detain him under the Mental Health Act, and we stressed that the most appropriate outcome should be an excellent voluntary mental health hostel, which was strongly supported by the SSD/health representatives at the conference.

The 'criminal justice' side, however, was obdurate that he must somehow be kept in hospital and, as Stan was apparently willing, if he could not be kept in the unit, then he should be transferred to, in effect, a long-term hospital.

It was evident that the issue had become 'political' and it was feared the media might become involved. The 'health' side asked my view, and this is still a matter of ambivalence to me. I had to excuse myself as I found myself in a situation of a conflict of interests. I pointed out that I lived in the city not far away and that I had daughters of the age of Stan's fantasy victims and, while I thought it unlikely that Stan would ever act out his fantasies, I could not live with myself if we got it wrong. I like to think that this was not too discriminating but, in effect, the weight of 'votes' swung firmly to the police view.

Stan was invited in to hear what was to be recommended. He expressed perfect willingness to be transferred, although he asked if there any training possibilities at the hospital as he had never liked his factory job and might like to try farming. The transfer was duly arranged and, to the best of my knowledge, he stayed there for a further three years, finally leaving and marrying a woman considerably older than himself.

This dilemma does not reflect too well on some of us who were there. Some might argue that we colluded with Stan to 'reinstitutionalise' him; that may be so, but it was a conundrum and a dilemma that at the time appeared irresolvable.

In part 'justification' and continuing unease about the above case, some years later, I had to respond to the anguished cry of a small village when a local severe learning disabled youth, who had long been teased by local children, had killed a seven-year-old child. Following a bullying teasing incident, he ran after them and cornered a seven-year-old-child and brutally killed her. The special tragedy of the situation was that the youth's family had been complaining about his increasing talk of and actual aggression, and earlier incidents had not in the villagers' views been taken seriously, as the local learning disabled service felt that he was being discriminated against. As the local 'social work educator', I was invited to a community meeting to try to explain 'what are you teaching your social workers'. On behalf of the discipline, university and as a member of the community, I had to involve myself in the family's and community's grief. Of course, this case was different and is perhaps a self-justifying apology for not taking a more energetic position in the case of Stan. Conversely, the 'warning' signs of talk of and increased aggression should have had greater consideration, as the most potent indicator of subsequent serious violence is earlier violence (Craig and Hodson 2000; Solimon and Reza 2001; Ash *et al.* 2003; McNeil and Binder 2005; Monahan *et al.* 2005).

The unexpected 'emergency'

Most of my pro bono mental health practice is linked to the university. Although I had no 'statutory' mandate, there was a tacit agreement that, should I require emergency provision, then it would be speedily forthcoming. This was a back-up position as the university being an inner city campus had occasional 'psychiatric emergencies' and the Registrar would ring me and ask me to deal with them. I was always ambivalent and downright anxious because, like any statutory social worker going to an emergency, it was always an open-ended situation and one never knew what one was going to have to deal with. On the other hand, it starkly highlighted how tough the work is and it gave a degree of street credibility with the students.

Following a regular late evening at the university, I had arrived home and was having a well-deserved large glass of wine when summoned to the telephone at 9 p.m. It was a near neighbour and colleague from another faculty who wanted advice 'because you've had more dealings with the police than I have and I've read your CND book (Taylor and Pritchard 1982) and you are the only person I know who can give us some advice'.

It transpired that a longstanding German friend had arrived unexpectedly and he had an unusual story to tell 'and as I know you speak German (not true really), we'd be very grateful if it was convenient for you to pop round'.

I was intrigued, not particularly pleased, but it was easier to visit then as I was fully booked for the next three days, so I went.

I met 'Karl', aged 31, who to my great relief spoke excellent English and was continental politeness personified. He came from a small town in Bavaria from a middle-class Catholic family, although both his parents were now dead. He viewed the 'Smiths' as his English aunt and uncle and, although they had not seen him for a decade, all family birthdays and festivals were remembered through cards and the occasional letter. He was a graduate and, despite two engagements, was unmarried. He had completed his National Service although this was something of a culture shock for him. The only 'unusual' thing about him was that he was socialist, in a part of Germany that is traditionally nationalist and somewhat right wing.

We started our meeting with glasses of excellent dry white wine as Dr Smith explained that, that morning, Karl had telephoned to ask whether he could come over because he needed somewhere safe. He would not explain over the telephone but swore that he had not done anything wrong, or criminal, but if they would allow him to visit, he would explain everything. Dr Smith went on, 'when you hear his story, with your knowledge of the CND and its sequel, you'll see why Karl was keen to seek your advice'.

Leaving Karl and myself to speak alone, armed with a second large glass of white wine, we settled down to explore this unexpected situation.

'I will have to go back a few years so that you can understand my present angst. The problem began when I was in the Officer Training Corps and some of the cadet officers were singing Nazi songs.' This is illegal in Germany and he found it offensive. The other young men, a minority, bullied the rest of the class and threatened to beat him up if he complained. He did complain 'as a good socialist to help the majority who were not like them' but they were as good as their word and Karl was badly beaten. The 'authorities' hushed up the incident and he was transferred out. 'But I will always remember them as I left, they told me they would come back some day and kill me – Gott sei Dank – God be praised, there are not many like that in Germany but, like your skinheads and football hooligans, they exist everywhere.'

Throughout, he delivered his narrative in a calm restrained way, but looked understandably very anxious. I hardly intervened other than on the rare occasion to help him find the right English word, but responded appropriately to any hint of emotion.

He had not heard from the neo-Nazis for some time; although his green/socialist views were unfashionable in his locale, he believed that his known political position had blocked his promotion in the commerce job he had, and this coincided with a sense of purposelessness that made him turn to teaching following his last broken engagement.

'Teaching gave me a sense of purpose to life – I could work for the future.' He had considered the priesthood again, but felt he needed to test out his vocation and was confident 'that God will be patient with me' until Karl could be unequivocally 'sure of God's call'.

Over the past three or four months following a letter to his local paper supporting protests against the 'anti-asylum seekers', a number of disturbing incidents had occurred. This culminated in his precipitate flight from his small town when he recognised people following him, noises on his telephone and some of his students making extreme right-wing remarks and he began to 'fear for my life'. When trying to get help from the authorities, he recognised a number of policemen who had been following him and/or who were either sympathetic to or actually belonged to the neo-Nazis. Therefore, he had to seek asylum and where else but in his 'second home and second favourite country, England'.

At first, he had gone to friends in another part of Germany but, after three days, he suddenly realised that he had been traced because he recognised one of his pursuers. He suddenly knew that 'they meant business and they would kill him'. He came to England because he knows he is safe here and England has a wonderful reputation for being a safe country but 'I don't like being thought a coward but I am one against many', and he saw part of the problem was that the authorities were embarrassed about any exposure of neo-Nazi activity.

The dilemma was what was I facing, a legitimate 'refugee' or a delusional situation? Despite the hour, I had to explore further, while expressing every concern at the understandable fears that he had, I wondered whether there might be an alternative explanation and 'whether he had been ill recently'. It transpired that Karl had had a breakdown when he was 24 and again about four years previously. He had recovered from both periods of serious anxiety, depression and excitement, and he admitted that he 'feared being taken over'. He had psychiatric treatment, psychopharmacology and support counselling, but his greatest help had been his priest, who was also a personal friend. Apart from this, there was little follow-up, although his priest encouraged him to continue his prophylactic medication but, about six months ago, partly because of side-effects, he had stopped taking his tablets.

He believed that the side-effects were a result of the neo-Nazis recruiting his doctor and began to fear 'but hope it was not true' that his priest friend was also being used by them – 'but I don't think he knew he was being used'.

By this time, I felt fairly confident that I was dealing with a young man with an acute episode of persecutory ideas and that he required treatment as soon as possible. Moreover, he explained how he had 'recognised the neo-Nazi – I saw a priest following me, I went into a library and he came in. I did not know his face but he could not disguise his hands', and this was the clinching diagnostic factor associated with a particular variation of schizophrenia called Capgras' syndrome, which, you will remember, is manifested by delusions about identity and impostors.

There now began a long discussion about whether Karl could trust me and whether he would be willing to see a psychiatrist colleague in the morning. Of course, I had to consider whether I should immediately contact the emergency ASW but, while it was clear to me that he was ill, he did not appear to be a risk to anyone and, at present, he was managing to contain his psychosis; the drama of an emergency admission might well undermine his parlous stability – but treatment he needed and must have. Fortunately, Karl agreed, providing I would go with him 'for I trust the English' and, despite the pressures on the department, I was fairly confident that I could get a consultant to see him.

It was now quite late and I spoke about having a nightcap, in part to act as a sedative for Karl.

I suddenly remembered the importance of checking out the safety of all and asked him whether he had taken any practical precautions to protect himself from an attack.

He had, he had carried 'what you say for an axt?' and yes I said 'an axe we call it in English'.

Panic, not Karl, but the social worker!

'But Karl you couldn't bring this through Heathrow, it's illegal.' 'Yes you are right, I left it in the toilet in Bonn.' I heaved a sigh of relief, but he went on 'but when I got to London I found almost the same axe maker.' Panic again.

Three large glasses of wine were not a good preparation for such an unexpected emergency as I had difficulty in thinking through what needed to be done. Did the presence of the axe change anything?

I proceeded 'But Karl, in England we are not allowed to carry any arms. We have no guns, we do not carry knives and are certainly not allowed to carry an axe. Do you have it with you now?'

He had. He reached for his briefcase and without any qualms handed it to me, 'of course I should have remembered, your police are very good they do not have guns, only at the airport, so please will you take this for me, for of course I do not want to break the law'.

Thankfully I took and placed it in my bag.

I said we must call the Smiths soon but, to give me a little more time and further 'normalise' the situation, I asked him to tell me about his teaching methods as I also was a teacher.

As he spoke, I wracked my brains to determine what to do next. Self-evidently, if there had been any effort on his part to keep the axe, I would have called in the statutory services, but the situation remained calm. He needed treatment, felt safe and was safe. There was no suggestion that he had exhibited any previous signs of violence (the key predictor in the vast majority of situations); indeed, if there had been any suggestion that he had actually fought, I think I would have sought a section, but he had recovered his calm after a period of some distress when he was explaining his fear about his doctor and priest.

Also, the Capgras delusion/illusion had occurred three days after leaving his own town, so proving there was no stress or pressure upon him; thus I felt he was safe and not a threat. Moreover, while I had promised Karl confidentiality about the details from the Smiths and I would not wish to alarm them, lest it alarm Karl, I would quietly test out whether they were happy for Karl to be with them.

The Smiths returned and I explained, with Karl's approval, that he had been under a lot of stress recently, and that he agreed with me that it would be best if he saw a doctor colleague of mine. The Smiths did not express any surprise and said 'I think that's wise Karl, for obviously some odd things have been happening to you, so if you can get you some help you ought to take advantage of it'.

So it was agreed and, to reinforce the normality of the situation, I accepted our host's offer of malt whisky, which I explained to Karl was a speciality and that, with Dr Smith's approval he might try two to show how varied malts could be. Dr Smith could not have been more accommodating and, though I knew I probably would not sleep, felt that Karl, safe in the bosom of the Smith household, would sleep soundly.

Was this the right decision?

I hope so; I think that, because I could take time and not be rushed about thinking of the next emergency, Karl could receive an appropriate mental health social work service, while acknowledging he was ill as per the Mental Health Act and did not need a place of safety, nor did his civil rights require any restriction for his or other people's safety.

What do you think?

I have taught from Karl's case and must confess that some psychiatrists think I should have admitted Karl; however about three in four think that Karl was treated appropriately. Indeed, the following day, he saw a psychiatrist who recommenced psychotropic drugs. He stayed a further two weeks with the Smiths and then was escorted back to Germany and met by colleagues, who also continued to treat him in the community.

This was one psychiatric emergency I would never forget.

As we draw to a close our pursuit of an evidence-based mental health social work, it must be admitted that you have been exposed to a considerable amount of varied information and approaches. It is hoped that, above all, working with distressed, disturbed and damaged people who have experienced a mental disorder is both feasible and can be very rewarding. If we can identify the client's key needs, the core stressors, and offer an appropriate bio-psychosocial integrated approach, we can bring considerable relief to them and enhance their repossession of their lives.

It is readily admitted that there are no grand, absolute answers, although we would all like to think there were. But the stimulus, yes and the joy, of working in this field, where truly, every person is different; we go on learning from them about other human beings, our society and about ourselves.

The controversy about mental disorder is likely to continue as these syndromes, of mood or psychotic disorders, become better understood; like the history surrounding 'autism', I suspect we will find that some conditions are largely biochemical but stress precipitated. Others will be largely psychosocial in origin but perhaps influenced by the person's biology. But above all, the effort to understand apparent disorders of the human mind will teach us to value that human capacity for thought and evaluation, which at its best brings together the art and science of mental health social work and all the disciplines concerned with the human condition.

Like medicine, mental health social work cures seldom, can improve often, but should comfort always. And in this union of mental health social work art and science, we can be confident that more is to be learned and be excited not downhearted by the fact that:

The old order changeth, yielding place to new. . .
Lest one good custom should corrupt the world.
                    (Tennyson, *The Passing of Arthur*)

so that we follow Francis Bacon when he says that 'If a man will begin with certainties, he shall end in doubts; but if he will be content to begin with doubts, he shall end in certainties.'

Finally, whenever the next grand theory comes along to 'explain' human behaviour, if it cannot be found reflected in the great poets and playwrights, then it is probably not all that important.

Go well.

Bibliography

Abdel-Khalek A and Lester D (2002) Can personality predict suicide? A study in two cultures. *International Journal of Social Psychiatry* 48: 231–9.

Abel KM, Webb RT and Appleby L (2005) Prevalence and predictors of parenting outcomes in a cohort of mothers with schizophrenia admitted for joint mother and baby psychiatric care in England. *Journal of Clinical Psychiatry* 66: 808–9.

Aber JL, Bennett NG, Conley DC and Li J (1997) The effects of poverty on child health and development. *Annual Review of Public Health* 18: 463–83.

Abraham J (2002) Trans-national industrial power, the medical profession and the regulatory state: adverse drug reactions and crisis over safety of Halcion in the Netherlands and the UK. *Social Science Medicine* 55: 1671–90.

Agbayewa MO, Marion SA and Wiggins S (1998) Socioeconomic factors associated with suicide in elderly populations. *Canadian Journal of Psychiatry* 43: 829–36.

Agerbo E, Nordentoft M and Mortensen PB (2003) Familial psychiatric and socioeconomic risk factors for suicide in young people: nest case–control study. *Evidence Based Mental Health* 6: 61–6.

Agid O, Shapira B and Lerer B (1999) Environment and vulnerability to major psychiatric illness: a case–control study of early parental loss in major depression, bipolar disorder and schizophrenia. *Molecular Psychiatry* 4: 163–72.

Agosti U, Nunes E and Levin F (2002) Rates of psychiatric co-morbidity amongst USA residents with a lifetime cannabis dependency. *American Journal Drug Alcohol Abuse* 28: 643–52.

Aihara H and Iki M (2002) Effects of socioeconomic factors on suicide from 1980 through 1999 in Osaka, Japan. *Journal of Epidemiology* 12: 439–49.

Al-Lamki (2000) Munchausen syndrome by proxy. *Saudi Medical Journal* 21: 482–6.

Andreasson S, Allebeck P and Rydberg U (1990) Schizophrenia in users and non-users of cannabis: longitudinal study in Stockholm county. *Acta Psychiatrica Scandinavica* 77: 454–6.

Angst J, Gamma A and Zhang H (2003) Recurrence of bipolar disorders and major depression: a life-long perspective. *European Archives of Psychiatry and Clinical Neurosciences* 253: 236–40.

Aoun S and Johnson L (2001) A consumer's perspective of a suicide intervention programme. *Australian and New Zealand Mental Health Nursing* 10: 97–104.

Appleby L (1997) *National Confidential Inquiry into Suicide and Homicide by People with Mental Illness*. London: Department of Health.

Appleby L, Shaw T, Amos T and Parsons R (1999) Suicide within 12 months of contact with mental health services. *British Medical Journal* 318: 1235–9.

Arendt M and Munk-Jorgensen P (2004) Heavy cannabis users seeking treatment – prevalence of psychiatric disorders. *Social Psychiatry and Psychiatric Epidemiology* 39: 97–105.

Arias B, Rosa A and Fanas LM (2002) Human genetic variation and mental disorder. *Neurotoxology Research* 4: 523–30.

Armstrong KL, Fraser JA, Dodds MR and Morris J (2000) Promoting secure attachment and maternal mood and child health in a vulnerable population: a randomised control trial. *Journal of Paediatrics and Child Health* 36: 555–62.

Ash D, Galletly C and Braben P (2003) Violence, self-harm, victimisation and homelessness in patients admitted to an acute inpatient unit in South Australia. *International Journal of Social Psychiatry* 49: 112–18.

ASWIG (2000) Approved Social Worker Interest Group. *Response to the Reform of the Mental Health Act 1983.* www.aswig.uk

Audit Commission (1996) *Misspent Youth: Youth Crime and the Criminal Justice System.* London: HMSO.

Audit Commission (1998) *Misspent Youth Re-Visited* London: HMSO.

Audit Commission (2004) *All Our Lives: Social Care in England and Wales 2002–03.* London: HMSO.

Baethge C, Grischka P, Smolka MN and Bauer M (2003) Effectiveness and outcome predictors in long-term lithium prophylaxis in unipolar major depressive disorder. *Journal of Psychiatric Neurosciences* 28: 355–61.

Bagley C and Ramsay R (1997) *Suicidal Behaviour in Adolescents and Adults: Research, Taxonomy and Prevention.* Aldershot: Ashgate.

Bagley C, Wood M and Young L (1994) Victim to abuser: mental health and behavioural sequels of the sexual abuse of males in childhood. *Child Abuse and Neglect* 18: 685–97.

Bahlmann M, Preuss UW and Soyka M (2002) Chronological relationship between personality disorder and alcohol dependence. *European Addiction Research* 8: 195–200.

Baker L (1997) *Homelessness and Suicide.* London: Shelter.

Baldwin DS (2000) Clinical experience with paroxetine in social anxiety disorder. *International Clinical Psychopharmacology* 15 (Suppl.): 19–24.

Baldwin DS (2004) Sexual dysfunction and antidepressants. *Journal of Psychopharmacology* 18 (Suppl.): A5.

Baldwin DS and Birtwhistle J (2002) *Depression: An Illustrated History.* Oxford: Blackwell Science.

Baldwin DS and Mayers A (2003) Sexual side-effects of antidepressant and anti-psychotic drugs. *Advances in Psychiatric Treatment* 9: 202–10.

Ball J, Kearney B, Wilhelm K and Barton B (2000) Cognitive behaviour therapy and assertion training groups for patients with depression and co-morbid personality disorders. *Behavioural Cognitive Therapy* 28: 71–85.

Banerjee S, Roy P and Nandi DN (2000) Psychiatric morbidity in a rural Indian community: changes over a 20 year interval. *British Journal of Psychiatry* 176: 351–6.

Banks P (1998) *Carer Support: Time for a Change?* London: King's Fund Cares Impact.

Barker DJP (2001) The malnourished baby and infant. *British Medical Bulletin* 60: 69–88.

Barker DJP, Ericksson JG, Forsen T and Osmond C (2002) The fetal origin of adult disease: strengths of effects and biological basis. *International Journal of Epidemiology* 31: 1235–9.

Barker P, Keady J, Croom S and Reynolds B (1998) The concept of 'serious mental illness': modern myths and grim realities. *Journal of Psychiatric and Mental Health Nursing* 5: 247–54.

Barnes M (2000) Users' views of mental health services. In Bilay D (ed.) *At the Core of Mental Health.* London: Pavilion, 363–85.

Barraclough B and Shepherd DM (1976) Birthday blues: the association of birthday with self-inflected death in the elderly. *Acta Psychiatrica Scandinavica* 54: 146–9.

Barraclough B and Shepherd D (1977) Public interest and private grief. *British Journal of Psychiatry* 131: 400–4.

Barraclough C, Haddock G, Lewis S and McGovern JM (2001) Randomised controlled trial of motivational interviewing, cognitive behaviour therapy and family intervention for patients with co-morbid schizophrenia and substance abuse. *American Journal of Psychiatry* 158: 1706–13.

Barrick TR, Mackay CE and Crow TJ (2005) Automatic analysis of cerebral asymmetry: an exploratory study of the relationship between brain torque and planum temporal asymmetry. *Neuroimaging* 24: 678–91.

Barrickman L (2003) AACAP guidelines on disruptive behavioural disorders. *Paediatric Clinics of North America* 50: 1000–17.

Bassuk EL, Mickelson K, Bissell HD and Perloff J (2002) Role of kin and non-kin support in mental health of low income women. *American Journal of Orthopsychiatry* 72: 39–49.

Battaglia M and Ogliari A (2005) Anxiety, panic attack: from human studies to animal research and back. *Neuroscience and Biobehaviour Review* 29: 169–79.

Bazire S (2001) *Psychotropic Drug Directory.* Salisbury: Quay Books.

BBC (2000) *News On-Line* 20 July 2000. *Officials back compulsory treatment orders.* London: BBC.

Bean P and Mounser P (1994) The community treatment order: proposals and prospects. *Journal of Social Policy* 23: 19–24.

Beautrais AL, Conner KR and Conwell Y (2003) Risk factors for suicide and medically serious suicide attempts among alcoholics: analysis of Canterbury Suicide Project. *Journal for the Study of Alcohol* 64: 551–4.

Beck A (1976) *The Prediction of Suicide.* Bowrie, MD: Charles Press.

Beck AT (1988) *Cognitive Therapy and Depression.* Chichester: Wiley.

Beck AT, Rush A, Shaw B and Emery G (1979) *Cognitive Therapy of Depression.* New York: Guilford Press.

Beck AT, Steer RA and Garrison B (1985) Hopelessness and eventual suicide: a ten-year prospective study of hospitalised patients with suicidal ideation. *American Journal of Psychiatry* 142: 559–63.

Beck AT, Steer RA, Beck JS and Newman CF (1993a) Hopelessness, depression, suicidal ideation and clinical diagnosis of depression. *Suicide and Life Threatening Behaviour* 23: 139–45.

Beck AT, Steer R and Brown G (1993b) *Cognitive Therapy of Substance Abuse.* New York: Guilford Press.

Beckett R, Beech A, Ford D and Fordham AS (1994) *Community-based Treatment Programmes for Sex Offenders: Evaluation of 7 Programmes.* London: Home Office.

Bellino S, Patria I and Bogelle E (2005) Major depression in patients with personality disorder: a clinical investigation. *Canadian Journal of Psychiatry* 50: 234–8.

Bender DS, Dolan RT, Skodol AE and Gunderson JS (2001) Treatment utilisation by patients with personality disorders. *American Journal of Psychiatry* 158: 295–302.

Bentall RP (1990) The illusion of reality: a review and integration of psychological research on hallucinations. *Psychological Bulletin* 107: 82–95.

Bentall R (1995) *Reconstructing Schizophrenia.* London: Routledge.

Bentall R (2003) *Madness Explained: Psychosis and Human Nature.* London: Allen.

Bentall RP, Claridge G and Slade DP (1989) The multi-dimensional nature of schizotypal traits: a factor analysis study with normal subjects. *British Journal of Clinical Psychology* 28: 363–78.

Bentall RP, Barker GA and Havers S (1991) Reality monitoring and psychotic hallucination. *British Journal of Clinical Psychology* 30: 213–22.

Berard RM (2001) Depression and anxiety in oncology: the psychiatrist's perspective. *Journal of Clinical Psychiatry* 62: 58–61.

Bergen HA, Martin G and Roeger L (2003) Sexual abuse and suicidal behaviour: a model constructed from a large community sample. *Journal of the American Academy of Child and Adolescent Psychiatry* 42: 1301–9.

Berger N (2004) Cannabis and schizophrenia. *Revue Médécine Liege* 59: 98–103

Berry L (2002) *The New Social Work: Perspectives from the General Social Care Council.* Annual Social Work Lecture, University of Southampton.

Bhui K, Brown P and Hardie T (1998) African-Caribbean men remanded in Brixton prison. Psychiatric and forensic characteristics and final outcome of court appearance. *British Journal of Psychiatry* 172: 337–44.

Bhui K, Stansfield S, Hull S and Feder G (2003) Inequalities of service to ethnic minorities. *British Journal of Psychiatry* 182: 105–16.

Bhui K, Stansfield S and Weich S (2005) Racial/ethnic discrimination and common mental disorders among workers: findings from the EMPIRIC study of ethnic minority groups in the UK. *American Journal of Public Health* 95: 496–501.

Bhurga D (1996) *Homelessness and Mental Illness.* Chichester: Wiley.

Bhurga D, Thompson N, Singh J and Fellow-Smith E (2003) Inception of deliberate self-harm in adolescents in West London. *International Journal of Social Psychiatry* 49: 247–50.

Bierer LM, Yehuda R and Siever LJ (2003) Abuse and neglect in childhood: relationship to personality disorder diagnosis. *CNS Spectrum* 8: 737–54.

Bindman J, Maingay S and Szmukler G (2003) The Human Rights Act and mental health legislation. *British Medical Journal* 182: 91–4.

Biondi M and Picardi A (2005) Increased maintenance of OCD remission after integrated serotonergic treatment and CBT compared with medication alone. *Psychotherapy Psychosomatic* 74: 123–8.

Bird L and Faulkener A (2000) *Suicide and Self Harm.* London: Mental Health Foundation.

Bird SM and Hutchinson SJ (2003) Male drugs-related deaths in a fortnight after release from prison: Scotland 1996–99. *Addiction* 98: 185–90.

Birtchnell J (1970) Psychiatric sequel to childhood bereavement. *British Journal of Psychiatry* 116: 572–5.

Birtchnell J (1981) In search of correspondence between age of psychiatric breakdown and parental age at death. Anniversary reactions. *British Journal of Medical Psychology* 54: 111–20.

Blakely TA, Collings SC and Atkinson J (2003) Unemployment and suicide. Evidence for a causal association? *Journal of Epidemiological Community Health* 57: 594–600.

Bodmer WF and McKie R (2000) *The Book of Man: The Quest to Discover our Genetic Heritage.* Oxford: Oxford University Press.

den Boer JR and Slaap SL (1998) Review of current treatment of panic disorders. *International Clinical Psychopharmacology* 13: 35–40.

Bohus M, Haaf B and Linehan MM (2000) Evaluation of in-patient dialectic behavioural therapy for borderline personality disorders: a prospective study. *Behaviour Research and Therapy* 38: 875–87.

Bolar JR and Mosher LR (2003) Treatment of acute psychosis without neuroleptics: two-year outcomes from the Soteria project. *Journal of Nervous and Mental Disorders* 191: 219–29.

Bollini P, Pampallona S, Orza MJ and Chalmers TC (1994) Anti-psychotic drugs: is more worse? A meta-analysis of the published RCTs. *Psychological Medicine* 24: 307–16.

Bools C, Neale B and Meadows R (1993) A follow-up of victims of fabricated illness (Munchausen syndrome by proxy). *Archives of Diseases of Children* 69: 625–30.

Bosinski HA (2003) Transsexual gender identity disorder: diagnostic and legal issues. *Urology* 42: 709–19.

Botnick MR, Heath KV, Cornelisse P and Hogg RS (2002) Correlates of suicide attempts in an open cohort of young men who have sex with men. *Canadian Journal of Public Health* 93: 59–62.

Bottomley A (1998) Depression in cancer and HIV infection: research findings and implications for effective antidepressant treatment. *European Journal of Cancer Care* 7: 181–91.

Bourgeois ML and Benezech M (2001) Criminal dangerousness, psychopathology and psychiatric co-morbidity. *Annales Medico-Psychologiques* 159: 475–86.

Bourget D and Labelle A (1992) Homicide, infanticide and filicide. *Psychiatric Clinics of North America* 15: 661–73.

Boydell J, Van Os J, Lambri M and Murray RM (2003) Incidence of schizophrenia in south-east London between 1965 and 1997. *British Journal of Psychiatry* 182: 45–9.

Bragin V, Chemodanova M and Aliev G (2005) Integrated treatment approach improves cognitive function in demented and clinically depressed patients. *American Journal of Alzheimer's Disorder and Other Dementias* 20: 21–6.

Breen N, Caine D and Coltheart M (2000) Models of face recognition and delusional misidentification: a review. *Cognitive Neuropsychology* 17: 55–71.

Breslau J, Kendler KS and Kessler RC (2005) Lifetime risk and persistence of psychiatric disorder across ethnic groups in the USA. *Psychological Medicine* 35: 317–27.

Bride BE and Real E (2003) Project assistance: a modified treatment community for homeless women living with HIV/AIDS and substance abuse. *Health and Social Work* 28: 166–8.

Brody JF (2001) Evolutionary recasting: ADHD, mania and its variants. *Journal of Affective Disorder* 65: 197–215.

Brotman LM, Klein RG, Kamboukos D and Sosinsky LS (2003) Preventive intervention for urban, low-income pre-schoolers at familial risk for conduct problems: a randomised pilot study. *Journal of Clinical Child Adolescent Psychology* 32: 246–57.

Brown GT, Day T, Henriques GR and Beck AT (2005) Cognitive therapy for preventing suicide attempts: a random controlled trial. *Journal of the American Medical Association* 294: 623–4.

Browne GW (1987) Social factors and the development and cause of depression in women. *British Journal of Social Work* Special Suppl.: 615–34.

Browne GW (2002) Social roles, context and evolution in the origins of depression. *Journal of Health and Social Behaviour* 43: 255–76.

Browne GW, Andrews B, Bifulco A and Veiel H (1990) Self-esteem and depression. *Social Psychiatry and Psychiatric Epidemiology* 25: 200–49.

Browne GW, Beck AT, Steer RA and Grisham JR (2000) Risk factors for suicide in psychiatric outpatients: a 20 year prospective study. *Journal of Consulting Clinical Psychology* 68: 371–7.

Brugha TS, Bebbington PE, Stretch T and Wykes J (1997) Predicting the short-term outcome of 1st episode and reoccurrence of clinical depression: a prospective study of life events and social support. *Journal of Clinical Psychiatry* 58: 298–300.

Brugha T, Jenkins R and Farrell M (2004) Risk factors and the prevalence of neurosis in ethnic groups in Great Britain. *Social Psychiatry and Psychiatric Epidemiology* 39: 939–46.

Brune M (2002) Toward an integration of interpersonal and biological processes. Evolutionary psychiatry as an empirically testable framework. *Psychiatry* 65: 48–57.

Bryson B (2003) *A History of Virtually Everything.* London: Penguin.

Buchanan N (1996) The use of Imolegrine in juvenile myoclonic epilepsy. *Seizure* 5: 49–51.

Burrows R (1997) *Homelessness and Social Policy.* London: Routledge.

Burton R (1590) *The Anatom of Melancholy.* Reprinted 1934. Oxford: Oxford University Press.

Buss D (2003) *Evolutionary Psychology: New Science of the Mind.* London: Allyn and Bacon.

Bustillo J, Lauriello J and Keith S (2001) The psychosocial treatment of schizophrenia: an update. *American Journal of Psychiatry* 158:163–75.

Butler A and Pritchard C (1986) *Mental Health Social Work.* London: Macmillan.

Bynner J, Elias P, McNight A, Pan H and Pierrre G (2002) *Young People's Changing Routes to Independence.* York: York Publishing.

Cahill J, Barker HM, Hardy G and Macaskill N (2003) Outcomes of patients completing and not completing cognitive therapy for depression. *British Journal of Clinical Psychology* 42: 133–43.

Cain ACC (2002) Children of suicide: the telling and the knowing? *Psychiatry* 65: 124–36.

Cairney J, Boyle M, Offord DR and Racine Y (2003) Stress, social support and depression in single and married mothers. *Social Psychiatry and Epidemiology* 38: 442–9.

Calfee JE (2000) The increasing necessity for market based pharmaceutical prices. *Pharmacoeconomics* 18: 47–57.

Cannon TD, Rosso IM, Hollister JM and Hadley T (2000) A prospective cohort study of genetic and perinatal influences in the aetiology of schizophrenia. *Schizophrenia Bulletin* 26: 351–66.

Cantor CH, Leenaars AA and Lester D (1997) Under-reporting of suicide in Ireland 1960–89. *Archives of Suicide Research* 3: 5–12.

Canvin K, Bartlett A and Pinfold V (2002) A 'bittersweet pill to swallow': learning from mental health services users' response to compulsory community care in England. *Health and Social Care in the Community* 10: 361–9.

Capp HB, Thyer BA and Bordnicks PS (1997) Evaluating improvement over the course of adult psychiatric hospitalisation. *Social Work and Health Care* 25: 55–66.

Cardno AG, Marshall EJ, Cold B and Murray RM (1999) Heritability estimates for psychiatric disorders: the Maudsley Twin psychosis series. *Archives of General Psychiatry* 56: 162–8.

Carpenter D and Brockington MI (1980) Study of mental illness of Asians, West Indians and Africans living in Manchester. *British Journal of Psychiatry* 137: 201–11.

Carr JA, Honey CR, Sinden M and Martzke JS (2003) A waitlist control-group study of cognitive, mood and quality of life after post-ventral pallidotomy in Parkinson's disease. *Journal of Neurosurgery* 99: 78–88.

Carter JW, Schulsinger F, Parnas J and Mednick SA (2002) A multivariate prediction model of schizophrenia. *Schizophrenia Bulletin* 28: 649–82.

Catty J, Burns T and Comas A (2001) Day centres for severe mental illness. *Cochrane Database Systematic Review* 2: CD0001710.

Cavanagh JT, Carson AJ, Sharpe M and Lawrie SM (2003) Psychological autopsy studies of suicide: a systematic review. *Psychological Medicine* 33: 395–405.

Cedereke M, Monti K and Ojehagen A (2002) Telephone contact with patients in the year after a suicide attempt: a randomised controlled study. *European Psychiatry* 17: 82–91.

Cerel J, Fristad MA and Weller RA (2000) Suicide-bereaved children and adolescents. II. Parental and family functioning. *Journal of the American Academy of Child and Adolescent Psychiatry* 39: 437–44.

Chance SA, Esiri MM and Crow TJ (2005) Macroscopic brain asymmetry is changed along the anterior–posterior axis in schizophrenia. *Schizophrenia Research* 74: 163–70.

Cheasty M, Clare AW and Collins C (1998) Relation between sexual abuse in childhood and adult depression: a case–control study. *British Medical Journal* 316: 198–201.

Chentsova-Dutton Y, Shortter S and Zisook S (2002) Depression and grief reaction in hospice caregivers pre death and 1 year afterwards. *Journal of Affective Disorders* 69: 380–97.

Chew-Graham CA, Mullin S, May CR and Cole H (2002) Managing depression in primary care: another example of the inverse care law? *Family Practitioner* 19: 632–7.

Chiesa M and Fonagy P (2003) Treatment for severe personality disorder: 36 month follow-up. *British Journal of Psychiatry* 183: 356–62.

Chiesa M, Bateman A and Friis S (2002) Patient characteristics, outcomes and costs of hospital-based treatment for people with personality disorders: comparing 3 different programmes. *Psychology and Psychotherapy* 75: 381–91.

Chilvers R, McDonald GM and Hayes AA (2002) Supported housing for people with severe mental disorder. *Cochrane Database Systematic Review* 4: CD000487.

Chioqueta AP and Stiles TC (2003) Suicide risk in outpatients with specific mood and anxiety disorders. *Crisis* 24: 105–12.

Cinnirella M and Loewenthal KM (1999) Religious and ethnic group influences on beliefs about mental illness: a qualitative interview study. *British Journal of Medical Psychology* 72: 505–24.

Clare A (1977) *Psychiatry in Dissent* London: Tavistock.

Claridge G, McCreey C, Bentall R and Popplewell D (1996) The factor structure of 'schyzotype' traits: a large replication study. *British Journal of Clinical Psychology* 35: 103–15.

Clark DM, Ehlers A, McManus F and Louis B (2003) Cognitive therapy versus fluoxetine in generalised social phobia: a randomised placebo-controlled trial. *Journal of Consulting Clinical Psychology* 71: 1058–67.

Clark LA, Vittengl JR, Kraft I and Jarrett RD (2003) Shared components of personality and psychosocial features predict depression after acute-phase cognitive therapy. *Journal of Personality Disorder* 17: 406–30.

Claus C and Lindberg L (1999) Serial murder as a 'Schahriar syndrome'. *Journal of Forensic Psychiatry* 10: 427–35.

Coffey C, Veit F, Wolfe R and Patton GC (2003) Mortality in young offenders: retrospective cohort study. *British Medical Journal* 326: 1064.

Coid J (1983) The epidemiology of abnormal homicide and murder followed by suicide. *Psychological Medicine* 13: 855–60.

Coid J, Kahtan N and Gault S (2000) Ethnic differences in admissions to secure forensic psychiatry services. *British Journal of Psychiatry* 177: 241–7.

Coid J, Petruckevitch A, Bebington P and Singleton W (2002a) Ethnicity differences in prison. *British Journal of Psychiatry* 181: 477–80.

Coid J, Petruckevitch A, Bebington P and Singleton W (2002b) Ethnic differences in prisoners: risk factors and psychiatric service use. *British Journal of Psychiatry* 181: 481–7.

Colom F, Vieta E, Reinares M and Gastro C (2003) Psycho-education efficacy in bipolar disorders: beyond compliance enhancement. *Journal of Clinical Psychiatry* 64: 1101–5.

Compton SN, Burns BJ, Helen LE and Robertson E (2002) Review of the evidence base for treatment of childhood psychopathology: internalising disorders. *Journal of Consulting Clinical Psychology* 70: 1240–66.

Conner KR, Beautrais AL and Conwell Y (2003) Risk factors for suicide and medically serious suicide attempts amongst alcoholics: analysis of Canterbury Suicide Project data. *Journal for the Study of Alcohol* 64: 551–4.

Cook EH (2001) Genetics of autism. *Child and Adolescent Psychiatry Clinics of North America* 10: 333–50.

Cope R (1989) The compulsory detention of African-Caribbeans under the Mental Health Act. *New Community* 15: 343–56.

Corby B (2000) Child abuse: towards a knowledge base. Buckingham: Open University Press.

Corre PG (2002) Is NICE being nice to patients with digestive cancers? *Gastrointestinal Oncology* 4: 1–4.

Corrigan PW, Watson AC and Hall LL (2005) Newspaper stories as measures of structural stigma. *Psychiatric Services* 56: 551–6.

Coulter A (1999) Sharing decisions with patients: is the information good enough? *British Medical Journal* 318: 22.

Coxe R and Holmes W (2001) A study of child abuse amongst child molesters. *Journal of Child Sexual Abuse* 10: 111–18.

Coyne JC, Thompson R and Pepper CM (2004) Role of life events in depression in primary medical versus psychiatric settings. *Journal of Affective Disorders* 82: 353–6.

Craig DE, Judd F and Hodgins G (2004) Therapeutic group programme for women with post-natal depression in rural Victoria. *Australasian Psychiatry* 13: 291–5.

Craig TK and Hodson S (2000) Homeless youth in London. 2. Accommodation, employment and health outcomes after one year. *Psychological Medicine* 30: 187–92.

Craig T (1995) *The Homeless Mentally Ill Initiative: An Evaluation of Four Clinical Teams*. London: Department of Health.

Craig TKJ (1996) *Off to a Bad Start: A Longitudinal Study of Homeless Young People in London*. London: Mental Health Foundation.

Craighead WE and Miklowitz DJ (2000) Psychosocial interventions for bipolar disorder. *Journal of Clinical Psychiatry* 13: 58–64.

Crow TJ (1997) Is schizophrenia the price homo sapiens pays for language? *Schizophrenia Research* 28: 127–41.

Curtin F and Schulz P (2004) Clonazepam and lorazepam in acute mania: a Bayesian meta-analysis. *Journal of Affective Disorders* 78: 201–8.

Cypriano LV, Rocha FDM and Souza GFJ (2000) Folie à deux: a clinical case record. *Psiquiatria Biológica* 8: 89–94.

D'Arcy PE (1998) Drug reactions and interactions: safety measures of the Drug Safety Committee of UK. *Journal of Pharmacology* 54: 44–7.

David AS and Cutting JC (eds) (1994) *The Neuro-psychology of Schizophrenia*. Hove: Lawrence Erlbaum.

Davidson D (2000) Managing Community Care. *Journal for Social Care, Health and Housing* 8: 32–4.

Davies J (1995) *Report of the Inquiry into the Circumstances leading to the death of Jonathan Newby.* Oxford: Oxford Health Authority.

Dazzan P and Bhugra D (2001) Use of Mental Health Act criteria in the decision-making process of compulsory admissions: a study of psychiatrists in South London. *Medicine in Social Science* 40: 336–44.

De Fauw N and Andriessen K (2003) Networking to support suicide survivors. *Crisis* 24: 29–31.

De Leo D, Conforti D and Carollo G (1997) A century of suicide in Italy: a comparison between old and young. *Suicide and Life Threatening Behaviour* 27: 239–49.

Dekovic M, Janssens JM and Van As AN (2003) Family predictors of antisocial behaviour in adolescence. *Family Process* 42: 223–35.

Delisi LE, Shaw S, Sherrington R and Crow TJ (2000) Failure to establish linkage on the X chromosome in 301 families with schizophrenia or schizoaffective disorders. *American Journal of Medical Genetics and Neuropsychiatric Genetics* 96: 335–41.

Democratic Health Network (1999) *Reform of the Mental Health Act: Government Proposals for Consultation.* 29 November 1999.

Department of Health (1992) *Report of the Michael Rooney Inquiry.* London: HMSO.

Department of Health (1995) *Child Protection: Messages from Research Studies in Child Protection.* London: HMSO.

Department of Health (1998) *Modernising Mental Health Services – Safe, Sound and Supportive.* London: Department of Health.

Department of Health (1999a) *Safer Services: Response to National Confidential Inquiry into Suicide and Homicide by People with Mental Illness.* London: Department of Health.

Department of Health (1999b) *Report of the Expert Committee: Review of The Mental Health Act 1983.* London: Department of Health.

Department of Health (2001) *Safety First: A five-year report of the National Confidential Inquiry into Suicide and Homicide by People with Mental Illness.* London: Department of Health.

Department of Health (2002) *Health and Personal Social Service Statistics.* London Department of Health Statistical Publications.

Desai RA, Liu-Mares W and Rosenheck RA (2003) Suicidal ideation and suicide attempts in a sample of homeless people with mental illness. *Journal of Nervous Mental Diseases* 191: 365–71.

Devrimci-Ozguven H and Sayil I (2003) Suicide attempts in Turkey: results of the WHO-EURO multi-centre study on suicidal behaviour. *Canadian Journal of Psychiatry* 48: 324–8.

Di Clemente CC, Carroll K, Miller WM and Donovan J (2002) A look inside treatment: therapeutic effects and treatment alliance. In Babor T and De Boca FK (eds) *Treatment Matching in Alcoholism.* Cambridge: Cambridge University Press, 215–35.

Diaz R (2000) *Mental Health and Homelessness.* London: Shelter.

Dinan TG (1997) *Biology of Mental Disorders.* London: Science Press.

Dobson F (1999) The Mental Health Act. *Community Care* 1293: 16.

Drake RE, Price JL and Drake ED (1996) *Dual Diagnosis of Major Mental Illnesses and Substance Misuse: New Directions for Mental Health Services.* San Francisco: Jossey-Bass.

Drake RE, Xie H and Shumway M (2004) Three-year outcomes of long-term patients with co-occurring bipolar and substance use disorders. *Biological Psychiatry* 56: 749–56.

Draper B and Anstey K (1996) Psychosocial stressors, physical illness and the spectrum of depression in elderly patients. *Australian and New Zealand Journal of Psychiatry* 30: 567–72.

Duckworth G and McBride H (1996) Suicide in old age: a tragedy of neglect. *Canadian Journal of Psychiatry* 41: 217–22.

Dugas MJ, Ladouceur R, Leger E and Boisvert JM (2003) Group CBT for generalised anxiety disorder: treatment outcome and long-term follow-up. *Journal of Clinical Consulting Psychology* 71: 821–5.

Duran-Tauleria DT, Rona PS, Chinn S and Burney P (1996) Influence of ethnic group on asthma history in children 1990–91: a cross-national survey study. *British Medical Journal* 313: 145–52.

Durkheim E (1868) *Le Suicide*. Translated by Spaudling JA and Simpson C 1952. London: Routledge.

Durressen A and Jorswieck R (1962) Towards a correction of Eysenck's report on psychoanalytical treatment results. *Acta Psychotherapia* 10: 329–42.

Duwe BV and Turetsky BI (2002) Misdiagnosis of schizophrenia in a patient with psychotic symptoms. *Neuropsychiatry, Neuropsychology and Behavioural Neurology* 15: 252–60.

Dyke DG, Hendryx MS, Short RA and McFarlane WR (2003) Service use amongst patients with schizophrenia in psycho-educational multiple-family group treatment. *Psychiatric Services* 53: 749–54.

Dyregrov K, Nordranger D and Dyregrov A (2003) Predictors of psychosocial distress after suicide, SIDS and accidents. *Death Studies* 27: 143–65.

Eaton WW and Harrison G (2000) Ethnic disadvantages and schizophrenia. *Acta Psychiatrica Scandinavica* 102 (Suppl. 47): 1–6.

Ebstein RF, Benjamin J and Belmaker RH (2000) Genetics of personality dimensions. *Current Opinion in Psychiatry* 13: 617–22.

Eckert LO, Sugar N and Fine D (2002) Characteristics of sexual assault in women with a major psychiatric diagnosis. *American Journal of Obstetrics and Gynecology* 186: 1284–8.

Edelstyn NMJ and Oybode F (1999) A review of the phenomenology and cognitive neuropsychological origins of the Capgras syndrome. *International Journal of Geriatric Psychiatry* 14: 48–9.

Ehlers A, Clark DM, Hackmann H and Mayou R (2003) A random controlled trial of cognitive therapy, self-help booklet and repeated assessments as early intervention for PTSD. *Archives of General Psychiatry* 60: 1024–32.

Elliott J and Denny P (2002a) Access to life-savings drugs. *New Statesman,* 7 November.

Elliott L and Denny P (2002b) US blocks cheap drug deal *Guardian*, 21 December.

Ellis HD and Lewis MB (2001) Capgras delusion: a window on face recognition. *Trends Cognitive Sciences* 5: 149-156

Enoch MA and Goldman D (2002) Problem drinking and alcoholism: diagnosis and treatment. *American Family Physician* 65: 441–50.

Ensminger ME, Hanson SG and Juon HS (2003) Maternal psychological distress: sons' and daughters' mental health and educational attainment. *Journal of the American Academy of Child and Adolescent Psychiatry* 42: 1108–15.

Evans BT and Pritchard C (2000) Cancer survival rates and GDP expenditure on health: a comparison of the USA with Denmark, Finland, France, Germany, Italy, Netherlands, Spain and Switzerland. *Public Health* 114: 336–9.

Evans DB, Tandon A, Murray CJ and Lauer JA (2001) Comparative efficiency of national health systems: cross-national economic analysis. *British Medical Journal* 323: 307–10.

Eynan R, Langley T, Tolomiczenko G and Goering P (2002) The association between homelessness and suicidal ideation and behaviour: results of a cross-sectional survey. *Suicide and Life Threatening Behaviour* 32: 418–27.

Eysenck HJ (1953) The effects of psychotherapy: an evaluation. *Journal of Consulting Psychology* 16: 38–44.

Eysenck HJ (1964) The effects of psychotherapy reconsidered. *Forschung Psychosomatik Medizin* 12: 38–44.

Fabrega H (2001) Cultural psychiatry: international perspectives. *Psychiatric Clinics of North America* 24: 595–608.

Falkov A (1996) *Study of Working Together. Part 8. Reports of Fatal Abuse and Parental Psychiatric Disorder: An Analysis of 100 Area Child Protection Committee Reviews.* London: HMSO.

Falloon IRH (1985) *Family Care of Schizophrenia.* London: Guilford Press.

Falloon IRH (1993) *Family Care of Schizophrenia.* London: Guilford Press.

Falloon IRH (1998) Optimal treatment for psychosis in an international multi-site demonstration project: Optimal Treatment Project Collaborators (OTPC). *Psychiatric Services* 50: 615–18.

Falloon IRH (2003) Implementation of evidence-based treatment for schizophrenic disorders: OTP Collaborative Group. *Seishin Shinkeigaku Zasshi* 105:1156–76.

Falloon IRH and Pedersen J (1985) Family management in the prevention of morbidity of schizophrenia: the adjustment of the family unit. *British Journal of Psychiatry* 147: 156–63.

Famularo R, Kinscherff R and Fenton T (1992) Psychiatric diagnosis of abusive mothers. A preliminary report. *Journal of Nervous Mental Diseases* 180: 658–61.

Farrington DP (1995) The development of offending and antisocial behaviour from childhood: key findings from the Cambridge Study in Delinquent Development. *Journal of Child Psychology and Psychiatry* 36: 929–64.

Fawcett JA (2003) Lithium combinations in acute maintenance treatment of unipolar and bipolar depression. *Journal of Clinical Psychiatry* 64: 32–7.

Feldman M and Brown R (2002) Munchausen by proxy in international context. *Child Abuse and Neglect* 26: 509–24.

Fernando S (1988) *Mental Health, Race and Culture.* London: Macmillan.

Fernando S, Ndeglia D and Wilson M (eds) (2000) *Forensic Psychiatry, Race and Gender.* London: Routledge.

Fombonne E, Wostear G, Harrington R and Rutter M (2001a) Maudsley long-term follow-up of child and adolescent depression. 2. Suicidality, criminality and social dysfunction in adulthood. *British Journal of Psychiatry* 179: 218–23.

Fombonne E, Wostear G, Cooper V, Harrington R and Rutter M (2001b) Maudsley long-term follow-up of child and adolescent depression. 1. Psychiatric outcomes in adulthood. *British Journal of Psychiatry* 179: 210–17.

Foot M (1978) *Nye Bevan 1945–1960.* Basingstoke: Macmillan.

Ford P, Cox M and Pritchard C (1997) 'Consumer' opinions of the Probation service: advice, assist and befriend and the reduction of crime. *Howard Journal* 36: 42–61.

Foreman DM, Foreman FD and Minty EB (2004) How should we measure social disadvantage in clinic settings? *European Child and Adolescent Psychiatry* 12: 308–12.

Foucault M (1965) *Madness and Civilisation.* New York: Random House.

Freedman R, Leonard S, Olincy A and Tsuang MT (2001) Evidence of multi-genetic inheritance of schizophrenia. *American Journal of Medical Genetics and Neuropsychiatric Genetics* 105: 794–800.

Freeman JP and Graham C (1999) *Compendium of Psychological Tests.* Chichester: Wiley.

Freemantle N (1999) Does the UK NHS need a fourth hurdle for pharmaceutical reimbursement to encourage more efficient prescribing? *Health Policy* 46: 25–65.

Fromouth FE (1988) The relationship of childhood sexual abuse with later psychological and sexual adjustment in a sample of college women. *Child Abuse and Neglect* 10: 5–15.

Fry PS and Barker LA (2002) Quality of relationships and structure properties of social support of female survivors of abuse. *Genetic Social and General Psychology Monograph* 128: 139–63.

Fu Q, Heath AC, Bucholz KK and Eisen SA (2002) Shared genetic risk of major depression, alcohol dependence and marijuana dependence: contribution to antisocial personality disorder. *Archives of General Psychiatry* 59: 1125–32.

Furedi F (2003) *Therapy Culture: Cultivating Vulnerability in an Uncertain Age.* London: Routledge.

Furnam B (1998) *It's Never Too Late to have a Happy Childhood: from Adversity to Resilience.* London: Brief Therapy Press.

Furukawa T, McGuire H and Barbui C (2003) Low dosage tricyclic antidepressants for depression. *Cochrane Database Systematic Review* CDO 003197.

Gabriels L, Cosyns P and Nuttins B (2003) Deep brain stimulation for treatment-refractory OCD, psychological and neuropsychological outcomes. *Acta Psychiatrica Scandinavica* 107: 275–84.

Gelder M, Mayou R and Cowen P (eds) (2001) *Shorter Oxford Textbook of Psychiatry.* Oxford: Oxford University Press.

Ghodsian M, Zajicek E, and Wlikind S (1984) A longitudinal study of maternal depression and child behaviour problems. *Journal of Child Psychology and Psychiatry and Allied Disciplines* 25: 91–109.

Gilberg CL (1992) Autism and autistic-like conditions: sub-class amongst disorders of empathy. *Journal of Child Psychology and Psychiatry* 33: 813–42.

Goffman E (1961) *Asylums.* Harmondsworth: Penguin.

Gold PB, Meisler N and Bailey L (2004) Employment outcomes for hard to reach persons with chronic and severe substance abuse disorders receiving assertive community treatment. *Substance Use and Misuse* 39: 2475–89.

Goodwin RD and Gotlieb IH (2003) Gender differences in depression: role of personality factors. *Psychiatric Research* 35: 135–42.

Goold P (1991) An Investigation into the Significance of Employment of Religious Beliefs in Schizophrenia. Unpubl. PhD thesis, University of Southampton.

Gossop M, Stewart D, Treacy S and Marsden J (2002) Prospective study of mortality among drug users during a 4 year period after seeking treatment. *Addiction* 97: 39–47.

Gostin LO (2000) Human rights of persons with mental disabilities. The European Convention on Human Rights. *International Journal of Law and Psychiatry* 23: 125–9.

Graham AJ, Macdonald AM and Hawkes CH (1997) British motor neuron disease twin study. *Journal of Neurology and Neurosurgery in Psychiatry* 62: 562–9.

Granholm E, Anthenelli R and Stoler M (2003) Brief integrated outpatient dual-diagnosis treatment reduces psychiatric hospitalisation. *American Journal of Addiction* 12: 306–13.

Green AI, Tohen M, Hamer RM and Cark WS (2004) First episode schizophrenia-related psychosis and substance disorders: acute response to olanzapine and haloperidol. *Schizophrenia Research* 66: 125–35.

Green MN (1998) Backward marking performance as an indicator of vulnerability to schizophrenia. *Acta Psychiatrica Scandinavica* 395: 34–40.

Greenberg DA, Hedge SE and Nicholl D (2001) Excess of twins among affected sibling pairs with autism: implications for the aetiology of autism. *American Journal of Human Genetics* 69: 1062–7.

Greenfield SF (2002) Women and alcohol disorders. *Harvard Review of Psychiatry* 10: 76–85.

Greenpeace (1980) From paradise to rubbish-tip. Campaign leaflet. Greenpeace.

Grgik M (2002) Children mental disorder as a result of parental misbehaviour or lack of authority. *Imago* 8: 321–6.

Gribbon J (2002) *Science: A History.* London: Penguin.

Grossman L, Martis B and Fichtner C (1999) Are sex offenders treatable? A research overview. *Psychiatric Services* 50: 349–61.

Grunze H and Moller HJ (2002) The place of antidepressants in the acute treatment of bipolar disorder. *Clinical Approaches to Bipolar Disorders* 1: 40–8.

Gumley A, O'Grady M, McNay L and Norrie J (2003) Early intervention for relapse in schizophrenia: results of a 12 month RCT of CBT. *Psychological Medicine* 33: 19–31.

Gunnell D, Middleton N and Frankel S (2003) Why are suicides rising in young men but falling in the elderly? *Social Science and Medicine* 57: 595–611.

Guthrie E, Kapur N, Mackway-Jones K, Chew-Graham C and Tomenson B (2001) Randomised controlled trial of brief psychological intervention after deliberate self poisoning. *British Medical Journal* 323: 135–8.

Haatainen KM, Tanskanen A, Kylma J and Viinamki H (2003) Life events are important in the course of hopelessness: a two-year follow-up study in a general population. *Social Psychiatry and Psychiatric Epidemiology* 38: 436–41.

Hall CM and Currow D (2005) Cannabinoids and cancer: causation, remediation and palliation. *Lancet Oncology* 6: 35–42.

Hall DE, Eubanks L, Meyyazhagan S, Kenny RD and Johnson SC (2000) Evaluation of covert surveillance in the diagnosis of Munchausen syndrome by proxy. *Paediatrics* 105: 1305–12.

Hall JP and Baker R (1971) Use of operant conditioning to re-instate speech in mute schizophrenics. *Behavioural Research and Therapy* 9: 326–9.

Hammen C, Shih J, Altman T and Brennan PA (2003) Interpersonal impairment and the prediction of depressive symptoms in adolescent children of depressed and non-depressed mothers. *Journal of the American Academy of Child and Adolescent Psychiatry* 42: 571–7.

Hammersley P, Dias A and Bentall RP (2003) Childhood trauma and hallucinations in bipolar affective disorders: preliminary investigation. *British Journal of Psychiatry* 182: 543–7.

Hankin BL, Fraely RC and Waldman ID (2005) Is depression best viewed as a continuum or discrete category? A taxometric analysis of childhood and adolescent depression in a population based study. *Journal of Abnormal Psychology* 114: 96–110.

Harkvy-Friedman JM, Kimhy D, Nelson EA and Mann JJ (2003) Suicide attempts in schizophrenia: the role of command auditory hallucinations for suicide. *Journal of Clinical Psychiatry* 64: 871–4.

Harris EC and Barraclough B (1997) Suicide as an outcome for mental disorder: a meta-analysis. *British Journal of Psychiatry* 170: 205–28.

Harris EC and Barraclough B (1998) Suicide as an outcome of mental disorder: a meta analysis. *British Medical Journal* 315: 286–7.

Harrison G (2002) Ethnic minorities and the Mental Health Act. *British Journal of Psychiatry* 180: 198–200.

Harrison G, Amin S, Sing SP, Croudace T and Jones P (1999) Outcome of psychosis in people of African-Caribbean origin: population based first episode. *British Journal of Psychiatry* 175: 43–9.

Harrison G, Gunnell D, Glazebrook C and Kwieceninski R (2001) Association between schizophrenia and social inequality. *British Journal of Psychiatry* 179: 346–50.

Hartl TL, Rosen C and Gusman F (2005) Predicting high-risk behaviours in veterans with PTSD. *Journal of Nervous Mental Disorders* 193: 464–72.

Hawton K, Roberts J and Goodwin G (1985) The risk of child abuse among mothers who attempt suicide. *British Journal of Psychiatry* 146: 415–20.

Hawton K, Harris L, Appleby L and Parrott H (2000) Effects of the death of Diana Princess of Wales on suicide and deliberate self harm. *British Journal of Psychiatry* 177: 463–6.

Hawton K, Harris L, Simkin S and Bond A (2001) Social class and suicidal behaviour: the association between social class and the characteristics of deliberate-self-harm. *Social Psychiatry and Psychiatric Epidemiology* 36: 437–43.

Hawton K, Houston K, Haw C and Harris L (2003) Co-morbidity of axis 1 and 11 disorders in patients who attempted suicide. *American Journal of Psychiatry* 160: 1494–500.

Hay DA, Martin NG, Foley D and Heath AC (2001) Phenotypic and genetic analyses of a short measure of psychosis proneness in a large-scale Australian twin study. *Twin Research* 4: 30–40.

Healy D and Whittaker C (2003) Anti-depressants and suicide: risk benefit conundrums. *Journal of Psychiatry and Neurosciences* 28: 331–7.

Heelawell D and Pentland B (2001) Relatives' reports of long term problems following traumatic brain injury. *Disability and Rehabilitation* 23: 300–5.

Henwood BD (1998) *Ignored and Invisible? Carers' Experience of the NHS*. London: Carers' National Association.

Herbert C, Levfevre H, Gignoux M and Launoy G (2002) Influence of social and occupational class and area of residence on management and survival in patients with digestive tract cancer. *Revue Epidemiologie Santé Publique* 50: 253–64.

Hermanowicz N (2002) A blind man with Parkinson's disease, visual hallucinations and Capgras syndrome. *Journal of Neuropsychiatry and Clinical Neurosciences* 14: 462–3.

Hetherington EM (2005) Divorce and the adjustment of children. *Paediatric Review* 26: 163–9.

Hill J, Pickles A and Bryatt M (2004) Juvenile versus adult onset depression: multiple differences imply different pathways. *Psychological Medicine* 34: 1483–93.

Hirschfeld RM, Montgomery SA, Amore M and Versiani M (2002) Partial response and non-response to antidepressant therapy: current approaches and treatment options. *Journal of Clinical Psychiatry* 63: 826–37.

HMSO (1983) *Mental Health Act 1983 – Chapter 20*. London: HMSO.

HMSO (1991) *The Health of the Nation: A Consultative Document for Health in England.* Green Paper. London: HMSO.

HMSO (1994) *The Report of the Inquiry into the Care and Treatment of Christopher Clunis (The Ritchie Report).* London: HMSO.

HMSO (1996) *Ethnicity and Health in England.* London: NHS Executive/NHS Ethnic Health Unit, HMSO.

Ho BC, Andreasen NC and Flaum M (2003) Progressive structural brain abnormalities and their relationship to clinical outcome: longitudinal magnetic resonance imaging study in schizophrenia. *Archives of General Psychiatry* 60: 585–90.

Hogan DP and Park JM (2000) Family factors and support in the development of very low-birth weight children. *Clinics in Perinatology* 27: 433–59.

Holinger D (1987) *Violent Death in the United States.* New York: Guildford.

Holmes J, Hever T, Hewitt L and Thapakar A (2002) A pilot twin study of psychological measures of ADHD. *Behaviour Genetics* 32: 389–95.

Holowka DW, King S and Brunet A (2003) Childhood abuse and dissociative symptoms in adult schizophrenia. *Schizophrenia Research* 76: 1–22.

Home Office (1994) *Criminal Statistics for England and Wales 1992.* London: HMSO.

Hopper K and Barrow SM (2003) Two genealogies of supported housing and their implications for outcome assessment. *Psychiatric Services* 54: 50–4.

House of Commons (1996) *Report of Comptroller and Auditor General: Health of the Nation – Progress Report HC 656.* London: Committee of Public Accounts.

House of Commons (2000) Select Committee on Health – Fourth Report. *Provision of NHS Mental Health Services – Legislative Change – Review of the Mental Health Act 1983* (http://www.parliament.the-stationery-office.co.uk/pa/cm199900/cmselec).

Howard J, Lennings CJ and Copeland J (2003) Suicidal behaviour in a young offender population. *Crisis:* 24: 98–104.

Howard LM, Thornicroft G and Appleby L (2004) Predictors of parenting outcome in women with psychotic disorders discharged from mother–baby units. *Acta Psychiatrica Scandinavica* 110: 347–55.

Hoyer J, Borchard B and Kunst H (2000) Diagnosis and disorder-specific therapy in sex offenders with mental disorders. *Verhaltenstherapie* 10: 7–15.

Hrobjartsson A and Gotzsche OC (2003) Placebo treatment versus no treatment. *Cochrane Database Systematic Review* CDO 003974.

Hull PR and D'Arcy C (2003) Isotretinoin use and subsequent depression and suicide: presenting the evidence. *American Journal of Clinical Dermatology* 4: 493–505.

Hunt IM, Robinson J, Bickley H and Appleby L (2003) Suicide in ethnic minorities within 12 months of contact with mental health services. *British Journal of Psychiatry* 183: 155–61.

Huprich SK (2003) Depressive personality and its relation to depressive mood, interpersonal loss and negative parental perceptions. *Journal of Nervous Mental Diseases* 191: 73–9.

Hurd RC (1999) Adults view their childhood bereavement experiences. *Death Studies* 23: 17–41.

Huxley P, Korer J and Tolley S (1987) The psychiatric caseness of clients referred to an urban social services department. *British Journal of Social Work* 17: 507–20.

Illich I (1971) *Medical Nemesis: The Medical Expropriation of Health.* London: Calder & Boyer.

ILO (2000) *Annual Statistics 2000.* Geneva: International Labour Office.

Ingraham LJ and Kety SS (2000) Adoption studies of schizophrenia. *American Journal of Medical Genetics/Seminars in Medical Genetics* 97: 18–22.

Inman W and Pearce G (1993) Prescriber profile and post-marketing surveillance. *Lancet* 342: 658–61.

Inoue Y and Mihara T (2001) Psychiatric disorders before and after surgery for epilepsy. *Epilepsia* 42 (Suppl. 6): 13–18.

Isacsson G, Holmgren P and Ahlner J (2005) Selective serotonin reuptake inhibitor antidepressants and the risk of suicide: a controlled forensic database study of 14,857 suicides. *Acta Psychiatrica Scandinavica* 111: 286–90.

Iwaniec D (1995) *The Emotionally Abused and Neglected Child: Identification, Assessment and Intervention.* Chichester: John Wiley.

Jamison KR (1995) *An Unquiet Mind: A Memoir of Moods and Madness.* New York: Picador.

Jamison KR (1996) *Touched with Fire: Manic-Depressive Illness and the Artistic Temperament.* New York: Simon & Schuster.

Jane-Llopis E, Honman C, Jenkins R and Andrews JR (2003) Predictors of efficacy in depression preventative programmes: a meta analysis. *British Journal of Psychiatry* 183: 384–97.

Jenkins R (2001) *Churchill.* Basingstoke: Macmillan.

Jenkins R, Bebbington P, Brugha TS and Meltzer H (1998) British psychiatric morbidity surveys. *British Journal of Psychiatry* 173: 4–7.

Jick SS, Kremers HM and Vasilakis-Scaramozza C (2000) Isotretinoin use and risk of depression, psychotic symptoms, suicide and attempted suicide. *Archives of Dermatology* 136: 1231–6.

Johansson JC, Jannsson M, Linner L and Schalling M (2001) Genetics of affective disorder. *European Neuropsychopharmacology* 11: 385–92.

Johnson JG, Cohen P, Skodal A and Brook JJ (1999) Personality disorder in adolescents and risk of major mental disorder and suicidality in adulthood. *Archives of General Psychiatry* 56: 805–11.

Jones K (1959) *Social Policy and Mental Health.* London: Routledge & Kegan Paul.

Jones R (1999) *Mental Health Act Manual,* 6th edn. London: Sweet and Maxwell.

Jones RD (2001) Depression and anxiety in oncology: the oncologist's perspective *Journal of Clinical Psychiatry* 62: 52–5.

Jones R, Gruer L, Gilchrist G and Oliver J (2002) Recent contact with health and social services by drug misusers in Glasgow who died of a fatal overdose in 1999. *Addiction* 97: 1517–22.

Jordan JR (2001) Is suicide bereavement different? A reassessment of the literature. *Suicide and Life Threatening Behaviour* 31: 91–102.

Joy CB, Adams EE and Rice K (2004) Crisis intervention for people with severe mental illness. *Cochrane Database Systematic Review* 18: CD001087.

Judge K and Benzeval M (1993) Health inequalities: new concerns about the children of single mothers. *British Medical Journal* 306: 677–80.

Kahn RS, Wilson K and Wise PH (2005) Intergenerational health disparities: socioeconomic status, women's health conditions and child behaviour problems. *Public Health Report* 120: 399–408.

Kahn SA and Faros S (2003) Reasons for not acting on suicidal ideas. *Journal of the Colleges of Physicians and Surgeons Pakistan* 13: 37–9.

Kahng JK and Mowbray CT (2005) What affects self-esteem of persons with psychiatric disabilities: role of causal attributions of mental illness. *Psychiatry Rehabilitation Journal* 28: 354–61.

Kalant H (2004) Adverse effects of cannabis on health: an update of the literature since 1996. *Progress in Neuropsychopharmacology* 28: 849–63.

Kallen K (2001) The impact of maternal smoking during pregnancy on delivery. *European Journal of Public Health* 11: 329–33.

Kane JM (1996) Factors which can make patients difficult to treat. *British Journal of Psychiatry* 169 (Suppl. 31): 10–15.

Katschnig H (2002) Kraepelins', Blueler's and Schneider's concept of schizophrenia. Their relevance to the stigma process. *Neuropsychiatry* 16: 11–19.

Kawahara Y, Ito K and Shin K (2005) RNA editing and death of motor neurons. *Nature* 427: 801.

Keller F and Schuler B (2002) Psycho-educational groups for families of in-patients with affective disorder. *Psychiatrica Praxis* 29: 130–5.

Kempe CH, Silverman FN, Steele BF, Droegemueller W and Silver HK (1962) The battered child syndrome. *Journal of the American Medical Association* 181: 17–24.

Kempe H and Kempe CH (1978) *Child Abuse*. London: Fontana.

Kendler KS, Myers J and Prescott CA (2000) Parenting and adult mood, anxiety and substance use disorders in female twins. An epidemiological, multi-informant, retrospective study. *Psychological Medicine* 30: 281–94.

Kerr A (2003) Governing genetics: reifying choice and progress. *New Genetics Society* 22: 111–26.

Kessing LV, Agerbo E and Mortensen PB (2003) Does the impact of major stressful life events on the risk of developing depression change throughout life? *Psychological Medicine* 33: 1177–84.

Kessing LV, Agerbo E and Mortensen PB (2004) Major stressful life events and other risk factors for first admission mania. *Bipolar Disorder* 6: 122–9.

Kim CH, Chang JW, Koo MS and Lee HS (2003) Anterior cingulotomy for refractory obsessive–compulsive-disorder. *Acta Psychiatrica Scandinavica* 107: 283–90.

Kim EY and Miklowitz DJ (2004) Expressed emotion as a predictor of outcome among bipolar patients undergoing family therapy. *Journal of Affective Disorders* 82: 343–52.

King EA, Baldwin DS, Sinclair JM and Campbell MJ (2001) The Wessex Recent In-patient Study 2: case-controlled study of 59 in-patient suicides. *British Journal of Psychiatry* 178: 537–42.

Kingdon DG (1996) Social policy and homelessness. In Bhurga D (ed.) *Homelessness and Mental Illness*. Chichester: Wiley, 34–56.

Kingdon D and Turkington D (2002) *The Case Study Guide to Cognitive Behaviour Therapy of Psychosis*. Chichester: Wiley.

Klar AS (2002) Chromosome 1:11 provides the best evidence for supporting the genetic aetiology of schizophrenia and bipolar affective disorders. *Genetics* 160: 1745–7.

Kleindienst N and Griel W (2003) Lithium in the long-term treatment of bipolar disorders. *European Archives of Psychiatry and Clinical Neurosciences* 25: 120–5.

Kleine P (1978) *Fact and Fantasy in Freudian Psychology*. Chichester: Wiley.

Klysner R, Bent-Hansen J, Hansen HL and Petersen HE (2003) Efficacy of citalopram in the prevention of recurrent depression in elderly patients: placebo-controlled study of maintenance therapy. *British Journal of Psychiatry* 181: 29–35.

Kmietowicz Z (2003) Gap between classes in life expectancy is widening. *British Medical Journal* 327: 68–9.

Kolmos I and Bach E (1987) Sources of error in registering suicide. *Acta Psychiatrica Scandinavica* 36: 23–43.

Korbin JE (1986) Childhood histories of women imprisoned for fatal child maltreatment. *Child Abuse and Neglect* 8: 387–92.

Koskinen O, Pukkila K and Rasanen P (2002) Is occupation relevant in suicide? *Journal of Affective Disorders* 70: 197–203.

Kuipers E (1996) The management of difficult to treat patients with schizophrenia using non-drug therapies. *British Journal of Psychiatry* 169 (Suppl. 31): 41–51.

Kumar P and Clarke M (1994) *Clinical Medicine*, 3rd edn. London: Balliere & Tindall.

Kung HC, Pearson JL and Liu X (2002) Risk factors for male and female suicide descendants ages 15–64 in the USA: results from National Mortality Follow-back Survey. *Social Psychiatry and Psychiatric Epidemiology* 38: 419–26.

Ladouceur CD, Dahl RE and Casey BJ (2005) Altered neonatal processing in pediatric anxiety, depression and co-morbid anxiety–depression. *Journal of Abnormal Child Psychology* 33: 165–77.

Laing R (1960) *The Divided Self*. London: Tavistock.

Laing R and Esterton D (1968) *Family, Madness, and Insanity*. Harmondsworth: Penguin.

Lamming Report (2003) *Report on the Death of Victoria Climbié*. London: Social Services Inspectorate.

Langlois S and Morrison P (2002) Suicide deaths and suicide attempts. *Health Reports* 13: 9–22.

Lau BWK (1989) Why do patients go to traditional healers? *Journal of the Royal Society of Health* 3: 92–5.

Lau BWK and Pritchard C (2001) Suicide of older people in Asian societies: an international comparison. *Australasian Journal on Ageing* 20: 196–202.

Lau WB (1996) Psychosocial context of health and illness. *Journal of the Royal Society of Health* 115: 220–4.

Lazarus AA (1976) *Multi-Model Therapy*. New York: Springer.

Lee DA, Randall F and Bentall RP (2004) Delusional discourse: an investigation comparing the spontaneous casual attributions of paranoid and non-paranoid individuals. *Psychology and Psychotherapy* 77: 525–40.

Leff J (1992) Over the edge: stress and schizophrenia. *New Scientist* 4 January: 30–4.

Leffley HP and Johnson DL (1990) *Families as Allies in the Treatment of the Mentally Ill*. New York: American Psychiatric Press.

Leffy J and Vaughan C (1998) *Expressed Emotion in Families*. London: Guilford Press.

Lelliott P and Audini B (2003) Trends in the use of Part II of the MHA 1983 in seven English local authority areas. *British Journal of Psychiatry* 182: 68–70.

Lenroot R, Busillio JR and Keith SR (2003) Integrated services for people with schizophrenia. *Psychiatric Services* 54: 1499–507.

Lester D (ed.) (2001) *Suicide Prevention: Resources for the Millennium*. Philadelphia: Routledge.

Lewis AJ (1955) Health as a social concept. *British Journal of Sociology* 4: 109–24.

Li Z, Meredith MP and Hoseyni MS (2001) A method to assess the proportion of treatment effect explained by surrogate endpoints. *Statistics in Medicine* 20: 3175–88.

Linden M and Barnow S (1997) The wish to die in very old persons: a psychiatric problem?. Results from the Berlin Ageing Study. *International Psychogeriatrics* 9: 902–13.

Lindsey D and Trocme N (1994) Have child protection efforts reduced child homicide? An examination of data from Britain and the USA. *British Journal of Social Work* 24: 715–32.

Linehan MM (1993) *Cognitive Behavioural Therapy for Borderline Personality Disorder and Skills and Manual for Treating Borderline Personality Disorder*. New York: Guildford.

Linehan MM, Dimeff LA, Reynolds S and Kivlahan DR (2002) Dialectic behaviour therapy versus comprehensive validation therapy plus 12-step for the treatment of opioid dependent women with borderline personality disorders. *Drug and Alcohol Dependence* 67: 13–26.

Lipman EL, McMillan HL and Boyle MT (2001) Childhood abuse and psychiatric disorder in single and married mothers. *American Journal of Psychiatry* 158: 73–88.

Llerena A, Caceres MC and Penas-Lledo EM (2002) Schizophrenia stigma amongst medical and nursing students 2. *European Psychiatry* 17: 298–99.

Luchins DJ (2004) At issue: will the term brain disease reduce stigma in mental illness? *Schizophrenia Bulletin* 30: 1043–8.

Ludwig AM (1994) Mental illness and creativity in female American writers. *American Journal of Psychiatry* 151: 1650–6.

Luecken LJ (2000) Attachment and loss during childhood experiences are associated with adult hostility, depression and social support. *Journal of Psychosomatic Research* 49: 85–91.

Lyon J, Dennison C and Wilson A (1996) *Tell Them So They Listen: Messages from Young People in Custody.* London: Stationery Office.

McCabe R and Priebe S (2002) Are therapeutic relationships in psychiatry explained by the patients symptoms? *European Psychiatry* 18: 220–5.

McCabe R, Ronan-Wanner UU, Hoffmann KJ and Priebe S (1999) Therapy, relationship and quality of life: association of two subjective constructs in schizophrenic patients. *International Journal of Social Psychiatry* 45: 276–83.

McClelland C and Crisp A (2001) Anorexia nervosa and social class. *International Journal of Eating Disorders* 29: 150–6.

McClure RJ, Davies PM, Meadows SR and Sibert JR (1996) Epidemiology of Munchausen's syndrome by proxy: non-accidental poisoning and suffocation. *Archives of Diseases in Childhood* 75: 57–61.

McDaniel JO, Purcell D and D'Augelli AR (2001) Relationship between sexual orientation: results of research findings. *Suicide and Life Threatening Behaviour* 31: 84–105.

MacDonald F, Paxton R and Allott R (2001) Improving GP's assessment and management of suicide risk. *International Journal of Health Care* 14: 133–88.

McDonald K (1993) Comparative homicide and the proper aims of social work. *British Journal of Social Work* 25: 489–98.

McGovern D and Cope R (1987) The compulsory detention of males in different ethnic groups with special reference to offender patients. *British Journal of Psychiatry* 150: 505–12.

McHolm A, McMillan H and Jamieson E (2003) The relationship between childhood physical abuse and suicidality amongst depressed women: results from a community sample. *American Journal of Psychiatry* 160: 933–8.

McKenna P, Willison JR, Lowe D and Neil-Dwyer G (1989) Cognitive outcome and quality of life one year after SAH. *Neurosurgery* 24: 361–8.

McKenzie K, Samele C, Van Horn E and Murray R (2001) Comparison of the outcome and treatment of psychosis in people of Caribbean origin living in the UK and British whites from the UK 700 trial. *British Journal of Psychiatry* 178: 160–5.

McKenzie K, Jones P, Lewis S, Williams M and Murray RM (2002) Lower prevalence of pre-morbid neurological illness in African-Caribbean than white psychotic patients in England. *Psychological Medicine* 32: 1285–91.

McKenzie K, van Os J, Samele C and Murray R (2003) Suicide and attempted suicide among young people of Caribbean origin with psychosis living in the UK. *British Journal of Psychiatry* 183: 40–4.

MacKirdy C and Shepherd D (2000) Capgras syndrome: possibly more common in the Maori of New Zealand? *Australian and New Zealand Journal of Psychiatry* 34: 865–8.

MacLeod AK, Williams JM and Linehan MM (1993) New developments in the understanding and treatment of suicidal behaviour. *Behavioural Psychotherapy* 20: 193–218.

McLloyd V (1990) The impact of economic hardship upon black families and their children: psychological distress, parenting and socioeconomic development. *Child Development* 61: 311–46.

McNeil DE and Binder RL (2005) Psychiatric emergency service use and homelessness, mental disorder and violence. *Psychiatric Services* 56: 699–704.

McSween JL (2002) The role of group interest, identity and stigma in determining mental health policy preferences. *Journal of Health Politics and Policy Law* 27: 773–800.

Madden DR (2002) The structure and function of glutamate receptor ion channels. *Nature Reviews: Neurosciences* 3: 91–101.

Madianou MG and Economou M (1994) Schizophrenia and family rituals: Measuring family rituals amongst schizophrenics and normals. *European Psychiatry* 9: 45–51.

Magnus SA and Mick SS (2000) Medical schools, affirmative action and the neglected role of social class. *American Journal of Public Health* 90: 1197–201.

Mahapatra SB and Hamilton M (1974) Examination of foreign psychiatrists: problems of language. *British Journal of Medical Education* 8: 271–4.

Maki P, Veijola J, Rasanen P and Isohanni M (2003) Criminality in the off-spring of anti-natally depressed mothers: 33-year follow-up of the Northern Finland 1966 birth cohort. *Journal of Affective Disorders* 74: 273–8.

Malhi GS, Matharu MS and Hales AS (2000) *Neurology for Psychiatrists.* London: Martin Dunitz.

Malm U, Ivarsson B and Falloon IR (2003) Integrated care in schizophrenia: a two-year randomised controlled study of two community based treatment programmes. *Acta Psychiatrica Scandinavica* 107: 415–23.

Malmberg ML and Fenton M (2001) Individual psychoanalytic psychotherapy for severe mental illness and schizophrenia. *Cochrane Database Systematic Review* 2: CD001360.

Marantz AG and Verghese J (2002) Capgras syndrome in dementia with Lewy bodies. *Journal of Geriatric Psychiatry and Neurology* 15: 239–41.

Margolese HC, Malchy L, Negrete J and Gill K (2004) Drug and alcohol use among patients with schizophrenia and related psychosis: levels and consequences. *Schizophrenia Research* 67: 157–66.

Maris RW (2002) Suicide. *Lancet* 360: 319–26.

Maris RW, Berman AL and Yufit RI (eds) (1992) *Assessment and Prediction of Suicide.* New York: Guilford Press.

Marley JA and Buila S (2001) Crimes against people with mental illness. Types, proportions and influencing factors. *Social Work* 46: 115–24.

Marshall WL (1997) Relationship between low self-esteem and deviant sexual arousal within non-familial child molesters. *Behavioural Modification* 21: 86–96.

Martens L and Addington AJ (2001) Psychological well-being of family members of an individual with schizophrenia. *Social Psychiatry and Social Epidemiology* 36: 128–33.

Martin JA (1984) Neglected fathers: limitations in diagnostic and treatment resources for violent men. *Child Abuse and Neglect* 8: 387–92.

Martinez C, Reitbrock S and Gunnell D (2005) Antidepressant treatment and the risk of fatal and non-fatal self-harm in first episode depression: a nested case–control study. *British Medical Journal* 330: 373–4.

Marwaha S and Livingston G (2002) Stigma, racism or choice. Why do depressed ethnic elders avoid psychiatrists? *Journal of Affective Disorders* 72: 257–65.

Massett HA, Greenup M and Maibach EW (2002) Public perceptions about prematurity: a national survey. *American Journal of Preventative Medicine* 24: 120–7.

Meadows R (1977) Munchausen syndrome by proxy: the hinterland of child abuse. *Lancet* 2: 343–5.

Meadows R (1994) Munchausen syndrome by proxy. *Journal of Clinical Forensic Medicine* 1: 121–7.

Meadows R (2002) Different interpretations of Munchausen syndrome by proxy. *Child Abuse and Neglect* 26: 501–8.

Mermelstein HT and Lesko L (1992) Depression in patients with cancer. *Psycho-Oncology* 1: 199–215.

Merrill KA, Tolbert VE and Wade WA (2003) Effective cognitive treatment for depression in a community mental health centre: a benchmarking study. *Journal of Clinical Consulting Psychology* 71: 404–9.

Messerschmitt P (2002) Adult outcome of children with attention deficit hyperactivity disorder. *Revue Practicien* 52: 2009–12.

Meyerowitz JJ (2001) Sex research at the borders of gender: transvestites, transsexuals and Alfred Kinsey. *Bulletin of the History of Medicine* 75: 72–90.

Michel A, Ansseau M, Legros JJ and Morment C (2002) The transsexual: what of the future? *European Psychiatry* 17: 353–60.

Middleton L (1999) Could do better. *Professional Social Work* November 26–29.

Miklowitz DJ (2004) The role of family systems in severe and recurrent psychiatric disorders: a developmental psychopathological view. *Developmental Psychopathology* 16: 667–88.

Miklowitz DJ, George E and Suddath RL (2003a) A randomised study of family-focused psycho-education and pharmacotherapy in the outpatient management of bipolar disorder. *Archives of General Psychiatry* 60: 904–13.

Miklowitz DJ, Richards JA and Sacher JA (2003b) Integrated family and individual therapy for bipolar disorders: results of a treatment development study. *Journal of Clinical Psychiatry* 64: 182–91.

Miles A (1987) *The Mentally Ill in Contemporary Society*. Oxford: Basil Blackwell.

Miller WR and Rollnick S (1991) *Motivational Interviewing – Preparing People to Change Addictive Behaviours*. New York: Guilford Press.

Millett K (1991) *The Loony Bin Trip*. London: Virago Press.

Miranda J, Chung YJ, Green BL and Belin S (2003) Treating depression in predominately low-income young minority women. A randomised controlled study. *Journal of the American Medical Association* 290: 57–68.

Modestin J, Oberson D and Erni T (1998) Possible antecedents of DSM III personality disorders. *Acta Psychiatrica Scandinavica* 97: 160–6.

Molinuevo JL, Valldeoriola F and Valls-Sole J (2003) Usefulness of neurophysiologic techniques in stereotactic subthalamic nucleus stimulation for advanced Parkinson's disease. *Clinical Neurophysiology* 114: 1793–999.

Monahan J, Steadman HJ and Silver E (2005) An actuarial model of violence risk assessment for persons with mental disorders. *Psychiatric Services* 56: 810–15.

Montoya A, Weiss AP, Price BH and Cosgrove GR (2002) Magnetic resonance imaging-guided stereotactic limbic leucotomy for treatment of intractable psychiatric disease. *Neurosurgery* 50: 1043–9.

Morgan HG, Jones EM and Owen JH (1993) Secondary prevention of non-fatal deliberate-self-harm: the Green Card study. *British Journal of Psychiatry* 163: 111–12.

Morris CD, Miklowitz DJ and Allen MH (2005) Care, satisfaction, hope and life functioning amongst adults with bi-polar disorder: First 1000 participants in Systematic Treatment Enhancement Programme. *Comprehensive Psychiatry* 46: 98–104.

Moss HB, Baron DA, Hardie TL and Vanyukov MM (2001) Preadolescent children of substance-dependent fathers with antisocial personality disorder: psychiatric disorders and problem behaviours. *American Journal of Addiction* 10: 269–78.

Mowbray C, Oyseman D, Bybee D and MacFarlane P (2001) Parenting of mothers with a severe mental illness. Different effects of diagnosis, clinical history and other mental health variables. *Social Work Research* 26: 225–40.

Muller-Oerlinghausen B, Berghofer A and Arhrens B (2003) The anti-suicidal and mortality reducing effect of lithium prophylaxis: consequence for guidelines in clinical psychiatry. *Canadian Journal of Psychiatry* 48: 433–9.

Mulvaney F, O'Callaghan E, Takei N and Larkin C (2001) Effect of social class at birth on risk and presentation of schizophrenia: case–control study. *British Medical Journal* 323: 1398–401.

Myer JE (1988) The treatment of the mentally ill in Nazi Germany. *Psychological Medicine* 18: 35–52.

Myers WC and Monaco L (2000) Personality disorder and psychopathy in juvenile sexual homicide offenders. *Journal of Forensic Sciences* 45: 698–701.

Narr K, Thompson P and Sharma T (2001) Three-dimensional mapping of gyral shape and cortical asymmetries in schizophrenia: gender effects. *American Journal of Psychiatry* 158: 244–55.

Neeleman J and Wessley S (1999) Ethnic minority suicide: a small geographical study in south London. *Psychological Medicine* 29: 429–36.

Neeleman J, Mak V and Wessley S (1997) Suicide by age, ethnic group, coroner's verdict and country of birth. A three-year survey of inner London. *British Journal of Psychiatry* 171: 463–7.

Newcomb M and Lock T (2001) Intergenerational cycle of maltreatment: a popular concept obscured by methodological limitations. *Child Abuse and Neglect* 25: 1219–40.

NICE (2000) *Clinical Recommendations 2000*. London: National Institute for Clinical Excellence.

NICE (2002) *Guidance on the Use of Newer (Atypical) Antipsychotic Drugs for the Treatment of Schizophrenia*. London: National Institute for Clinical Excellence.

NICE (2005) *Digest of Clinical Recommendations*. London: National Institute for Health and Clinical Excellence.

Nishiguchi N, Matsushita S, Suzuki K and Higuchi S (2001) Association between 5HT2A receptor gene promoter region polymorphism and eating disorders in Japanese patients. *Biological Psychiatry* 50: 123–8.

Noell JW and Ochs LM (2001) Relationship of sexual orientation to substance abuse, suicidal ideation and suicide attempts. *Journal of Adolescent Health* 29: 31–6.

Nolan KA, Volavka J and Saito T (2000) An association between a polymorphism of the trytophan hydroxylase gene and aggression in schizophrenia and schizoaffective disorder. *Psychiatric Genetics* 10: 109–15.

Norstrom T and Skog OJ (2001) Alcohol and mortality: methodological and analysis issues in aggregate analysis. *Addiction* 96 (Suppl.): S5–17.

Noyes P (1991) *Child Abuse – A Study of Inquiry Reports.* London: HMSO.

Noyes R (2001) Co-morbidity in generalised anxiety disorder. *Psychiatric Clinics of North America* 24: 41–55.

O'Connell P and Grimbly C (2002) *A Mental Health Research Project for Centrepoint.* London: King's Fund.

O'Leary J (1997) *Beyond help? Improving Service Provision for Street Homeless People with Mental Health, Alcohol and Drug Dependency Problems.* London: National Homeless Alliance.

Obafunwa JO and Busuttil A (1994) A review of completed suicide in the Lothian and Borders region of Scotland. *Social Psychiatry and Psychiatric Epidemiology* 29: 100–6.

Odell S and Commander M (1999) A follow-up study of people with a severe mental illness treated by a specialist homeless team. *Psychiatric Bulletin* 23: 139–42.

Office of the Deputy Prime Minister (2003) *Supporting People Fund.* London: ODPM (www.spkweb.org.uk).

Okin RL and Pearsall D (1993) Patient's perception of the quality of their life 11 years after discharge from a state hospital. *Hospital and Community Psychiatry* 44: 236–40.

ONS (2005) *Health Statistics 2003.* London: Office of National Statistics.

d'Orban P (1990) Female homicide. *Irish Journal of Psychological Medicine* 7: 64–70.

Owen C, Tennet C and Jones M (1994) Cancer patients' attitude to final events in life: wish for death, attitudes to cessation of treatment, suicide and euthanasia. *Psycho-oncology* 3: 1–9.

Padmavathi R, Rajkumar S and Srinivasan TN (1998) Schizophrenic patients who were never treated: a study in an Indian urban community. *Psychological Medicine* 28: 1113–17.

Page AC and Hooke YR (2002) Outcome for depression and over-anxious inpatients before and after cognitive behavioural therapy: a naturalist comparison. *Journal of Mental Disorders* 191: 653–9.

Pallis DY and Stoffelmyer BE (1978) Social attitudes and treatment amongst psychiatrists. *British Journal of Medical Psychology* 46: 75–81.

Paradise J (2001) Current concepts of preventing child sexual abuse. *Current Opinions in Paediatrics* 13: 402–407.

Park G (2002) *Someone and Anyone: Assessment Practice in Voluntary Sector Services for Homeless People in London.* London: King's Fund.

Park MJ, Tyer P, Elseworth E and MacDonald A (2002) The measurement of engagement in the homeless mentally ill: the Homeless Engagement and Acceptance Scale. *Psychological Medicine* 32: 855–61.

Parker G, Roy K, Wilheim K and Hadzi-Pavlovic P (1999) Exploration of links between early parenting and personality type disorders. *Journal of Personality Disorders* 13: 361–74.

Parkin A (2000) Contrasting agendas in the reform of mental health law – the Expert Committee and the Green Paper. *Web Journal of Current Legal Issues.*

Patel V (2000) International representation in psychiatry: survey of six leading journals. *British Journal of Psychiatry* 178: 406–9.

Paul JP, Catania J, Pollack L and Stall R (1992) Suicide attempts among gay and bisexual men: lifetime prevalence and antecedents. *American Journal of Public Health* 92: 1338–45.

Paykel ES (2001) Evolution of life event research in psychiatry. *Journal of Affective Disorders* 62: 141–9.

Pedler M (1999a) *Mind the Law – Mind's Evidence to the Government's Mental Health Act Review Team.* London: Mind Publications.

Pedler M (1999b) Green Paper published. *Community Care* 18–24 November.

Pekkala E and Merinder L (2002) Psycho-education for schizophrenia. *Cochrane Database Systematic Review* 2: CD002831.

Peterson EM, Luoma JB and Dunne E (2002) Suicide survivors' perceptions of the treating clinician. *Suicide and Life Threatening Behaviour* 32: 158–66.

Pfeffer CR, Karus D and Jiang H (2000) Child survivors of parental death from cancer or suicide: depressive and behavioural outcomes. *Psycho-oncology* 9: 1–10.

Pharoah FM, Rathbone J and Steiner DG (2003) Family intervention for schizophrenia. *Cochrane Database Systematic Review* 17: CD000088.

Phillips MR, Pearson V, Li F and Yang L (2002) Stigma and expressed emotion: a study of people with schizophrenia and their family members in China. *British Journal of Psychiatry* 181: 488–93.

Pilgrim D and Rogers A (1998) *A Sociology of Mental Health and Illness.* Buckingham: Open University Press.

Pilling S, Bebbington P, Kuipers E and Morgan C (2002) Psychological treatments in schizophrenia. II. Meta-analysis of randomised controlled trials of social skills training and cognitive remediation. *Psychological Medicine* 32: 783–91.

Pilmann F (2001) Social rank and depression: an example of 'evolutionary psychopathology'. *Fortschung Neurologische Psychiatrica* 69: 268–77.

Pinker S (1998) *How the Mind Works.* London: Penguin Group.

Pirkis J, Burgess P and Dunt D (2001) Self-reported needs for care among persons who have suicidal ideation or who have attempted suicide. *Psychiatric Services* 52: 381–3.

Plant R (1968) *Casework and Moral Theory.* London: Routledge & Kegan Paul.

Platt S (1984) Unemployment and suicidal behaviour: a review of the literature. *Social Science and Medicine* 19: 93–115.

Platt S, Biile-Brahe U and Kerkhof A (1992) Parasuicide in Europe: the WHO-EURO multi-centre study on parasuicide. 1. Introduction and preliminary analysis. *Acta Psychiatrica Scandinavica* 85: 97–104.

Polimeni J and Reiss JP (2003) Evolutionary perspectives on schizophrenia. *Canadian Journal of Psychiatry* 48: 34–9.

Popper K and Eccles J (1984) *The Self and its Brain: Arguments for Interactionalism.* Chichester: Macmillan.

Porter R (1993) *The Faber Book of Madness.* London: Faber.

Porter S, Woodworth M and Boer D (2003) Characteristics of sexual homicides committed by psychopathic and non-psychopathic offenders. *Law and Human Behaviour* 27: 459–70.

Post RM, Denicoff K, Leverich GS and Nolen WA (2003) Morbidity in 258 bipolar outpatients followed for 1 year. *Journal of Clinical Psychiatry* 64: 680–90.

Pote HL and Orrell MW (2002) Perceptions of schizophrenia in multi-cultural Britain. *Ethnic Health* 7: 7–20.

Potkin SG, Alphs L, Hsu C and Green A (2003) Predicting suicidal risk in schizophrenic and schizoaffective patients in a prospective 2-year trial. *Biological Psychiatry* 15: 444–52.

Powell C (1995) *A Soldier's Way: An Autobiography.* New York: Random House.

Price BH, Baral I, Cosgrove GR and Cassem EH (2001) Improvement in severe self-mutilation following limbic leucotomy: five case series. *Journal of Clinical Psychiatry* 62: 925–32.

Prins H (2005) *Deviants: Patients or Offenders?* 6th edn. London: Routledge.

Pritchard C (1988) Suicide, gender and unemployment in the British Isles 1975–85. *Social Psychiatry and Psychiatric Epidemiology* 23: 85–9.

Pritchard C (1990) Suicide, unemployment and gender variations in the Western world 1974–1986: Are females in Anglophone countries protected from suicide? *Social Psychiatry and Psychiatric Epidemiology* 25: 73–80.

Pritchard C (1991) Levels of risk and psycho-social problems of families on the 'at risk of abuse' register: some indicators of outcome two years after case closure. *Research, Policy and Planning* 9, 19–26.

Pritchard C (1992a) Youth suicide in Australia and New Zealand 1973–87: a comparison with the Western world. *Australian and New Zealand Journal of Psychiatry* 26: 609–17.

Pritchard C (1992b) Youth suicide, gender and unemployment in the UK 1973–88. *British Journal of Psychiatry* 160: 750–5.

Pritchard C (1992c) Children's homicide as an indicator of effective child protection. A comparative study of Western European statistics. *British Journal of Social Work* 22: 663–84.

Pritchard C (1992d) Is there a link between suicide in young men and unemployment? A comparison of the UK with other European countries. *British Journal of Psychiatry* 160: 750–6.

Pritchard C (1992e) What can we afford for the National Health Service? A comparison of UK government expenditure 1973/74–1992/93 and a contrast with France, Germany and Italy. *Social Policy and Administration* 26: 40–54.

Pritchard C (1994) Psychiatric targets in 'Health of the Nation': regional suicide in Britain by age and gender. Changes in regional employment prospects – precursors of failure? *Journal of the Royal Society of Health* 5: 23–35.

Pritchard C (1995) Sudden-infant-death-syndrome, child homicide and child malignancies: connections or coincidences? *Social Work and Social Science Review* 5: 195–227.

Pritchard C (1996a) The influence of culture upon suicide: comparison of suicide in the People's Republic of China and the developed world by age and gender. *Acta Psychiatrica Scandinavica* 31: 362–7.

Pritchard C (1996b) New patterns of suicide by age and gender in the United Kingdom and the Western world 1974–1992: an indicator of social change? *Social Psychiatry and Psychiatric Epidemiology* 31 227–34.

Pritchard, C. (1996c) Search for an indicator of effective child protection in a re-analysis of child homicide in the major Western world countries 1973–1992. A response to Lindsey and Trocme, and McDonald. *British Journal of Social Work* 26: 545–64.

Pritchard C (1999) *Suicide – the Ultimate Rejection? A Psycho-social Study.* Buckingham: Open University Press.

Pritchard C (2000) Evaluating Bevan House (Specialist Mental Health Placement). Unpublished Report to the Society of St Dismas, Southampton.

Pritchard C (2001) *Family–Teacher–Social Work Alliance in Reducing Truancy and Delinquency.* RDS Paper 78. London: Home Office.

Pritchard C (2002) Children's homicide and road deaths in England and Wales and the USA: an international comparison 1974–97. *British Journal of Social Work* 32: 495–502.

Pritchard C (2004) *The Child Abusers.* Buckingham: Open University Press.

Pritchard C and Amunullah S (2006) Suicide and 'other external cause' deaths in Islamic countries: a comparative analysis with UK and Western world a repository for 'hidden suicides'. *British Journal of Psychiatry* (in press).

Pritchard C and Bagley C (2000) Multi-criminal and violent groups among child sex offenders: a heuristic typology in a 2-year cohort of men in two English counties. *Child Abuse and Neglect* 24: 579–86.

Pritchard C and Bagley C (2001) Suicide and murder in child murderers and child sexual abusers. *Journal of Forensic Psychiatry* 12: 269–86.

Pritchard C and Baldwin D (2000) Effects of age and gender on elderly suicide rates in Catholic and Orthodox countries: an inadvertent neglect? *International Journal of Geriatric Psychiatry* 15: 904–10.

Pritchard C and Baldwin D (2002) Elderly suicides in Asian and English-speaking countries. *Acta Psychiatrica Scandinavica* 105: 271–5.

Pritchard C and Butler A (2000a) Criminality, murder and the cost of crime in coterminous cohorts of 'excluded-from-school' and 'looked-after' adolescents as young adults (16–24). *International Journal of Adolescent Medicine and Health* 12: 223–44.

Pritchard C and Butler A (2000b) Victims of crime, murder and suicide in coterminous cohorts of 'excluded-from-school' and 'looked-after' adolescents as young adults (16–24). *International Journal of Adolescent Medicine and Health* 12: 275–94.

Pritchard C and Butler A (2003) Child homicide in the USA 1974–97: an international comparison – grounds for concern. *Journal of Family Violence* 18: 341–50.

Pritchard C and Clooney D (1994) *Fractured Lives and Fragmented Policies: The Homeless on the South Coast.* Bournemouth: Bournemouth Churches Housing Association.

Pritchard C and Cox M (1990) Analysis of young adult clients in probation and social service caseloads. *Research Policy and Planning* 8: 1–8.

Pritchard C and Evans BT (1996) Comparison of deaths in England and Wales and the developed countries 1973–92 and new malignancies in England and Wales 1971–88. *Public Health* 110: 49–59.

Pritchard C and Evans B (1997) Population density and cancer mortality by age and gender in England and Wales and the Western world 1963–1993. *Public Health* 111: 215–20.

Pritchard C and Evans BT (2001) An international comparison of 'youth' (15–24) and young-adult (25–34) homicide 1974–94: highlighting the USA anomaly. *Critical Social Policy* 11: 83–93.

Pritchard C and Galvin K (2006) Comparison of 'all cause' and cancer deaths in England and Wales and the USA 1979–2000 and a review of GDP expenditure on health. *Public Health* (in press).

Pritchard C and Hansen L (2005a) Child, adolescent and youth suicide and undetermined deaths in England and Wales compared with Australia, Canada, France, Germany, Italy, Japan, Netherlands, Spain and the USA 1974–1999. *International Journal of Adolescent Medicine and Health* 17: 239–53.

Pritchard C and Hansen L (2005b) Comparison of suicide in people aged 65–74 and 75+ by gender in England and Wales and the major Western countries 1974–1999. *International Journal of Geriatric Psychiatry* 20: 17–25.

Pritchard C and King E (2004) Comparison of child-sex-abuse-related v mental-disorder-related suicide in a six year regional cohort of suicides. *British Journal of Social Work* 34: 181–97.

Pritchard C and Lewis C (2006) Comparison of violent deaths in three continents: the extremes of abuse. *Child Abuse and Neglect* (in press).

Pritchard C and Stroud J (1999) Men and women who kill and men who abuse children. A study of the psychiatric–child abuse interface. In Bagley C and Mallick K (eds) *Child Sexual Abuse and Adult Offenders: New Theory and Research.* Aldershot: Ashgate, 255–84.

Pritchard C and Sunak S (2005) *Etiology and Epidemiology of Amyotropic Lateral Sclerosis.* Report to the Board of Public Health, Massachusetts.

Pritchard C and Taylor R (1978) *Social Work: Reform or Revolution?* London: Routledge & Kegan Paul.

Pritchard C and Wallace S (2006) Suicide and other violent deaths in the USA and the September 11th tragedy: an international comparison. *Archives of Suicide Research* (in press).

Pritchard C and Ward IR (1974) Family dynamics of school-phobics: a multi-variate analysis. *British Journal of Social Work* 4: 61–94.

Pritchard C and Williams R (2001) A three-year comparative longitudinal study of a school-based social work and family service to reduce truancy, delinquency and school-exclusion. *Journal of Law and Family Welfare* 23: 1–21.

Pritchard C, Lang D and Neil-Dwyer G (1997a) Has efficiency gone too far? A fiscal analysis as the context for practice. *Southampton Health Journal* 13: 18–22.

Pritchard C, Cox M and Dawson A (1997b) A comparison of suicide and 'violent death' amongst a five-year cohort of male probationers and general population: evidence of accumulative socio-psychiatric vulnerability. *Journal of the Royal Society of Health* 117: 175–80.

Pritchard C, Williams R and Bowen D (1998) A consumer study of young people's views of their educational social worker: engagement v non-engagement as an indicator of effective intervention. *British Journal of Social Work* 28: 915–38.

Pritchard C, Foulkes L, Lang DA and Neil-Dwyer N (2001) Psychosocial outcomes for patients and carers after aneurysmal subarachnoid haemorrhage. *British Journal of Neurosurgery* 15: 456–63.

Pritchard C, Baldwin D and Mayers A (2004a) Changing patterns of adult (45–74) neurological deaths in the major Western countries 1979–1997. *Public Health* 118: 268–83.

Pritchard C, Foulkes L, Lang DA and Neil-Dwyer N (2004b) Prospective comparative study of 'enhanced' versus 'treatment-as-usual' following subarachnoid haemorrhage. *British Journal of Neurosurgery* 18: 158–68.

Pritchard C, Chapman L, Davies A and Neil-Dwyer G (2004c) Psychosocioeconomic outcomes in acoustic neuroma patients and their carers related to tumour size. *Clinical Otolaryngology* 29: 1–7.

Qin P, Agerbo E and Mortensen PB (2003) Suicide risk in relation to socioeconomic, demographic, psychiatric and familial factors: a national-register based study of all suicides in Denmark 1981–1997. *American Journal of Psychiatry* 160: 765–72.

Rai-Atkins R, Jama AA, Wright N and Katbamna S (2002) *Best Practice in Mental Health: Advocacy for African, Caribbean and South Asian Communities.* London: Policy Press.

Ramsbotham D (2001) What price imprisonment? 16th Annual Lecture of the Faculty of Law, University of Southampton, February 21.

Rankin P, Bentall RP and Kinderman P (2005) Perceived relationships with parents and paranoid delusions: comparisons of currently ill, remitted and normal participants. *Psychopathology* 38: 16–25.

Raulin C, Rauh J and Togel B (2001) Folie à deux in the laser age. *Hautartz* 52: 1094–7.

Read J (1998) Child abuse and severity of disturbance amongst adult psychiatric patients. *Child Abuse and Neglect* 22: 359–68.

Read J and Argyle N (1999) Hallucinations, delusions and thought disorder among adult psychiatric inpatients with a history of child abuse. *Psychiatric Services* 50: 1467–72.

Reder P and Duncan S (1997) Adult psychiatry – a missing link in the child protection network. *Child Abuse Review* 6: 35–40.

Reinares M and Vieta E (2004) Impact of psychosocio-education on family caregivers of bipolar patients. *Psychotherapy Psychosomatics* 73: 312–319.

Rendall JM, Gigisman HJ, Keck P and Geddes JR (2003) Olanzapine alone or in combination for acute mania. *Cochrane Database Systematic Review* CD 004040.

Renshaw J (1987) Care in the community: individual care planning and care management. *British Journal of Social Work* 17: 36–51.

Rentrop M, Themi T and Forstl H (2002) Delusional misidentification: symptoms and neurological models. *Fortschritte Neurologie Psychiatrie* 70: 313–20.

Ret IM, Samuels JF, Eaton W and Nestadt G (2002) Adult antisocial personality traits are associated with low parental care and maternal over-protection. *Acta Psychiatrica Scandinavica* 106: 126–31.

Retterstol N (1993) *Suicide: A European Perspective.* Cambridge: Press Syndicate.

Richards T (1998) Partnerships with patients. *British Medical Journal* 316: 85–6.

Rieber RE (1999) Hypnosis, false memory and multiple personality: a trinity of affinity. *History of Psychiatry* 10: 3–11.

Rihmer Z (1999) Dysthymic disorder: implications for diagnosis and treatment. *Current Psychiatry* 12: 69–75.

Riordan S, Smith H and Humphreys JS (2002) Conditionally discharged restricted patients and the need for long-term medium security. *Medicine, Science and Law* 42: 339–43.

Rizvi SL and Linehan MM (2001) Dialectical behaviour therapy for personality disorders. *Current Psychiatry Reports* 3: 64–9.

Robinson C and Williams V (2002) Carers of people with learning disabilities and their experience of the 1995 Carers Act. *British Journal of Social Work* 32: 169–83.

Rock BD and Cooper M (2000) Social work in primary care: a demonstration student unit utilising practice research. *Social Work and Health Care* 31: 1–17.

Rose D (2001) *User's Voices: The Perspectives of Mental Health Service Users on Community and Hospital Care.* London: Sainsbury Centre for Mental Health.

Rossol S (2001) Alcohol and liver. *Verdauungskrankheiten* 1: 1–18.

Rowlands O (1998) *Informal Carers: An Independent Study carried out on behalf of the Department of Health General Household Survey.* London: Stationery Office.

Royal College of Psychiatry (2005) *Curriculum for Membership of the RCPsych.* London: Royal College of Psychiatry.

Runeson B and Asberg M (2003) Family history of suicide among suicide victims. *American Journal of Psychiatry* 160: 1525–6.

Russell B (2000) *A History of Western Philosophy.* London: Routledge.

Rutter M (1999) Psychosocial adversity and child psychopathology. *British Journal of Psychiatry* 174: 480–93.

Rutter M (2000) Genetic studies of autism: from the 1970s into the millennium. *Journal of Abnormal Child Psychology* 28: 3–14.

Rutter M (2003) The interplay of nature, nurture and developmental influences: the challenge ahead for mental health. *Archives of General Psychiatry* 60: 203–5.

Rutter M and Soucar E (2002) Youth suicide and sexual orientation. *Adolescence* 37: 289–99.

Rutter M, Bailey A and Le Conteur A (1994) Autism and known medical conditions: myth and substance. *Journal of Child Psychology and Psychiatry* 35: 311–22.

Rutter M, Silberg L, O'Connor T and Simonoff E (1999) Genetics and child psychiatry. II. Empirical research findings. *Journal of Child Psychology and Psychiatry* 40: 19–55.

Ryan KD, Kilmer RP, Cace AM and Hoyt DR (2000) Psychological consequences of child maltreatment in homeless adolescents. Untangling the unique effects of maltreatment and family environment. *Child Abuse and Neglect* 24: 333–52.

Ryan P (2003) Mental health: links between empowerment and the effects of stigma on service users and their families. *Research Matters* 15: 37–42.

St Aubyn G (1992) *Queen Victoria: A Portrait.* London: Athenaeum.

Sattar G (2003) The death of offenders in England and Wales. *Crisis* 24: 17–23.

Saxena S, Eliahoo J and Majeed A (2002) Socioeconomic and ethnic group differences in self-reported health status and use of health services by children and young people in England. *British Medical Journal* 325: 520–3.

Schneider J (1993) Care programming in mental health: assimilation and adaptation. *British Journal of Social Work* 23: 383–403.

Schneidmann ES (1985) *Definition of Suicide.* New York: Wiley International.

Schulze B and Angermeyer MC (2002) Changing perspectives: stigma from the point of view of people with schizophrenia, their families and mental health professionals. *Neuropsychiatrie* 16: 78–86.

Schulze B and Angermeyer MC (2003) Subjective experiences of stigma: focus group study of schizophrenic patients, their relatives and mental health professionals. *Social Science and Medicine* 56: 299–312.

Scott JP (1993) Homelessness and mental illness. *British Journal of Psychiatry* 162: 314–24.

Scott MJ and Stradling JG (1991) The cognitive behavioural approach with depressed clients. *British Journal of Social Work* 21: 533–44.

Sedgwick P (1982) *Psycho Politics.* London: Pluto Press.

Seebohm Report (1968) *Report on Personal Social Services.* London: Department of Health and Social Security, HMSO.

Seifert D (2000) GnRH analogues. A new treatment of sex offenders. *Sexuologie* 7: 1–11.

Seiger K, Dorge P, Wainwright U and Kamps I (2001) Folie à deux: a rare psychiatric disease. *Notartz* 17: 14–17.

Seligman MEP (1975) *Learned Helplessness: On Depression, Development and Death.* San Francisco: Freedman.

Sharma V (2001) The effect of ECT on suicide risk in patients with mood disorders. *Canadian Journal of Psychiatry* 46: 707–9.

Shaw J, Appleby L, Amos T and Parsons R (1999) Mental disorder and clinical care of people convicted of homicide: national clinical survey. *British Medical Journal* 318: 1240–4.

Shepherd M (1994) Maternal depression, child care and the social work role. *British Journal of Social Work* 24: 33–51.

Shepherd M (2002) Mental health and social justice and gender. *British Journal of Social Work* 32: 779–98.

Shilling C (1996) *The Body and Social Theory.* London: Macmillan.

Shooter M (2002) *Presidential Address RCPsych.* Royal College of Psychiatrists Meeting, University of Southampton.

Short R, Ching-Chang S and Yoshimoto T (2003) Surgical outcome of 31 patients with carcinapharyngomiolias. *Journal of Neurosurgery* 96: 704–13.

Siever LJ, Torgensen S, Gunderson JG and Kendler KS (2002) The borderline diagnosis. III. Identifying endophenotypes for genetic studies. *Biological Psychiatry* 51: 964–8.

Silberstein P, Lawrence R and Schnier R (2002) A case of neurosyphilis with a florid Jarisch–Herxheimer reaction. *Journal of Clinical Neuroscience* 9: 689–90.

Silove D (1998) Is posttraumatic stress disorder an over learned survival response: an evolutionary hypothesis. *Psychiatry* 61: 181–90.

Silveria ER and Ebrahim S (1998) Social determinates of psychiatric morbidity and well-being in immigrant elders in west London. *International Journal of Geriatric Psychiatry* 13: 801–12.

Simon LMJ, Sales B, Kaszniak A and Khan M (1992) Characteristics of child molesters. *Journal of Interpersonal Violence* 7: 211–25.

Singh GK, Miller BA, Hankey BF and Edwards BK (2004) Persistent area socioeconomic disparities in US incidence of cervical cancer, mortality, stage and survival 1975–2000. *Cancer* 101: 1051–7.

Singh I (2003) Thought for the Day. *Today* programme. BBC Radio 4.

Skinner R and Cleese J (1994) *Families and How to Survive Them.* Chichester: Macmillan.

Smale G (1984) *Self-Fulfilling: Self-Defeating Strategies and Behavioural Change.* London: Routledge & Kegan Paul.

Smit F, Bolier L and Cuijpers P (2003) Cannabis use as a probably causative factor in the later development of schizophrenia. *Nederlands Tijdschrift Geneesked* 147: 2178–83.

Smith K and Leon L (2001) *Turned Upside Down: Developing Community-based Crisis Services for 16–25 year olds.* London: Mental Health Foundation.

Social Exclusion Unit (1998a) *Reducing Teenage Pregnancy.* London: Stationery Office.

Social Exclusion Unit (1998b) *Truancy and Social Exclusion.* London: Stationery Office.

Social Exclusion Unit (1998c) *Homelessness and Social Exclusion.* London: Stationery Office.

Soliman AE and Reza H (2001) Risk factors and correlates of violence among acutely ill adult psychiatric inpatients. *Psychiatric Services* 52: 75–80.

Souery D, Rivelli SK and Mendlewicz J (2000) Molecular genetics and family studies in affective disorders: state of the art. *Journal of Affective Disorders* 62: 45–51.

Southall S, Plunket M, Falkov A and Samuels M (1997) Covert video recordings of life-threatening child abuse: lessons for child protection. *Paediatrics* 100: 735–60.

Southgate C (2000) Sestina for Karen and Ros and Sue, Richard and Peter and Simon, and many others. In Southgate C. *Beyond the Bitter Wind – Poems 1982–2000.* London: Shoestring Press.

Spataro SJ, Mullen PE and Moss SA (2005) Impact of child sexual abuse on mental health: prospective study in males and females. *British Journal of Psychiatry* 186: 76.

Special Hospitals' Treatment Resistant Research Group (1996) Schizophrenia, violence, clozapine and risperidone: a review. *British Journal of Psychiatry* 169 (Suppl. 31): 21–30.

Spicker JO (1995) *Social Policy: Themes and Approaches.* New York: Prentice Hall/Harvester Wheatsheaf.

Spirito S and Overholser J (2003) The suicidal child: assessment and management of adolescents after a suicide attempt. *Child and Adolescent Psychiatric Clinics of North America* 12: 649–65.

Spratt C and Callan J (2003) Reflective critique and collaborative practice in evaluation: promoting change in medical education *Medical Teaching* 25: 82–8.

Stevens A and Price J (2000) *Evolutionary Psychiatry: A New Beginning*, 2nd edn. London: Brunner-Routledge.

Stoltenberg ST and Burmeister M (2000) Recent progress in psychiatric genetics: some hope but no hype. *Human Molecular Genetics* 12: 927–33.

Stroud J (1997) Mental disorder and the homicide of children: a review. *Social Work and Social Science Review* 6: 149–62.

Stroud J (2001) European child homicide studies: quantitative studies and a preliminary report on complementary qualitative research. *Social Work Europe* 7: 31–7.

Stroud J (2003) Psycho-social antecedents of women who have killed children. Unpubl. PhD thesis, Goldsmiths, University of London.

Stubner S, Volkl G and Soyka M (1998) Differential diagnosis of dissociative disorder (multiple personality disorder). *Nervenartz* 69: 440–5.

Swanson CJ, Bures M and Schoepp D (2005) Metabotropic glutamate receptor as novel targets for anxiety and stress disorders. *Nature Reviews: Neurosciences* 4: 132–44.

Szasz T (1960) The myth of mental illness. *American Psychologist* 15: 113–18.

Szasz TS (1970) *Ideology and Insanity: Essays on the Psychiatric Dehumanisation of Man.* New York: Syracuse.

Szasz TS (2002) *Liberation by Oppression: A Comparative Study of Slavery and Psychiatry.* London: Transaction Publishers.

TADS (2003) Treatment for Adolescents with Depression Study (TADS): rationale, design, methods. *Journal of the American Academy of Child and Adolescent Psychiatry* 42: 531–42.

Takeuchi H, Hiroe T, Kanai T and Furukawa A (2003) Childhood parental separation experiences and depressive symptomatology in acute major depression. *Psychiatric Clinical Neurosciences* 57: 215–25.

Tandon R and Jibson MD (2003) Efficacy of newer generation anti-psychotics in the treatment of schizophrenia. *Psycho-Neuro-Endocrinology* 28: 9–26.

Targosz S, Bebbington P, Lewis G and Meltzer H (2003) Lone mothers, social exclusion and depression. *Psychological Medicine* 33: 715–22.

Tarrier N and Barraclough S (1992) Family interventions for schizophrenia. *Behavioural Modification* 14: 408–40.

Tarrier N, Lewis S, Haddock G, Bental R and Dunn G (2004) CBT in first-episode and early schizophrenia: 18 month follow-up study of a randomised controlled trial. *British Journal of Psychiatry* 184: 231–9.

Taylor FC, Ascione R, Rees K, Narayan P and Angelini GD (2003) Socioeconomic deprivation is a predictor of poor post-operative cardiovascular outcomes in patients undergoing coronary artery bypass grafting. *Heart* 89: 1062–6.

Taylor PJ and Gunn J (1999) Homicides by people with mental illness: myth and reality. *British Journal of Psychiatry* 174: 9–14.

Taylor R and Pritchard C (1982) *The Protest Makers: The British Anti-nuclear Campaign Twenty Years on 1958–78.* Oxford: Pergamon Press.

Teichman TY, Bar-El Z and Elizur A (2003) Cognitive, interpersonal and behavioural predictors in patients and spouse depression. *Journal of Affective Disorders* 74: 247–56.

Tennant C (2002) Life events, stress and depression: a review of recent findings. *Australian and New Zealand Journal of Psychiatry* 36: 173–82.

Tenny G, Wheatley R, Samuels S and Southall S (1994) Covert surveillance in Munchausen's syndrome by proxy. *British Medical Journal* 308: 1100–2.

Tessa C, Mascalchi M and Domenici R (2002) Permanent brain damage following acute poisoning in Munchausen's by proxy. *Neuropaediatrics* 32: 90–2.

Testa M, Vanzile-Tamsin W and Livingston JA (2004) Role of victim and perpetrator intoxication in sexual assault outcomes. *Journal of the Study of Alcohol* 65: 320–9.

Tharyan P and Adams CE (2002) Electroconvulsive therapy for schizophrenia. *Cochrane Database Systematic Review* CD000076.

Thoits PN (2005) Differential labelling of mental illness by social status: a new look at an old problem. *Journal of Health and Social Behaviour* 46: 102–19.

Thomas P, Romme M and Hammelijnck J (1996) Psychiatry and the politics of the underclass. *British Journal of Psychiatry* 169: 401–4.

Thompson C, Ostler K, Peveler RS, Baker N and Kinmouth A (2001a) Dimensional perspective on the recognition of depressive symptoms in primary care: the Hampshire project 3. *British Journal of Psychiatry* 179: 317–23.

Thompson C, Syddall H, Rodin I, Osmond C and Barker DJP (2001b) Birth weight and the risk of depression in later life. *British Journal of Psychiatry* 179: 450–5.

Thompson W and Pritchard C (1987) *Prejudice and Discrimination amongst Southampton Citizens: Grounds for Optimism.* Report to the Equal Opportunities Committee, Southampton City Council.

Tilson HA (1998) Developmental neurotoxicology of endocrine disrupters: identifying information gaps and research needs. *Environmental Health Perspective* 106: 807–11.

Tohen M, Chengappa NR, Supopes T and Brier A (2002) Efficacy of olanzapine in combination with valporate or lithium in the treatment of mania in patients partly non-responsive to valporate or lithium monotherapy. *Archives of General Psychiatry* 59: 62–9.

Torgersen S (2000) Genetics of patients with borderline personality disorders. *Psychiatric Clinics of North America* 23: 1–9.

Towl G (1999) Self-inflicted deaths in prisons in England and Wales from 1988–1996 (1999). *British Journal of Forensic Practice* 1: 28–33.

Trefferes PD and Rinne-Albers MA (2005) Selective serotonin reuptake inhibitors (SSRIs) are not indicated for children and adolescents with depression. *Nederlands Tijdscherarch Geneeskdam* 149: 1314–17.

UNICEF (1999) *The State of the World's Children.* Geneva: United Nations.

United Nations (1948) *Declaration of Human Rights.* New York: UN.

US Bureau of Statistics (2004) *USA Annual Statistics 2003.* Washington, DC: US Bureau of Statistics.

Utting W (1997) *People Like Us: Review of Safeguards for Children Living away from Home.* London: HMSO for the Department of Health.

Van den Bree MBM (1998) Genetic influences in antisocial personality and drug use disorders. *Drug and Alcohol Dependence* 49: 177–87.

Van der Wurff FB, Stek ML, Hoogendijk WL and Beekman AT (2003) ECT for the depressed elderly. *Cochrane Database Systematic Review* CDO 003593.

Veen ND, Selten J, Van der Tweel I and Kahn RS (2004) Cannabis use and age onset of schizophrenia. *American Journal of Psychiatry* 161: 501–6.

Verdoux H (2002) Long-term psychiatric and behavioural consequence of prenatal exposure to drugs. *Therapie* 57: 181–5.

Vieregge P, Schoffke KA and Frederich HJ (1992) Parkinson's disease in twins. *Neurology* 42: 1453–61.

Vitek K, Bakay RA, Freeman A and DeLong MR (2003) Randomised trial of pallidotomy versus medical therapy for Parkinson's disease. *Annals of Neurology* 53: 558–69.

Waern M, Rubenowitz E and Wilhelmson K (2003) Predictors of suicide in the old elderly. *Gerontology* 49: 328–34.

Wagner T, Krampe H and Ehenreich H (2004) Substantial decrease of psychiatric co-morbidity in chronic alcoholics with integrated outpatient treatment: results of a prospective study. *Journal of Psychiatric Research* 38: 619–35.

Wagstaff AJ, Cheer SM, Matheson A and Ormrod D (2002) Paroxetine: an update of its use in psychiatric disorders in adults. *ADIS Drug Evaluation* 62: 655–703.

Walford G, Kennedy MT, Manwell MKC and McKune N (1990) Father-perpetrators of child sex abuse who commit suicide. *Irish Journal of Psychological Medicine* 7: 144–5.

Walker Z and Stevens T (2002) Dementia with Lewy bodies: clinical characteristics and diagnostic criteria. *Journal of Geriatric Psychiatry and Neurology* 15: 188–94.

Wallace C, Mullen PE and Burgess P (2004) Criminal offending in schizophrenia over a 25 year period marked by de-institutionalisation and increasing prevalence of co-morbid substance abuse disorders. *American Journal of Psychiatry* 161: 716–27.

Walsh E, Moran P, Scott C and Fahy T (2003) Prevalence of violent victimisation in severe mental illness. *British Journal of Psychiatry* 183: 233–8.

Wancata J (2002) Stigma: a commentary from a gerontopsychiatry perspective. *Neuropsychiatrie* 16: 115–16.

Wang PW, Ketter T, Becker OV and Nowakowska C (2003) New anticonvulsant medication uses in bipolar disorder. *CNS Spectator* 8: 930–2.

Warner, R. (2000) *The Environment of Schizophrenia.* London: Routledge.

Waslick BD, Walsh BT, Greenhill L and Lieber D (1999) Open trial of fluoxetine in children and adolescents with dysthymic disorder or double depression. *Journal of Affective Disorders* 56: 227–36.

Wasserman D, Varni A and Eklund G (1994) Male suicides and alcohol consumption in the former USSR. *Acta Psychiatrica Scandinavica* 89: 306–13.

Wasylenki D, Goering PN and Lemire D (1993) The hostel out-reach programme: assertive case management for homeless mentally ill people. *Hospital and Community Psychiatry* 44: 848–53.

Webster R (1995) *Why Freud was Wrong: Science and Psychoanalysis.* London: Harper Collins.

Webster R (1998) *The Great Children's Home Scandal.* London: Harper Collins.

Weintraub D, Eskander ML and Stern MD (2003) Psychiatric complications in Parkinson's disease. *American Journal of Geriatric Psychiatry* 11: 844–51.

Weisman AG, Lopez SR, Ventura J and Hwang S (2000) Comparison of psychiatric symptoms in Anglo-American and Mexican American patients with schizophrenia. *Schizophrenia Bulletin* 26: 817–22.

Welch SS and Linehan MM (2002) High-risk situations associated with parasuicide and drug use in borderline personality disorder. *Journal of Personality Disorder* 16: 561–9.

Wertheimer A (1991) *A Special Scar: Family Survivors of Suicide.* Basingstoke: Macmillan.

WHO (1979a) *International Classification of Diseases*, 9th edn. Geneva: World Health Organization.

WHO (1979b) *World Annual Health Statistics.* Geneva: World Health Organization.

WHO (1992) *Annual World Health Statistics.* Geneva: World Health Organization.

WHO (2000) *The ICD.10 Classification of Mental and Behavioural Disorders.* Geneva: World Health Organization.

WHO (2001–5) *World Annual Statistics.* Geneva: World Health Organization. www.who. whosis.org

Wiklander M, Samuelsson M and Asberg M (2003) Shame reactions after suicide attempt. *Scandinavian Journal of Caring Sciences* 17: 293–300.

Wild N (1988) Suicide of perpetrators after disclosure of child sexual abuse. *Child Abuse and Neglect* 12: 119–21.

Wildes JE, Harkness KL and Simons AD (2002) Life events, number of social relationships and 12 month naturalistic course of major depression in a community sample of women. *Depression and Anxiety* 16: 104–13.

Wilkinson D, Holmes C, Stammers S and North J (2002) Prophylactic therapy with lithium in elderly patients with unipolar depression. *International Journal of Geriatric Psychiatry* 17: 619–22.

Williams JW Jr, Barrett J and Oxman T (2000) Treatment of dysthemia and minor depression in primary care: a randomised controlled trial in older adults. *Journal of the American Medical Association* 284: 1519–26.

Wilson EO (1975) *Sociobiology: The New Synthesis.* Cambridge, MA: Harvard University Press.

Wilson EO (1998) *Consilience: The Unity of Knowledge.* London: Little Brown.

Wilson EO (2002) *The Future of Life.* London: Little Brown.

Wilson G (1998) *The Great Sex Divide: A Study of Male–Female Differences.* London: Peter Owen.

Wirdefeldt K, Gratz M and Schalling M (2004) No evidence of hereditability in Parkinson's disease in Swedish twins. *Neurology* 63: 305–11.

Wolf T and Muller-Oerlinghausen B (2002) The influence of successful prophylactic drug treatment of cognitive dysfunction in bipolar disorders. *Bipolar Disorders* 4: 263–70.

Wolfe N and Stuber J (2002) State mental hospitals and their host communities: the origins of hostile public reactions. *Journal of Behavioural Health Services Research* 29: 304–17.

Wolfersdorf M, Vogel R, Kornacher J and Wurst FM (2001) The aftermath of suicide of a psychiatric inpatient – experiences in hospitals with relatives as suicide survivors. *Psychiatrica Praxis* 28: 341–4.

Woodward M, Nursten J and Badger D (2000) Mental disorder and homicide: a review of epidemiological research. *Epidemiologia Psichiatria Sociale* 9: 171–89.

Woodworth M and Porter S (2002) In cold blood: characteristics of criminal homicides as a function of psychopathy. *Journal of Abnormal Psychology* 111: 436–45.

Wrightson KJ and Wardle J (1997) Cultural variation in health locus of control. *Ethnicity and Health* 2: 13–20.

Wyatt G, Loeb T, Solis B and Carmona J (1999) The prevalence and circumstances of child sexual abuse across a decade. *Child Abuse and Neglect* 23: 45–60.

Yeung A, Neault N, Howarth S and Nierenberg A (2002) Screen for major depression in Asian-Americans: a comparison of the Beck and the Chinese Depression Inventory. *Acta Psychiatrica Scandinavica* 105: 252–7.

Zachary MJ, Mulvihill MN and Goldfrank LR (2002) Domestic abuse in the emergency department: can a risk profile be defined? *Academy of Emergency Medicine* 8: 796–803.

Zammit S, Allebeck P, Andreasson S, Lundberg I and Lewis G (2002) Self-reported cannabis use as a risk factor for schizophrenia in Swedish conscripts of 1969: historical cohort study. *British Medical Journal* 325: 1199–201.

Zaretsky A (2003) Targeted psychosocial interventions for bipolar disorder. *Bipolar Disorder* 5 (Suppl. 2): 80–7.

Zink T and Sill M (2004) Intimate partner violence and job instability. *Journal of the American Women's Association* 59: 32–5.

Index

304 *Index*

and 31; dilemmas in 241–3; dynamics of 97–9; endogenous depression 28–9; Freud's view of 98; genetic weighting of mood disorders 77–8; interpersonal relationships and 99; manic depression 36; mild depression 28–9; moderate to mild 31; mood, depressive episodes and 30; practice assessment and intervention, modality for 109–10; problems with drugs? 107–9; Prozac SSRI controversy 102–7; reactive depression 28–9; recurrent brief depression (RBD) 96; severe depression (with and without psychotic symptoms) 31–2; social work assessment, areas of 109; social work with people with mood disorders 95–121; subclinical depressions (SCD) 96; suicidal behaviour, association with 107; symptoms 31; unipolar mood disorder 95–7; *see also* mania; mental disorder; personality disorders; schizophrenias; suicide and DSH
Descartes, René 19, 20, 50
Deviants: Patients or Offenders? (Prins, H.) 93
diagnosis: diagnostic rigidity 74–5; substance abuse and schizophrenia, dual diagnosis 127–9; value of 51
dialectic behaviour therapy (DBT) 69, 111, 186
diazepams 107–8
dissociative (conversion) disorders 28
Dixon Inquiry 239
Dobson, Frank 209–10
dopamine 100, 101
Drug Abuse and Mental Health Administration, US 24
Dryden, John 18
Durkheim, Emile ix, 16, 24, 150
dysthymia 104–5

early parental loss (EPL) 99
eating disorders 27
Eccles, Sir John 22
ego-dynamic theories 8–9, 13–14, 98, 145–6
electroconvulsive therapy (ECT) 143, 206
emotional disorders, childhood onset 28
environmental 'triggers' 99, 118, 128, 130
epilepsy 41, 118–19, 144–5
ethnicity 54–6
Euripedes 5–6

European Convention on Human Rights 211–12
European Human Rights Act 94
evidence-based practice 7, 48–9, 73, 94, 266; ASW, complexity of role of 215–16; bio-psychosocial treatment 118–19; biological endowment and environment, interaction of 9–10; environment and biological endowment, interaction of 9–10; interdisciplinary research and integrated conclusions 75–8; knowledge, evidence-based 105, 198; long-term psychotherapy 145–6; mood stabilisers, recommendation of 118; need for 7–9; practice-related research and 14–15; resource implications 52–3
evolutionary psychologists 75–8
examples/experience *see* practice experiences
Eysenck, Hans 146

first-line atypical anti-psychotic drugs 131–2
Fox, George xii
Freud, Sigmund 105; on depression 98

Galbraith, J.K. 89
Gates of Perception (Huxley, A.) 37, 41
gender 56–7
General Medical Council 197–8
George III 3
The Gift (Titmuss, R.) 87
Gribbon, John 21
Guinan, Pat 212

habit and impulse disorders 28
Hamilton, Professor Max x, 11, 15, 87, 141
Hamlet (Shakespeare, W.) xi, 4, 12–13, 18, 97, 149–50
health, definition of 19
The Health of the Nation (1991 Green Paper) 208
Healy, Dr Derek 102–3
Hinduism 5, 16, 42
A History of Western Philosophy (Russell, B.) 20
homelessness, stigma of 237
Homelessness Act (2002) 221
Hood, Thomas 149, 150, 167
Housing Act (1990) 221
Housing Benefit 224, 235
housing *see* accommodation

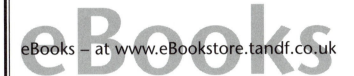